RECENT ADVANCES IN

Haematology

RECENT ADVANCES IN HAEMATOLOGY

Contents of Number 7
Edited by A. V. Hoffbrand, M. K. Brenner

Current and prospective gene therapy protocols and their application to haematological disease
R. C. Moen
Detection of minimal residual disease in leukemia and lymphoma
D. Campana
The genetic basis of myelodysplasia
D. Culligan, A. Jacobs, R. A. Padua
New drug treatment for acute myeloblastic leukemia
M. R. Wollman, J. Mirro Jr
Ras and GAP
D. C. S. Huang, J. F. Hancock
Cell adhesion in the hematopoietic system
M. W. Makgoba, A. Bernard
Immunotherapy of leukemia
M. K. Brenner
Bone marrow transplantation for hemoglobinopathy and sickle cell disease
M. Walters, D. Matthews, K. M. Sullivan
The management of HIV infection
M. C. I. Lipman, M. A. Johnson
Hepatitis C and the haematologist
G. M. Dusheiko, B. Wonke, S. M. Donohue
Oral iron chelation therapy
F. N. Al-Refaie, A. V. Hoffbrand
Familial thrombophilia
F. E. Preston, E. Briët
The molecular biology of factor VIII and von Willebrand factor
E. G. D. Tuddenham

ISBN 0443 046891

You can place your order by contacting your local medical bookseller or the Sales Promotion Department, Churchill Livingstone, Robert Stevenson House, 1–3 Baxter's Place, Leith Walk, Edinburgh EH1 3AF, UK

Tel: (0131) 556 2424; Telex: 727511 LONGMN G; Fax: (0131) 558 1278

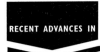

RECENT ADVANCES IN

Haematology

Edited by

M. K. Brenner MA MB PhD FRCP MRCPath
Director, Division of Bone Marrow Transplantation, and
Member, Department of Hematology/Oncology,
St Jude Children's Research Hospital, Memphis, Tennessee;
Professor, Department of Pediatrics and Department of Medicine,
University of Tennessee, USA

A. V. Hoffbrand MA DM FRCP FRCPath FRCP(Edin) DSc
Professor of Haematology and Honorary Consultant,
Royal Free Hospital and School of Medicine, London, UK

NUMBER EIGHT

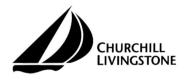

NEW YORK EDINBURGH LONDON MADRID MELBOURNE SAN FRANCISCO AND TOKYO 1996

CHURCHILL LIVINGSTONE
Medical Division of Pearson Professional Limited

Distributed in the United States of America by
Churchill Livingstone Inc., 650 Avenue of the Americas,
New York, N.Y. 10011, and by associated companies,
branches and representatives throughout the world.

© Pearson Professional Ltd 1996

All rights reserved; no part of this publication may be
reproduced, stored in a retrieval system, or transmitted
in any form or by any means, electronic, mechanical,
photocopying, recording or otherwise, without either
the prior written permission of the Publishers
(Churchill Livingstone, Robert Stevenson House,
1–3 Baxter's Place, Leith Walk, Edinburgh EH1 3AF)
or a licence permitting restricted copying in the
United Kingdom issued by the Copyright Licensing
Agency Ltd, 90 Tottenham Court Road, London W1P 9HE.

First published 1996

ISBN 0443 052379
ISSN 0143-697X

British Library Cataloguing in Publication Data
A catalogue record for this book is available from the
British Library.

Library of Congress Cataloging in Publication Data
A catalog record for this book is available from the
Library of Congress.

The publisher's policy is to use paper manufactured from sustainable forests

Page layout: Gerard Heyburn, Janet Smith

Printed in Singapore

Contents

1. Regulation of apoptosis in normal hemopoiesis and hematological disease — 1
   D. Campana, J. L. Cleveland
2. The clinical use of haemopoietic growth factors — 21
   A. P. Haynes, A. E. Hunter, N. H. Russell
3. Treatment of childhood ALL — 45
   J. M. Chessells
4. New therapies for chronic lymphocytic leukemia — 65
   C. A. Koller, M. J. Keating
5. Gaucher disease — 83
   A. Zimran, E. Beutler
6. Treatment of acute myeloid leukaemia in elderly patients — 119
   M. Baudard, R. Zittoun
7. Paroxysmal nocturnal haemoglobinuria — 137
   P. Hillmen
8. Automated blood cell counters — 159
   J. M. England
9. Transplantation for patients without HLA identical siblings — 191
   J. Hows, B. Bradley
10. Inhibitors and the control of thrombosis — 213
    S. R. Stone, R. W. Carrell
11. Stimulation of fetal hemoglobin synthesis using pharmacological agents — 231
    G. P. Rogers
12. Human stem cell biology and therapy — 247
    K. Auditore-Hargreaves, M. Krieger, C. Jacobs, S. Heimfeld, R. J. Berenson
13. Gene transfer into human hemopoietic progenitor cells — 263
    M. K. Brenner, J. M. Cunningham, B. P. Sorrentino, H. E. Heslop

Index — 287

Preface

These are exciting times for haematologists because advances in molecular and cellular biology have led not only to increased understanding of the mechanisms of diseases, but also offer an accelerating array of possibilities for their prevention and treatment. It is hoped that despite the financial exigencies of managed care in the United States and of the purchaser/provider separation in the UK, clinical research structures can be preserved so that patients can benefit from these advances. In the current volume, we have included chapters that describe some of the major advances that are currently being made in the understanding of the biology and pathology of malignant and non-malignant blood disorders. The volume also provides up to date clinical reviews of the most (cost) effective means of treating major haematological diseases. We hope that this volume will be useful both for haematologists in training and for established clinical and research haematologists who wish to update their knowledge in labaoratory and clinical aspects of the subject.

As always, we are most grateful to our authors for their excellent contribvutions, despite many competing calls on their time. Finally, we would like to thank our editorial staff at Cuhurchill Livingstone for their assistance in the editing and preparation of this volume.

Malcom Brenner, MA MB, PhD, FRCP, MRCPath
A Victor Hoffbrand, MA, DM, FRCP, FRCPath, FRCP(Edin), DSc

Contributors

Karen Auditore-Hargreaves PhD
CellPro, Incorporated, Bothell, Washington, USA

Marion Baudard MD
Assistant, Service d'Hématologie, Hôpital Hôtel-Dieu de Paris, Paris, France and Fellow, Laboratory of Cell Biology, National Cancer Institute, NIH, Bethesda, Maryland, USA

Ronald J. Berenson MD
Mercer Island, Washington, USA

Ernest Beutler MD
Chairman, Department of Molecular Experimental Medicine, The Scripps Research Institute, La Jolla, California, USA

Ben Bradley MB ChB PhD MA FRCPath
Professor of Transplantation Immunology, University of Bristol, Southmead Health Services, Bristol, UK

Malcolm K. Brenner MB PhD FRCP MRCPath
Director, Division of Bone Marrow Transplantation, St Jude Children's Research Hospital, Memphis Tennessee, USA

Dario Campana MD PhD
Associate Member, Department of Haematology/Oncology, St Jude Children's Research Hospital, Associate Professor of Paediatrics, University of Tennessee, Memphis Tennessee, USA

Robin W. Carrell PhD FRCPath
Professor and Head, Department of Haematology, MRC Centre, University of Cambridge, Cambridge, UK

J.L. Cleveland
Associate Member, Department of Biochemistry, St Jude Children's Research Hospital, Memphis Tennessee, USA

Judith M. Chessells MD FRCP FRCPath DObst RCOG
Professor of Haematology and Oncology, Leukaemia Research Fund, Institute of Child Health, London, UK

CONTRIBUTORS

J.M. Cunningham MD
Assistant Member, Division of Experimental Haematology, St Jude Children's Research Hospital, Memphis Tennessee, USA

John M. England PhD MRCPath
Department of Haematology, Watford General Hospital, Watford, UK

A.P. Haynes DM MRCP MRCPath
Lecturer in Haematology, City Hospital, Nottingham, and University of Nottingham, UK

S. Heimfeld PhD
CellPro, Incorporated, Bothell, Washington, USA

Helen E. Heslop MD FRACP FRCPA
Associate Member, Division of Bone Marrow Transplantation, St Jude Children's Research Hospital, Memphis Tennessee, USA

Peter Hillmen MB ChB MRCP MRCPath PhD
Haematological Malignancy Diagnostic Service, Institute of Pathology, General Infirmary at Leeds, Leeds, UK

A. Victor Hoffbrand DM FRCP FRCPath DSc
Professor of Haematology, Department of Haematology, Royal Free Hospital, London, UK

Jill Hows MB BS MD MSc FRCPath
Professor of Clinical Haematology, Department of Transplantation Sciences, University of Bristol, Southmead Health Services, Bristol, UK

A.E. Hunter MRCP MRCPath
Consultant Haematologist, City Hospital, Nottingham, UK

C. Jacobs PhD MD
CellPro, Incorporated, Bothell, Washington, USA

Michael J. Keating MD
M.D. Anderson Cancer Center, University of Texas, Houston, Texas, USA

Charles A. Koller MD
Associate Professor of Medicine, Department of Haematology, M.D. Anderson Cancer Center, University of Texas, Houston, Texas, USA

Monica S. Krieger PhD
CellPro, Incorporated, Bothell, Washington, USA

Griffin P. Rodgers MD
Chief, Molecular Hematology Section, NIDDK/NIH, Bethesda, Maryland, USA

N.H. Russell MD FRCP FRCPath
Reader in Haematology, City Hospital, Nottingham, and University of Nottingham, UK

B.P. Sorrentino
Assistant Member, Division of Experimental Haematology, St Jude Children's Research Hospital, Memphis Tennessee, USA

Stuart R. Stone PhD
Department of Haematology, MRC Centre, University of Cambridge, Cambridge, UK

A. Zimram
Department of Molecular Experimental Medicine, The Scripps Research Institute, La Jolla, California, USA

R. Zittoun
Professor and Head, Service d'Hématologie, Hôpital Hôtel-Dieu de Paris, Paris, France

1

Regulation of apoptosis in normal hemopoiesis and hematological disease

D. Campana   J. L. Cleveland

The term apoptosis was first applied by Kerr et al (1972) to describe a temporal series of morphologic changes occurring in dying cells, including cell shrinkage and nuclear fragmentation, which are distinct from the cell swelling and lysis that accompany cell death by necrosis. Another characteristic feature of apoptosis is that dying cells are rapidly eliminated by phagocytes, thus restricting the disruption of surrounding living tissue (reviewed by Howie et al 1994).

Apoptosis or 'programmed cell death' plays a central role in embryogenesis, morphogenesis and regulation of normal cell turnover in multicellular organisms. Apoptosis is an integral part of all developmental programs, including those of the musculoskeletal system where it affects the formation of feet and wing from limb buds; the reproductive system, where it determines the involution of the Mullerian ducts in males; and the nervous system, where > 50% of neurons are eliminated by apoptosis through competition for neurotrophic factors (reviewed by Koury 1992, Howie et al 1994). Variable apoptotic rates are also likely to regulate the homeostasis of proliferating tissues, and thus participate in the control of hemopoiesis and lymphopoiesis. Changes in propensity to apoptosis have been clearly linked to oncogenesis (reviewed by Korsmeyer 1992, Packham & Cleveland 1995), and most anticancer drugs appear to induce this process (reviewed by Hickman 1992, Reed 1995). Thus, knowledge of the molecular mechanisms that regulate apoptosis has important clinical implications.

Our understanding of the molecular events that trigger and accompany apoptosis, and the role that this process plays in normal development, oncogenesis and therapy has increased dramatically over the last decade. In this review, we discuss the molecular processes that control apoptosis, and the role of apoptosis in normal and malignant lymphohemopoiesis. We also describe some of the methods currently used to detect and enumerate apoptotic cells.

INDUCERS OF APOPTOSIS

At certain stages of cell differentiation, apoptosis may occur by default, unless cell viability is supported by survival factors produced by other cells (Raff 1992). Therefore, one important inducer of apoptosis is the removal of essential trophic factors. For example, growth factor deprivation causes atrophy of hormone-dependent tissues via induction of apoptosis, as has been observed in the endometrium, prostate and adrenal cortex deprived of progesterone, testosterone and ACTH, respectively (reviewed by Koury 1992, Howie et al 1994). Apoptosis following removal of trophic factors in lymphohemopoietic cells has been extensively documented. Growth factor- and cytokine-dependent hemopoietic cell lines undergo rapid apoptosis when cultured in the absence of the required factor (Duke & Cohen 1986, Williams et al 1990, Koury & Bondurant 1990, Rodriguez-Tarduchy et al 1990, McConkey et al 1991, Nunez et al 1990), and normal and leukemic immature lymphoid cells rapidly die by apoptosis in vitro (Manabe et al 1992, 1994b). Although the critical survival factors for the latter cells have not yet been identified, it is known that they are produced by the bone marrow microenvironment. Indeed, bone marrow-derived stromal layers effectively suppress apoptosis of immature lymphoid cells in vitro (Manabe et al 1992). Apoptosis induced by factor deprivation has also been shown in cultures of B-cell chronic lymphocytic leukemia (CLL) cells (McConkey et al 1991, Buschle et al 1993). Apoptosis in these cells can be suppressed by cytokines such as interferon-γ (Buschle et al 1993), interferon-α (Panayotidis et al 1994), interleukin-4 (IL-4; Dancescu et al 1992, Panayotidis et al 1993) and IL-13 (Fluckiger et al 1994a) and by ligation of CD40 (Fluckiger et al 1994b).

Apoptosis can not only occur by default but it can also be triggered by exogenous stimuli. Thus, dimerization or oligomerization of some cell surface receptors triggers apoptosis. For example, apoptosis of immature T-cells is rapidly induced by ligation of T-cell receptor/CD3 (Smith et al 1989) and of Fas/Apo1 (reviewed by Nagata & Golstein 1995; also see below). In B-cells, death can be induced by engagement of surface immunoglobulins (Cuende et al 1993), and ligation of CD38 (Kumagai et al 1995).

Apoptosis is also induced by exposure to high temperature (Migliorati et al 1992), to ionizing and UV radiation (Sellins & Cohen 1987), and to a wide variety of cytotoxic drugs. Virtually all cytotoxic drugs used in the treatment of cancer appear to involve apoptosis in their mechanism of action (reviewed by Hickman 1992, Reed 1995). Therefore, relative propensity to apoptosis may explain differences in the susceptibility of different cancers to chemotherapy. One of the most extensively studied family of drugs that induces apoptosis are glucocorticoids (Wyllie 1980). Glucocorticoid-mediated apoptosis, and indeed several forms of programmed cell death, is prevented by inhibitors of protein synthesis, such as cycloheximide, and of transcription, such as actinomycin D, as well as by zinc, a blocker of the endonucleases which cleave chromatin into oligonucleosomal fragments (Wyllie et al 1984, Cohen & Duke 1984). Activation of these endonucleases by glucocorticoids appears to be allosteric and does not involve their de novo synthesis (Hickman 1992). Resistance to glucocorticoids does not seem to be simply a consequence of the lack of surface receptors, since the leukemic line CEM C1 expresses functional receptors yet glucocorticoid fails to trigger the apoptotic cascade (Zawydiwski et al 1983).

Topoisomerase I and II inhibitors are also effective inducers of apoptosis. For example, HL-60 and KG1a myeloid leukemia cell lines undergo rapid apoptosis after treatment with etoposide, a topoisomerase II inhibitor, and camptothecin, a topoisomerase I inhibitor (Kauffman 1989, Del Bino & Darzynkiewicz 1991). Interestingly, etoposide-induced apoptosis is not suppressed by inhibitors of protein synthesis but is suppressed by an inhibitor of RNA synthesis suggesting an uncommon mechanism of action (Kauffman 1989). Finally, apoptosis induced by DNA-reactive drugs (such as cisplatin, nitrogen mustard, chlorambucil, melphalan and BCNU), antimetabolites (such as methotrexate) and phase-specific agents (such as araC and taxol) has also been reported (reviewed by Hickman 1992, Reed 1995). We have recently shown that the purine analogue 2-chloro-2'-deoxyadenosine (2CdA) induces apoptosis in leukemic lymphoblasts (Kumagai et al 1994), which, in this respect, are analogous to cells in B-CLL and hairy cell leukemia (Carson et al 1992, Robertson et al 1993).

A particularly interesting area of research with potential clinical applications is the identification of agents that specifically trigger apoptosis in defined cell subpopulations. A paradigm of this concept is the observation that IL-4, a cytokine with pleiotropic activities, induces apoptosis in leukemic lymphoblasts (Manabe et al 1994a), but not in normal hemopoietic progenitor cells (Paul 1991). In our study, IL-4 was cytotoxic to most cases of B-lineage acute lymphoblastic leukemia (ALL), including all six cases with the t(9;22) or the t(4;11) chromosomal features which are often associated with a fatal outcome. These findings support current clinical testing of IL-4 in cases of high-risk ALL resistant to conventional therapy. Other cytokines, such as IL-10 (Fluckiger et al 1994b) and IL-5 (Mainou-Fowler et al 1994) have been shown to induce apoptosis in B-CLL cells, and represent potentially useful agents to include in clinical trials.

MORPHOLOGIC AND BIOCHEMICAL EVENTS OF APOPTOSIS

Despite the diversity of signals which can induce apoptosis, the resulting biochemical and morphological changes are largely overlapping, suggesting common effector pathways. Apoptosis often, but not always, requires RNA and/or protein synthesis. Therefore, it has been considered a programmed 'suicide' process, since the cell actively participates in its own destruction. Apoptosis rapidly proceeds through distinct morphologic changes (Kerr et al 1972, Evan et al 1992, Howie et al, 1994). Initially, cell volume decreases owing to loss of water and ions, and cell density increases. However, cell membranes, including the nuclear envelope and mitochondrial membranes, remain intact. Therefore, cells are impermeable to vital dyes such as trypan blue and propidium iodide until the later stages of the process. Marked changes occur in the nucleus, as chromatin condenses, marginates to the nuclear envelope and, ultimately, forms dense membrane-bound micronuclei. Concomitantly, the cell surface membrane ruffles and blebs and the nucleus breaks into fragments. Finally, the cell disintegrates into 'apoptotic bodies', which are phagocytosed by tissue macrophages. Interestingly, these phagocytes apparently recognize specific cell surface molecules expressed only in cells undergoing apoptosis. Since membrane integrity is largely retained and dying cells are rapidly eliminated, no intracellular contents are released, and inflammatory reactions are avoided. In normal tissues undergoing a high rate of apoptosis (e.g. thymus), or during chemotherapy, the number of apoptotic cells detectable by morphology or by histochemical labeling of fragmented DNA is low (i.e. < 1%), owing to the speed of the process (generally 30 to 60 minutes) and the efficient phagocytosis of dead cells (Howie et al 1994).

Apoptosis commonly involves the activation of endonucleases, which generate single-stranded DNA breaks preferentially between nucleosomes. This results in genomic DNA fragments of 180 base pairs (bp) or multiples, causing the characteristic 'ladder' appearance after gel electrophoresis (Fig. 1). The early formation of 50 to 300 bp fragments caused by the release of chromatin loop domains has also been demonstrated (Oberhammer et al 1993). The identity of the endonucleases is still uncertain, but several candidates have been identified. One is an 18 kD DNase isolated from thymocytes, termed Nuc 18, which is Ca^{2+} and Mg^{2+}-dependent (Gaido & Cidlowski 1991). Another putative apoptotic endonuclease is DNase II, which is not Ca^{2+} and Mg^{2+}-dependent (Barry & Eastman 1993). A third candidate is the Ca^{2+} and Mg^{2+}-dependent enzyme DNase I (Peistch et al 1993). Although typical, DNA cleavage is not an absolute requirement for apoptosis, as this can occur in some cells without DNA laddering, and enucleated cells retain their ability to undergo cytosolic changes typical of apoptosis (Jacobson et al 1994).

Cell death induced by ligation of the Fas/Apo1 antigen has been used to investigate the biochemical events that accompany apoptosis. Ligation of Fas/Apo1 induces rapid protein tyrosine kinase activity and phosphorylation of several unidentified intracellular substrates (Eischen et al 1994). This signal transduction event appears to be directly linked to apoptosis, since apoptosis was markedly reduced when cells were incubated with tyrosine kinase inhibitors before ligation of Fas/Apo1. Activation of proteases may also be part of the apoptotic pathway. Lahti et al (1995) showed that ligation of Fas/Apo1 in leukemic T-cell lines induced a dramatic increase in mRNA, steady-state protein levels and enzyme activity of PITSLRE kinase, a protein kinase of the $p34^{cdc2}$-family of cell cycle related kinases. In addition to induction of PITSLRE transcription and translation, proteolysis of larger isoforms contributed to the increase of a 50 kD PITSLRE isoform. This phenomenon was also observed during glucocorticoid-induced apoptosis indicating that it is a common biochemical event in the apoptotic pathway. Suppression of apoptosis by protease inhibitors in the myeloid cell line HL-60 and in normal thymocytes was also observed by Bruno et al (1992). Finally, recent results

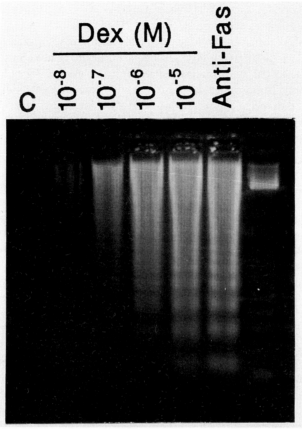

Fig. 1 Detection of apoptosis by DNA gel electrophoresis. T-cell acute lymphoblastic leukemia CEM-C7 cells were treated with dexamethasone (Dex) at the indicated concentrations for 72 hours or with anti-Fas antibody (100 ng/ml; UBI) for 6 hours. Cells were then lysed and DNA processed as described in the text. The typical DNA ladder of multiples of 180 base pairs is evident. Virtually no fragmented DNA was extracted from untreated cells (C). The lane on the far right contains the molecular weight marker of multiples of 123 base pairs.

have suggested a potential role for reactive oxygen species (i.e. the superoxide ion, hydrogen peroxide and the hydroxyl radical) in apoptosis (Hockenbery et al 1993, Buttke & Sandstrom 1994).

MOLECULAR REGULATION OF APOPTOSIS

Apoptosis occurs in virtually all organisms, and the fundamental evolutionary pathways that regulate this process are conserved. For example, the nematode *Caenorhabditis elegans* has been used extensively to identify genes that regulate apoptosis during development. *C. elegans* has 1090 somatic cells, 131 of which are programmed to die by apoptosis at specific developmental stages (reviewed by Ellis et al 1991). Analysis of mutant worms with abnormal numbers of cells has led to the identification of three *ced* (cell death abnormal) genes (3, 4 and 9) as key regulators of apoptosis (Ellis et al 1991). Mutations that induce loss of *ced-9* function increase cell death (Hengartner et al 1992), whereas those that induce a gain of function produce extra cells during development (Hengartner & Horvitz 1994). Interestingly, *ced-9* is structurally related and functionally homologous to the mammalian anti-apoptotic gene *bcl-2* (Hengartner & Horvitz 1994). Importantly, *bcl-2* can partially rescue *ced-9* function in *ced-9*-deficient worms (Vaux et al 1992). By contrast, *ced-3* and *-4* promote cell death; their loss of function produces worms with additional cells (reviewed by Ellis et al 1991). *Ced-3* is structurally similar to a class of mammalian proteases, typified by the IL-1β-converting enzyme (ICE), a cysteine-protease that cleaves *pro-IL-1β* to its active form (Yuan et al 1993). Transient expression of murine ICE or ced-3 induces apoptosis in fibroblasts (Miura et al 1993). Conversely, expression of crmA, a virus-encoded inhibitor of cystein proteases, blocks ICE- and *ced-3*-induced death (Yuan et al 1993). Moreover, a role for cysteine proteases in apoptosis during development has been implied by studies showing that crmA can block death of neuronal cells following nerve growth factor withdrawal (Gagliardini et al 1994).

Mammalian genes that modulate apoptosis represent an expanding family (Table 1). One of the most extensively studied regulators of apoptosis is *bcl-2*. Enforced expression of *bcl-2* generally suppresses apoptosis in lymphohemopoietic cells and neurons (Vaux et al 1988, Nunez et al 1990), although exceptions, e.g. Apo1/Fas-induced cell death, have been reported (Nagata & Golstein 1995). Bcl-2 is an integral membrane protein that is found in outer mitochondrial membranes, endoplasmic reticulum and nuclear membrane (Hockenbery et al 1990, Monaghan et al 1992, Nguyen et al 1993). However, membrane localization is apparently not essential for Bcl-2 function, as a mutant form of Bcl-2 lacking membrane anchor sequences retains, albeit partially, anti-apoptotic activity (Hockenbery et al 1993). Although no specific biochemical function has been assigned to Bcl-2, it can function as an

Table 1 Proteins that regulate apoptosis in mammalian cells

Inducers	Suppressors
Bax	Bcl-2*
$Bcl-X_s$	$Bcl-X_L$
Bad	A1
Bak	Mcl-1
E2F*	BAG
NUR77	pRb*
p53*	
ICE, Nedd-2 (cycteine proteases)	
c-Myc	
ODC	
Cyclin A	
$p34^{cdc2}$	

* Prolonged cell survival resulting from alterations of these proteins has been implicated in oncogenesis.

antioxidant (Hockenbery et al 1993). Bcl-2 activity requires formation of heterodimers with the related protein Bax, which accelerates apoptosis and antagonizes Bcl-2 function (Oltvai et al 1993). Therefore the equilibrium in the formation of Bcl-2:Bax heterodimers (suppressors of death) and Bax:Bax homodimers (activators of death) appears to be central in the molecular regulation of apoptosis (Yin et al 1994). In addition, several other Bcl-2-related family members, which also regulate apoptosis, have recently been identified. These include the suppressors of death Bcl-X_L (Boise et al 1993), Mcl-1 (Kozopas et al 1993), A1 (Lin et al 1993) and BAG (Takayama et al 1995), and additional death inducers Bcl-X_S (a spliced version of Bcl-X_L; Boise et al 1993), Bad (Yang et al 1995) and Bak (Farrow et al 1995, Chittenden et al 1995, Kiefer et al 1995). All Bcl-2 family members physically interact through their shared motifs (reviewed in Oltvai & Korsmeyer 1994). Interestingly, there is some specificity in these interactions, as, for example, Mcl-1 only dimerizes with Bax, and Bad preferentially associates with Bcl-X_L (Oltvai & Korsmeyer 1994). The critical function of some of these molecules during lymphohemopoietic development has been conclusively demonstrated. Deletion of Bcl-2 or of Bcl-X_L leads to fulminant apoptosis in the developing thymus of Bcl-2 -/- knock-out mice (Veis et al 1993), or in all hemopoietic lineages in Bcl-X_L -/- mice (Motoyama et al 1995).

REGULATORS OF CELL PROLIFERATION ALSO MODULATE APOPTOSIS

A balance between cell proliferation and cell death controls the homeostasis of tissues and organs. Therefore, several proteins associated with cell proliferation can induce apoptosis if overexpressed or expressed at inappropriate times. These include c-Myc (reviewed in Packham & Cleveland 1995), E2F-1 (Wu & Levine 1994), cyclin A (Hoang et al 1994) and p34^{cdc2} (Shi et al 1994), all of which can promote inappropriate entry of cells into the S phase of the cell cycle, and cause subsequent apoptosis.

The expression of c-Myc is rapidly induced by mitogenic stimulation of normal cells, and is downregulated by withdrawal of serum or specific growth factors. c-Myc promotes cell cycle progression and inhibits differentiation (Packham & Cleveland 1995). The first direct demonstration that c-Myc could promote apoptosis came from experiments with 32D.3 cells, a murine myeloid cell line whose viability and growth is absolutely dependent on IL-3 (Askew et al 1991). Withdrawal of IL-3 from the cells leads to a rapid downregulation of c-Myc expression, which precedes accumulation of cells in the G_0/G_1 phase of the cell cycle and their death by apoptosis. Remarkably, enforced c-Myc expression has dramatic consequences on this regulatory network and induces immediate cell death in the absence of IL-3 (Askew et al 1991). Subsequent observations in fibroblasts have indicated that induction of apoptosis is a common fate for cells with deregulated c-Myc (Evan et al 1992). Similar observations have been made with E2F (Qin et al 1995).

Since both c-Myc and E2F function as transcription factors, and this activity is required for induction of apoptosis, it is suspected that transcriptional targets of either gene serve as mediators in the apoptotic pathway. Recently, several of the proposed transcriptional targets of c-Myc have been tested as mediators of apoptosis. In 32.3D cells, ornithine decarboxylase (ODC), a direct transcriptional target of c-Myc, is an effector of c-Myc-induced apoptosis. Enforced expression of ODC enzyme activity induces apoptosis, albeit not as effectively as c-Myc, while DFMO, an inhibitor of ODC enzyme activity, inhibits rates of c-Myc-induced apoptosis (Packham & Cleveland 1994).

The transcription factor p53 functions as a G_1 check point of the cell cycle (Kastan et al 1992, Lane 1992). Overexpression of p53 blocks cells in G_1 and p53 is also induced following DNA damage (Kastan et al 1992). This results either in G_1 arrest, which allows DNA repair before S phase entry, or induces apoptosis, depending on the extent of DNA damage, the presence of survival factors and/or cell type. For example, p53 is required for apoptosis of thymocytes induced by ionizing radiation or etoposide, yet is not necessary for death induced by dexamethasone (Clarke et al 1993, Lowe et al 1993). Additionally, p53 contributes to apoptosis of some myeloid cell lines following IL-3 withdrawal (Gottlieb et al 1994, Yonish-Rouach et al 1991), but not in erythroid progenitors following erythropoietin withdrawal (Kelley et al 1994). In summary, p53 functions as a safety mechanism that opposes entry of cells in S phase before DNA repair occurs, blocking the propagation of potentially oncogenic mutations or genetic instability (Lane 1992). Notably, however, apoptosis can occur in lymphocytes of p53 deficient mice after irradiation (Strasser et al 1994). Therefore, p53 is not essential for apoptosis caused by DNA damage.

APOPTOSIS IN LYMPHOHEMATOPOIESIS

Extensive cell death occurs during thymocyte maturation when up to 90% of immature T-cells are deleted by apoptosis during the processes of positive and negative selection that shape the T-lymphocyte compartment (reviewed by King & Ashwell 1993). Apoptosis of immature T-cells is induced by ligation of CD3 with specific antibodies (Smith et al 1989).

An important mediator of apoptosis in the immune system is Fas/Apo1, a transmembrane receptor that is a member of the tumor necrosis factor (TNF) and nerve growth factor (NGF) receptor superfamily (reviewed by Nagata & Golstein 1995). The FAS/Apo1 ligand is structurally homologous to the TNF/NGF family of molecules (Nagata & Golstein 1995). Fas/Apo1 is expressed on many cell types including immature and activated T-cells, activated B-cells, natural killer (NK) cells, monocytes, myeloid cells and fibroblasts. Evidence for a physiological role of this molecule, however, has been chiefly provided in studies of T-cell development and function. It has been established that the interaction between Fas/Apo1 and its ligand is an important regulator of T-cell selection (Nagata & Golstein 1995). This function is well demonstrated by the observation that mice homozygous for *lpr*, a germline mutation that results in loss of function of the murine Fas, develop a systemic lupus erythematosus-like autoimmune disease (reviewed by Nagata & Golstein 1995). This is caused by a failure in negative selection of self-reactive T-lymphocytes, as Fas is required for death induced by engagement of the T-cell receptor (Nagata & Golstein 1995). Fas/Apol also appears to participate in the effector functions of the immune system, and it has been shown to be involved in T-cell mediated cytotoxicity (Owen-Schaub et al 1992).

Additional evidence that apoptosis is an integral part of T-cell differentiation comes from the work of Akbar et al (1993) who showed that transition of CD45RA+ 'naive' T-cells to activated CD45RO+ cells was associated with decreases in Bcl-2 expression and propensity to undergo apoptosis. Apoptosis of CD45RO+ primed/memory T-cells in vitro could be prevented by exogenous stimuli such as IL-2 or co-culture with fibroblasts. Moreover, CD45RO+ T cells that express CD8 and expand during viral infections also have low levels of Bcl-2 and a tendency to undergo apoptosis (Akbar et al 1994). These cells are rapidly eliminated by tissue macrophages, which ingest apoptotic cells, recognized through surface molecules which include $\alpha_v\beta_3$ integrin (the vitronectin receptor), CD36 and thrombospondin (Akbar et al 1994).

Death by apoptosis is probably the fate of normal B-cell precursors that do not productively rearrange their immunoglobulin genes and fail to differentiate further along the B-cell pathway (reviewed by Cohen 1991). Moreover, self-reactive B-cells can be, like T-cells, deleted by apoptosis. Experiments in transgenic mice have shown that self-reactive B-lymphocytes are eliminated if they encounter membrane-bound self-antigens at early stages of development in the bone marrow (Hartley et al 1993). Elimination of these cells occurs by apoptosis and it is markedly suppressed by targeted overexpression of the Bcl-2 gene. Self-reactive B-cells can also be eliminated via apoptosis in peripheral lymphoid organs, where they are excluded from the normal migration pathways into the lymphoid follicles (Cyster et al 1994). B-cells undergo further selection in the germinal center according to their affinity for antigens presented by follicular dendritic cells (Liu et al 1989). The basis for this selection is the tendency of B-cells at this stage of differentiation to initiate apoptosis, perhaps determined by their extremely low Bcl-2 expression (Liu et al 1991). Indeed, isolated germinal center B-cells rapidly die by apoptosis, unless their surface immunoglobulins are cross-linked; other stimuli that rescue these cells from apoptosis include ligation of CD40 and of CD23 (Liu et al 1991). Moreover, Gregory et al (1991) showed that Epstein-Barr virus (EBV) infection protects B-cells from apoptosis through the expression of virus-coded proteins. EBV-positive Burkitt's lymphoma clones that express only one of these proteins (EBNA 1) remain sensitive to apoptosis, not unlike normal germinal center B-cells. However, clones in which eight EBV latent proteins are activated become resistant to induction of apoptosis.

Apoptosis also plays a key role in the homeostatic control of hemopoietic progenitor cells. The role of apoptosis in the movement of prenatal hemopoiesis sites and hemoglobin switching have been postulated (Koury 1992). Growth factors that suppress apoptosis of immature myeloid lines in culture include IL-3 (Rodriguez-Tarduchy et al 1990), granulocyte-macrophage colony stimulating factor (GM-CSF; Williams et al 1990), granulocyte-colony stimulating factor (G-CSF; Williams et al 1990) and macrophage-colony stimulating factor (M-CSF; Tushinski et al 1982). Whether normal myeloid progenitors require constant exposure to these factors for viability has not yet been ascertained. The myeloid cell line HL-60 undergoes apoptosis after differentiation in vitro by exposure to retinoic acid (Martin et al 1990). It has been shown that levels of Bcl-2 protein expression decrease during HL-60 differentiation and during normal myeloid maturation (Delia et al 1992). Peripheral blood neutrophils and eosinophils also undergo apoptosis when maintained for prolonged periods of time in culture (Cotter et al 1994). In vivo, apoptotic neutrophils are cleared by phagocytes, an event that operates through a recognition system similar to that outlined above for virally infected lymphocytes (Savill et al 1990).

Peripheral blood monocytes undergo apoptosis after 24 hours of culture in the absence of stimuli such as IL-1β, tumor necrosis factor or GM-CSF (Mangan & Wahl 1991). Infection of bone marrow-derived macrophages with the parasite *Leishmania donovani* inhibits apoptosis, probably through the induction of cytokines such as TNF and GM-CSF (Moore & Matlashewski 1994).

Erythropoietin (EPO) has been shown to suppress apoptosis in erythroid progenitor cells. Koury and Bondurant (1990) have proposed a model of erythropoiesis (which they postulate could extend to other hemopoietic cells) in which progenitor cells reach a stage of development at which they become dependent on growth factors for survival. In erythroid cells, the EPO-dependent stage would include the erythroid colony-forming units (CFU-E) and the immature erythroblasts. In this model, individual cells require different amounts of growth factor to survive. Therefore, the amount of available growth factor determines the number of surviving progenitor cells. In erythroid development, only a minority of the EPO-dependent progenitors survives due to the limited amounts of EPO available. When these levels increase (e.g. because of anemia), the number of surviving progenitors increases, whereas when EPO-levels decrease (e.g. because of hypertransfusion) very few EPO-dependent progenitors survive (Koury 1992).

APOPTOSIS AND ONCOGENESIS

Defective expression of molecules that induce apoptosis at critical stages of differentiation may contribute to the development of neoplasia by prolonging cell survival (Fig. 2). For example, removal of the apoptosis inducer p53 by gene deletion in mice is followed by the development of numerous tumors, and inactivating mutations of the p53 gene have been observed in many types of cancer. Conversely, overexpression of molecules that suppress apoptosis has also been associated with the development of neoplasia. Transgenic mice with *bcl-2* under transcriptional control of immunoglobulin enhancer sequences display marked hyperplasia and accumulate small resting B-cells

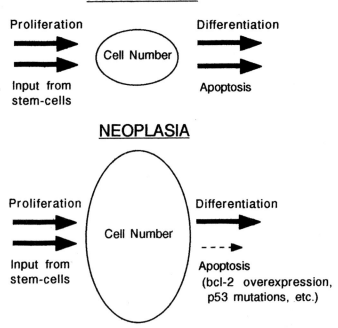

Fig. 2 Apoptosis and the development of neoplasia. The number of cells at a transitional stage of differentiation (e.g. myeloid and lymphoid progenitor cells, activated lymphoid cells) depends on events that increase cell numbers, such as input from stem cells and proliferation, and events which decrease cell numbers, such as differentiation and apoptosis. The homeostasic balance between these events may be broken by alterations of genes that regulate apoptosis, leading to neoplasia.

with extended survival in vitro (McDonnell & Korsmeyer 1991). After a long latency period, these mice develop clonal B-cell lymphomas, often associated with c-*myc* translocations (McDonnell et al 1989). There are notable discrepancies in Bcl-2 expression between follicular B-cell non-Hodgkin's lymphoma cells, which exhibit high levels of Bcl-2, and their normal counterparts, proliferating germinal center cells, which appear to be Bcl-2 negative.

Discrepancies in Bcl-2 expression between leukemic lymphoblasts in ALL and their normal counterparts, normal B-cell progenitors of the bone marrow, have also become apparent (Campana et al 1993a). In our recent study, flow cytometric measurements of Bcl-2 in leukemic lymphoblasts from 43 cases of B-lineage ALL were markedly heterogeneous, but were clearly higher than those detected in normal bone marrow $CD10^+$ B-lymphoid progenitors and $CD19_v^+$ peripheral blood B-lymphocytes (Coustan-Smith et al 1996). Likewise, levels of Bcl-2 in all nine T-ALL cases studied were higher than those found in thymic immature $CD1a^+$ cells, and, in four cases, they were also higher than those observed in peripheral blood T-lymphocytes (Coustan-Smith et al 1996). Overexpression of Bcl-2 may therefore contribute to leukemogenesis via prolongation of the life-span of progenitor cells, which could facilitate further genetic alterations leading to neoplasia. Overexpression of Bcl-2 may also explain the ability of specific leukemic lymphoblasts to grow outside the bone marrow microenvironment. The molecular mechanisms leading to overexpression of Bcl-2 in ALL cells are still unknown and none of the cases in our series had the chromosomal translocation 14;18, known to deregulate *bcl*-2 expression in NHL.

Enforced c-*myc* expression promotes neoplastic transformation both in vitro and in vivo (reviewed by Packham & Cleveland 1995). Transgenic mice carrying c-*myc* under the transcriptional control of immunoglobulin enhancer sequences, an allele that resembles the translocation found in Burkitt's lymphoma and targets deregulated c-*myc* expression to the B-cell compartment, are prone to B-cell lymphomas (reviewed by Packham & Cleveland 1995). Alterations in c-Myc levels or structure observed in human cancer may also modulate c-Myc-induced apoptosis. Since c-Myc induces apoptosis, the association of activation of c-*myc* and the development of neoplasia appears paradoxical. Indeed, enforced c-*myc* expression by itself does not cause tumors in transgenic mice (reviewed by Packham & Cleveland 1995). Genes which co-operate with c-*myc* to accelerate tumorigenesis have been identified by infection with recombinant retroviruses, cross-breeding transgenic mice strains and by insertional mutagenesis, and include *bcl*-2 (Nunez et al 1990). Bcl-2 suppresses c-Myc-induced apoptosis without inhibiting c-Myc-induced cell cycle progression (Bissonette et al 1992). Therefore, at least in part, c-Myc-mediated tumorigenesis can be considered the result of activation of c-Myc-induced cell cycle progression and apoptosis, and the specific suppression of apoptosis by co-operating oncogenes (Packham & Cleveland 1995). However, additional events are apparently required for tumorigenic conversion, as tumor formation in transgenic mice harboring both deregulated c-*myc* and *bcl*-2 requires additional somatic mutations, which have not yet been identified.

METHODS TO DETECT AND MEASURE APOPTOSIS

The activation of apoptosis can be revealed by the appearance of cells with fragmented nuclei, which can be observed in the tissue culture vessels by use of an inverted microscope, by examination of smears and cytocentrifuge preparations or by electron microscopical analysis of fixed cells. Nuclear fragmentation can also be visualized with DNA-binding fluorochromes such as DAPI, ethidium bromide and Hoechst 33342. Other approaches provide early direct evidence of apoptosis including DNA fragmentation assays and flow cytometry.

DNA fragmentation assay

Many methods to visualize DNA fragmentation by gel electrophoresis have been reported. Here we briefly describe a technique that has yielded consistent results in our laboratory (Fig. 1) – a modification of the protocol described by Sellins & Cohen (1987). Mononuclear cells (0.5–2 x 10^6) are centrifuged at 500 x g for 10 minutes and the cell pellet is lysed with 0.5 ml of hypotonic lysing buffer (10 mM Tris, pH 7.4; 1 mM EDTA; 0.2% Triton X-100). Lysates are then centrifuged at 11 000 x g for 10 minutes to separate intact from fragmented chromatin, and the genomic DNA precipitated for 16–48 hours at -20°C in 50% isopropanol and 0.5 M NaCl. The precipitates are then centrifuged at 11 000 x g for 10 minutes, air-dried, resuspended in TE buffer (10 mM Tris, pH 7.4; 1 mM EDTA) and heated at 55°C for 10 minutes. The loading buffer (15 mM EDTA; 2% sodium dodecyl sulfate; 50% glycerol; 0.5% orange G) is added to the samples at a 1:5 (vol:vol) ratio, and the mixture heated to 65°C for 10 minutes. The samples and the molecular size marker (e.g. 123 bp DNA ladder; Gibco BRL) are loaded into the dry wells of a 1.5% agarose gel, electrophoresed for 30 minutes at 20 V, then TBE buffer (0.09 M Tris borate; 0.002 M EDTA) is added until the gel is completely immersed. Electrophoresis is continued for 3–4 hours at 20 V, after which the gels are incubated in TBE buffer containing DNase-free RNase A (Boehringer Mannheim Corp.) at 37°C for 3 hours to digest RNA, stained with ethidium bromide (2 µg/ml) for 15 minutes, washed and photographed. In this assay, intact chromatin and oligonucleosomal fragments are separated by centrifugation. Therefore, in the absence of apoptosis, the gel lane with the corresponding supernatant DNA appears empty (Fig. 1).

Flow cytometry

Several strategies have been used to detect and quantitate apoptosis by flow cytometry. Changes in the light scattering properties of the cells accompany early morphologic changes characteristic of apoptosis. These changes consist of decreased forward and increased orthogonal light scatter signals (Swat et al 1991, Campana et al 1993b). Therefore, apoptotic cells form a distinct cluster in a dot plot histogram. If the population analyzed is a mixture of different cell types, subsets can be identified by simultaneously labeling cells with antibodies. To enumerate viable cells in our experiments, we design 'gates' in the light-scattering dot plot around the area where the vast majority of leukemic cells or lymphoid progenitors are found at the initiation of the experiments, excluding apoptotic cells. The parameters of such 'gates' are recorded and subsequently applied in counting the number of non-apoptotic cells present in the culture. These numbers are then corrected according to the percentage of cells expressing a given phenotype in the sample studied.

Low DNA stainability, caused by DNA fragmentation and diffusion of low molecular weight DNA product from the cells, is typical of cells undergoing apoptosis (Fig. 3; Nicoletti et al 1991, Telford et al 1992, Darzynkiewicz et al 1992). We have used the following method to assess DNA content and detect cells with hypodiploidy. We perform cell fixation and permeabilization using 0.25% para-formaldehyde and 0.2% Tween 20, respectively. Cells are then treated with DNAse-free RNAse (11.25 Kunitz Units) and labeled with

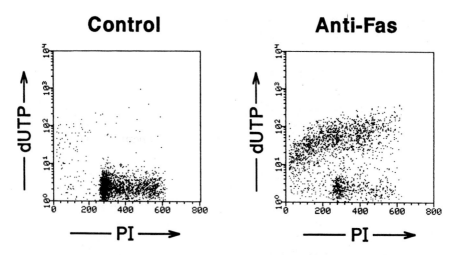

Fig. 3 Detection of apoptosis by flow cytometry. T-cell acute lymphoblastic leukemia CEM-C7 cells were treated with anti-Fas antibody (100 ng/ml; UBI) for 6 hours. Cells were then permeabilized and incubated with digoxigenin-labeled dUTP followed by an antibody to digoxigenin labeled with fluorescein isothiocyanate (see text). Cells were also counterstained with propidium iodide (PI) to reveal DNA content. Induction of apoptosis by ligation of Fas is revealed by the emergence of dUTP labeled cells (Y axis) and by the appearance of cells with hypodiploid DNA content (X axis). Note that some dUTP-positive cells retain an apparently normal DNA content, indicating that dUTP labeling is more sensitive than PI labeling for detecting apoptosis.

7-actinomycin D (7-AAD; 25 mg/ml; Sigma) or propidium iodide (PI; 10 mg/ml; Calbiochem) for at least 30 minutes (Campana et al 1993b). Cells are then analyzed by flow cytometry using a FACScan equipped with the CellFit software (Becton Dickinson).

Another approach to measure apoptosis by flow cytometry is the detection of fragmented DNA by incorporating tagged nucleotides. Gavrieli et al (1992) described the TUNEL (terminal deoxynucleotidyl transferase (TdT)-mediated dUTP-biotin nick end labeling) and Wisjman et al (1993) reported a similar method for in situ end-labeling (ISEL) of DNA stand breaks. These methods were originally applied to detect apoptotic cells in tissue sections, but can be adapted to study apoptosis in cell suspensions. We have successfully used the technique described by Gold et al (1993) with minor modifications. In this method, cells are fixed and permeabilized as described above, followed by incubation with fluorescein 12-dUTP and unconjugated dATP, dCTP and dGTP, in the presence of DNA polymerase I (or TdT; all available from Sigma). After overnight incubation at 37°C, the reaction is stopped by adding EDTA and cells are analyzed by flow cytometry. Apoptotic cells are labeled by the fluoresceinated-dUTP.

Labeling of total DNA content with propidium iodide and of fragmented DNA can be performed simultaneously. In this case, however, best results are obtained by replacing fluoresceinated-dUTP with digoxigenin-labeled dUTP

(Oncor). This, in turn, needs to be visualized with a fluorescein-labeled antibody to digoxigenin (Fig. 3; Darzynkiewicz et al 1992).

KEY POINTS FOR CLINICAL PRACTICE

- Apoptosis plays a central role in embryogenesis, morphogenesis and regulation of normal cell turnover in multicellular organisms. Apoptotic rates participate in the control of hemopoiesis and lymphopoiesis.

- Apoptosis often requires RNA and/or protein synthesis and has been considered a programmed 'suicide' process. The number of apoptotic cells detectable in tissues is low due to the speed of the process and the efficient phagocytosis of apoptotic cells.

- The stimuli that induce apoptosis are diverse but the resulting biochemical and morphological changes are largely overlapping, indicating common effector mechanisms.

- Virtually all cytotoxic drugs used in the treatment of cancer appear to involve apoptosis in their mechanism of action. Therefore, propensity to apoptosis may explain differences in the curability of different cancers by chemotherapy. A novel area of research with potential clinical applications is the identification of agents that specifically trigger apoptosis in defined cell subpopulations.

- Defective expression of molecules that induce apoptosis, or overexpression of molecules that suppress apoptosis at critical stages of differentiation, may contribute to the development of neoplasia by prolonging survival of defective cells.

- Several suppressors and inducers of apoptosis have been identified. The molecular mechanisms that regulate cell death may be as complex as those that control cell proliferation.

REFERENCES

Akbar A N, Borthwick N, Salmon M et al 1993 The significance of low bcl-2 expression by CD45RO T cells in normal individuals and patients with acute viral infections. The role of apoptosis in T cell memory. J Exp Med 178: 427–438

Akbar A N, Savill J, Gombert W et al 1994 The specific recognition by macrophages of CD8+, CD45RO+ T cells undergoing apoptosis: a mechanism for T cell clearance during resolution of viral infections. J Exp Med 180: 1943–1947

Askew D S, Ashmun R A, Simmons B C et al 1991 Constitutive c-myc expression in an IL-3-dependent myeloid cell line suppresses cell cycle arrest and accelerates apoptosis. Oncogene 6: 1915–1922

Barry M A, Eastman A 1993 Identification of deoxyribonuclease II as an endonuclease involved in apoptosis. Arch Biochem Biophys 300: 440–448

Bissonnette R P, Echeverri F, Mahboubi A et al 1992 Apoptotic cell death induced by c-*myc* is inhibited by *bcl*-2. Nature 359: 552–554

Boise L H, Gonzalez-Garcia M, Postema C E et al 1993 bcl-x, a bcl-2-related gene that functions as a dominant regulator of apoptotic cell death. Cell 74: 597–608

Bruno S, Del Bino G, Lassota P et al 1992 Inhibitors of proteases prevent endonucleolysis accompanying apoptotic death of HL-60 leukemic cells and normal thymocytes. Leukemia 6: 1113–1120

Buschle M, Campana D, Hoffbrand A V et al 1993 Interferon-γ inhibits apoptotic cell death in B-cell chronic lymphocytic leukemia. J Exp Med 177: 213–218

Buttke T M, Sandstrom P A 1994 Oxidative stress as a mediator of apoptosis. Immunol Today 15: 7–10

Campana D, Coustan-Smith E, Manabe A et al 1993a Prolonged survival of B-lineage acute lymphoblasic leukemia cells is accompanied by overexpression of bcl-2 protein. Blood 81: 1025–1031

Campana D, Manabe A, Evans W E 1993b Stroma-supported immunocytometric assay (SIA): a novel method for testing the sensitivity of acute lymphoblastic leukemia cells to cytotoxic drugs. Leukemia 7: 482–488

Carson D A, Wasson D B, Esparza L M et al 1992 Oral antilymphocyte activity and induction of apoptosis by 2-chloro-2'-arabino-fluro-2' -deoxyadenosine. Proc Natl Acad Sci USA 89: 2970–2974

Chittenden T, Harrington E A, O'Connor R et al 1995 Induction of apoptosis by the bcl-2 homologue Bak. Nature 374: 733–736

Clarke A R, Purdie C A, Harrison D J et al 1993 Thymocyte apoptosis induced by p53-dependent and independent pathways. Nature 362: 849–852

Cohen J J 1991 Programmed cell death in the immune system. Adv Immunol 50: 55–85

Cohen J J, Duke R C 1984 Glucocorticoid activation of a calcium-dependent endonuclease in thymocyte nuclei leads to cell death. J Immunol 132: 38–42

Cotter T G, Fernandes R S, Verhaegen S et al 1994 Cell death in the myeloid lineage. Immunol Rev 142: 93–112

Couston-Smith E, Kitanaka A, Pui C-H et al 1996 Clinical relevance of bcl-2 expression in childhood acute lymphoblastic leukemia. Blood (in press)

Cuende E, Ales-Martinez J E, Ding L et al 1993 Programmed cell death by bcl-2-dependent and independent mechanisms in B lymphoma cells. EMBO J 12: 1555–1560

Cyster J G, Hartley S B, Goodnow C C 1994 Competition for follicular niches excludes self-reactive cells from the recirculating B-cell repertoire. Nature 371: 389–395

Dancescu M, Rubio-Trujillo M, Biron G et al 1992 Interleukin 4 protects chronic lymphocytic leukemic B cells from death by apoptosis and upregulates Bcl-2 expression. J Exp Med 176: 1319–1326

Darzynkiewicz Z, Bruno S, Del Bino G et al 1992 Features of apoptotic cells measured by flow cytometry. Cytometry 13: 795–808

Del Bino G, Darzynkiewicz S 1991 Camptothecin, teniposide, or 4'-(9-acridinylamino)-3-methansulfon-m-anisitidine, but not mitoxantrone or doxorubicin, induce degradation of nuclear DNA in the S-phase of HL-60 cells. Cancer Res 51: 1165–1169

Delia D, Aiello A, Soligo D et al 1992 Bcl-2 proto-oncogene expression in normal and neoplastic human myeloid cells. Blood 79: 1291–1298

Duke R C, Cohen J J 1986 IL-2 addiction: withdrawal of growth factor activates a suicide program in dependent T cells. Lymphokine Res 5: 289–299

Eischen C M, Dick C J, Leibson P J 1994 Tyrosine kinase activation provides an early and requisite signal for Fas-induced apoptosis. J Immunol 153: 1947–1954

Ellis R E, Yuan J, Horvitz H R 1991 Mechanisms and functions of cell death. Annu Rev Cell Biol 7: 663–698

Evan G I, Wyllie A H, Gilbert C S et al 1992 Induction of apoptosis in fibroblasts by c-myc protein. Cell 69: 119–128

Farrow S N, White J H M, Martinou I et al 1995 Cloning of a bcl-2 homologue by interaction with adenovirus E1B 19K. Nature 374: 731–733

Fluckiger A C, Briere F, Zurawski G et al 1994a IL-13 has only a subset of IL-4-like activities on B chronic lymphocytic leukaemia cells. Immunology 83: 397–403

Fluckiger A C, Durand I, Banchereau J 1994b Interleukin-10 induces apoptotic cell death of B-chronic lymphocytic leukemia cells. J Exp Med 179: 91–99

Gagliardini V, Fernandez P A, Lee R K et al 1994 Prevention of vertebrate neuronal death by the crmA gene. Science 263: 826–828

Gaido M L, Cidlowski J A 1991 Identification, purification and characterization of a calcium-dependent endonuclease (NUC18) from rat thymocytes. NUC18 is not histone H2B. J Biol Chem 266: 18580–18585
Gavrieli Y, Sherman Y, Ben-Sasson S A 1992 Identification of programmed cell death in situ via specific labeling of nuclear DNA fragmentation. J Cell Biol 119: 493–501
Gold R, Schmied M, Rothe G et al 1993 Detection of DNA fragmentation in apoptosis: application of in situ nick translation to cell culture systems and tissue sections. J Histochem Cytochem 41: 1023–1030
Gottlieb E, Haffner R, von Ruden T et al 1994 Down-regulation of wild-type p53 activity interferes with apoptosis of IL-3-dependent hematopoietic cells following IL-3 withdrawal. EMBO J 13: 1368–1374
Gregory C D, Dive C, Henderson S et al 1991 Activation of Epstein-Barr virus latent genes protects human B cells from death by apoptosis. Nature 349: 612–614
Hartley S B, Cooke M P, Fulcher D A et al 1993 Elimination of self-reactive B lymphocytes proceeds in two stages: arrested development and cell death. Cell 72: 325–335
Hengartner M O, Ellis R E, Horvitz H R 1992 Caenorhabditis elegans gene *ced*-9 protects cells from programmed cell death. Nature 356: 494–499
Hengartner M O, Horvitz H R 1994 Activation of *C. elegans* cell death protein ced-9 by an amino acid substitution in a domain conserved in Bcl-2. Nature 369: 318–320
Hickman J A 1992 Apoptosis induced by anticancer drugs. Cancer and metastasis reviews 11: 121–139
Hoang A T, Cohen K J, Barrett J F et al 1994 Participation of cyclin A in *myc*-induced apoptosis. Proc Natl Acad Sci USA 91: 6875–6879
Hockenbery D, Nunez G, Milliman C et al 1990 *Bcl*-2 is an inner mitochondrial membrane protein that blocks programmed cell death. Nature 348: 334–336
Hockenbery D M, Oltvai Z N, Yin X M et al 1993 *Bcl*-2 functions in an antioxidant pathway to prevent apoptosis. Cell 75: 241–251
Howie S E M, Harrison D J, Wyllie A H 1994 Lymphocyte apoptosis. Mechanisms and implications in disease. Immunol Rev 142: 141–156
Jacobson M D, Burne J F, Raff M C 1994 Programmed cell death and Bcl-2 protection in the absence of a nucleus. EMBO J 13: 1899–1910
Kastan M B, Zhan Q, el-Deiry W S et al 1992 A mammalian cell cycle checkpoint pathway utilizing p53 and GADD45 is defective in ataxia-telangiectasia. Cell 71: 587–597
Kauffman H 1989 Induction of endonucleolytic DNA cleavage in human acute myelogenous leukemia cells by etoposide, camptothecin and other cytotoxic anticancer drugs: a cautionary note. Cancer Res 49: 5870–5878
Kelley L L, Green W F, Hicks G G et al 1994 Apoptosis in erythroid progenitors deprived of erythropoietin occurs during the G1 and S phases of the cell cycle without growth arrest or stabilization of wild-type p53. Mol Cell Biol 14: 4183–4192
Kerr J F R, Wyllie A H, Currie A R 1972 Apoptosis: a basic biological phenomenon with wide-ranging implications in tissue kinetics. Br J Cancer 26: 239
Kiefer M C, Brauer M J, Powers V C et al 1995 Modulation of apoptosis by the widely distributed Bcl-2 homologue Bak. Nature 374: 736–739
King L B, Ashwell J D 1993 Signaling for death of lymphoid cells. Curr Opin Immunol 5: 368–373
Korsmeyer S J 1992 Bcl-2 initiates a new category of oncogenes: regulators of cell death. Blood 80: 879–886
Koury M J 1992 Programmed cell death (apoptosis) in hematopoiesis. Exp Hematol 20: 391–394
Koury M J, Bondurant M C 1990 Erythropoietin retards DNA breakdown and prevents programmed cell death in erythroid progenitor cells. Science 248: 378–381
Kozopas K M, Yang T, Buchan H L et al 1993 MCL-1, a gene expressed in programmed myeloid cell differentiation, has sequence similarity to bcl-2. Proc Natl Acad Sci USA 90: 3515–3520
Kumagai M, Manabe A, Coustan-Smith E et al 1994 Use of stroma-supported cultures of leukemic cells to assess antileukemic drugs. II. Potent cytotoxicity of 2-chloro-deoxyadenosine in acute lymphoblastic leukemia. Leukemia 8: 1116–1123
Kumagai M, Coustan-Smith E, Murry D J et al 1995 Ligation of CD38 suppresses human B lymphopoiesis. J Exp Med 181: 1101–1110
Lahti J M, Xiang J, Heath L S et al 1995 PITSLRE protein kinase activity is associated with apoptosis. Mol Cell Biol 15: 1–11

Lane D P 1992 Cancer. p53, guardian of the genome. Nature 358: 15–16

Lin E Y, Orlofsky A, Berger M S et al 1993 Characterization of A1, a novel hemopoietic-specific early-response gene with sequence similarity to *bcl*-2. J Immunol 151: 1979–1988

Liu Y J, Joshua D E, Williams G T et al 1989 Mechanism of antigen-driven selection in germinal centres. Nature 342: 929–931

Liu Y J, Mason D Y, Johnson G D et al 1991 Germinal center cells express bcl-2 protein after activation by signals which prevent their entry into apoptosis. Eur J Immunol 21: 1905–1910

Lowe S W, Schmitt E M, Smith S W et al 1993 p53 is required for radiation-induced apoptosis in mouse thymocytes. Nature 362: 847–849

McConkey D J, Aguilar-Santelises M, Hartzell P et al 1991 Induction of DNA fragmentation in chronic B-lymphocytic leukemia cells. J Immunol 146: 1072–1076

McDonnell T J, Deane N, Platt F M et al 1989 *bcl*-2-immunoglobulin transgenic mice demonstrate extended β cell survival and follicular lymphoproliferation. Cell 57: 79–88

McDonnell T J, Korsmeyer S J 1991 Progression from lymphoid hyperplasia to high-grade malignant lymphoma in mice transgenic for the t(14; 18). Nature 349: 254–256

Mainou-Fowler T, Craig V A, Copllestone J A et al 1994 Interleukin-5 increases spontaneous apoptosis of B-cell chronic lymphocytic leukemia cells in vitro independently of bcl-2 expression and is inhibited by IL-4. Blood 84: 2297–2304

Manabe A, Coustan-Smith E, Behm F G et al 1992 Bone marrow derived stromal cells prevent apoptotic cell death in B lineage acute lymphoblastic leukemia. Blood 79: 2370–2377

Manabe A, Coustan-Smith E, Kumagai M et al 1994a Interleukin-4 induces programmed cell death (apoptosis) in cases of high risk acute lymphoblastic leukemia. Blood 83: 1731–1737

Manabe A, Murti K G, Coustan-Smith E et al 1994b Adhesion-dependent survival of normal and leukemic human B lymphoblasts on bone marrow stromal cells. Blood 83: 758–766

Mangan D F, Wahl S M 1991 Differential regulation of human monocyte programmed cell death (apoptosis) by chemotactic factors and pro-inflammatory cytokines. J Immunol 147: 3408–3412

Martin S J, Bradley J G, Cotter T G 1990 HL-60 cells induced to differentiate towards neutrophils subsequently die via apoptosis. Clin Exp Immunol 79: 448–453

Migliorati G, Nicoletti I, Crocicchio F et al 1992 Heat shock induces apoptosis in mouse thymocytes and protects them from glucocorticoid-induced cell death. Cell Immunol 143: 348–356

Miura M, Zhu H, Rotello R et al 1993 Induction of apoptosis in fibroblasts by IL-1 β-converting enzyme, a mammalian homolog of the C. elegans cell death gene *ced*-3. Cell 75: 653–660

Monaghan P, Robertson D, Amos T A et al 1992 Ultrastructural localization of *bcl*-2 protein. J Histochem Cytochem 40: 1819–1825

Moore K J, Matlashewski G 1994 Intracellular infection by *Leishmania donovani* inhibits macrophage apoptosis. J Immunol 152: 2930–2937

Motoyama N, Wang F, Roth K A et al 1995 Massive cell death of immature hematopoietic cells and neurons in Bcl-x-deficient mice. Science 267: 1506–1509

Nagata S, Golstein P 1995 The fas death factor. Science 267: 1449–1456

Nguyen M, Millar D G, Yong V W et al 1993 Targeting of *Bcl*-2 to the mitochondrial outer membrane by a COOH-terminal signal anchor sequence. J Biol Chem 268: 25265–25268

Nicoletti I, Migliorati G, Pagliacci M C et al 1991 A rapid and simple method for measuring thymocyte apoptosis by propidium iodide staining and flow cytometry. J Immunol Meth 139: 271–279

Nunez G, London L, Hockenbery D et al 1990 Deregulated *Bcl*-2 gene expression selectively prolongs survival of growth factor-deprived hemopoietic cell lines. J Immunol 144: 3602–3610

Oberhammer F, Wilson J W, Dive C et al 1993 Apoptotic death in epthelial cells: cleavage of DNA to 300 and/or 50 kb fragments prior to or in the absence of internucleosomal fragmentation. EMBO J 12: 3679–3684

Oltvai Z N, Korsmeyer S J 1994 Checkpoints of dueling dimers foil death wishes. Cell 79: 189–192

Oltvai Z N, Milliman C L, Korsmeyer S J 1993 *Bcl*-2 heterodimerizes *in vivo* with a conserved homolog, *Bax*, that accelerates programmed cell death. Cell 74: 609–619

Owen-Schaub L B, Yonehara S, Crump III W L et al 1992 DNA fragmentation and cell death is selectively triggered in activated human lymphocytes by Fas antigen engagement. Cell Immunol 140: 197–205

Packham G, Cleveland J L 1994 Ornithine decarboxylase is a mediator of c-myc-induced apoptosis. Mol Cell Biol 14: 5741–5747

Packham G, Cleveland J L 1995 c-Myc and apoptosis. Biochim Biophys Acta, 1242: 11-28

Panayiotidis P, Ganeshguru K, Jabbar S A et al 1993 Interleukin-4 inhibits apoptotic cell death and loss of the bcl-2 protein in B-chronic lymphocytic leukaemia cells in vitro. Br J Haematol 85: 439–445

Panayiotidis P, Ganeshaguru K, Jabbar S A et al 1994 Alpha-interferon protects B-chronic lymphocytic leukaemia cells from apoptotic cell death in vitro. Br J Haematol 86: 169–173

Paul W E 1991 Interleukin-4: a prototypic immunoregulatory lymphokine. Blood 77: 1859–1870

Peitsch M C, Polzar B, Stephan H et al 1993 Characterization of the endogenous doxyribonuclease involved in nuclear DNA degradation during apoptosis (programmed cell death). EMBO J 12: 371–377

Qin X Q, Livingston D M, Kaelin W G, Jr. et al 1995 Deregulated transcription factor E2F-1 expression leads to S-phase entry and p53-mediated apoptosis. Proc Natl Acad Sci USA 91: 10918–10922

Raff M C 1992 Social controls on cell survival and cell death. Nature 356: 397–400

Reed J C 1995 Bcl-2: prevention of apoptosis as a mechanism of drug resistance. Hemato Onco Clin North Am 9: 451–473

Robertson L E, Chubb S, Meyn R E et al 1993 Induction of apoptotic cell death in chronic lymphocytic leukemia by 2-chloro-2^1 deoxyadenosine and 9-β-D-arabinosyl-2-fluoroadenine. Blood 81: 143–150

Rodriguez-Tarduchy G, Collins M, Lopez-Rivas A 1990 Regulation of apoptosis in interleukin-3-dependent hemopoietic cells by interleukin-3 and calcium ionophores. EMBO J 9: 2997–3002

Savill J, Dransfield I, Hoog N et al 1990 Vitronectin receptor mediated phagocytosis of cells undergoing apoptosis. Nature 343: 170–173

Sellins K S, Cohen J J 1987 Gene induction by γ-irradiation leads to DNA fragmentation in lymphocytes. J Immunol 139: 3199–3206

Shi L, Nishioka W K, Th'ng J et al 1994 Premature p34cdc2 activation required for apoptosis. Science 263: 1143–1145

Smith C A, Williams G T, Kinston R et al 1989 Antibodies to CD3/T-cell receptor complex induced death by apoptosis in immature T cell in thymic cultures. Nature 337: 181–184

Strasser A, Harris A W, Jacks T et al 1994 DNA damage can induce apoptosis in proliferating lymphoid cells via p53-independent mechanisms inhibitable by bcl-2. Cell 79: 329–339

Swat W, Ignatowicz L, Kisielow P 1991 Detection of apoptosis of immature CD4+8+ thymocytes by flow cytometry. J Immunol Meth 137: 79–87

Takayama S, Sato T, Krajewski S et al 1995 Cloning and functional analysis of BAG-1: a novel Bcl-2-binding protein with anti-cell death activity. Cell 80: 279–284

Telford W G, King L E, Fraker P J 1992 Comparative evaluation of several DNA binding dyes in the detection of apoptosis-associated chromatin degradation by flow cytometry. Cytometry 13: 137–143

Tushinski R J, Oliver I T, Guilbert L J et al 1982 Survival of mononuclear phagocytes depends on a lineage-specific growth factor that the differentiated cells selectively destroy. Cell 28: 71–81

Vaux D L, Cory S, Adams J M 1988 *Bcl*-2 gene promotes haemopoietic cell survival and cooperates with c-*myc* to immortalize pre-B cells. Nature 335: 440–442

Vaux D L, Weissman I L, Kim S K 1992 Prevention of programmed cell death in *Caenorhabditis elegans* by human *bcl*-2. Science 258: 1955–1957

Veis D J, Sorenson C M, Shutter J R et al 1993 *Bcl*-2-deficient mice demonstrate fulminant lymphoid apoptosis, polycystic kidneys, and hypopigmented hair. Cell 75: 229–240

Wijsman J H, Jonker R R, Keijzer R et al 1993 A new method to detect apoptosis in paraffin sections: in situ end-labeling of fragmented DNA. J Histochem Cytochem 41: 7–12

Williams G T, Smith C A, Spooncer E et al 1990 Haemopoietic colony stimulating factors promote cell survival by suppressing apoptosis. Nature 343: 76–79

Wu X, Levine A J 1994 p53 and E2F-1 cooperate to mediate apoptosis. Proc Natl Acad Sci USA 91: 3602–3606

Wyllie A H 1980 Glucocorticoid-induced thymocyte apoptosis is associated with endogenous endonuclease activation. Nature 284: 555–556

Wyllie A H, Morris R G, Smith A C et al 1984 Chromatin cleavage in apoptosis: association with condensed chomatin morphology and dependence on macromolecular synthesis. J Pathol 142: 67–77

Yang E, Zha J, Jockel J et al 1995 Bad, a heterodimeric partner for Bcl-x$_L$ and Bcl-2, displaces Bax and promotes cell death. Cell 80: 285–291

Yin X M, Oltvai Z N, Korsmeyer S J 1994 BH1 and BH2 domains of *Bcl*-2 are required for inhibition of apoptosis and heterodimerization with *Bax*. Nature 369: 321–323

Yonish-Rouach E, Resnitzky D, Lotem J et al 1991 Wild-type p53 induces apoptosis of myeloid leukaemic cells that is inhibited by interleukin-6. Nature 352: 345–347

Yuan J, Shaham S, Ledoux S et al 1993 The *C. elegans* cell death gene *ced*-3 encodes a protein similar to mammalian interleukin-1 β-converting enzyme. Cell 75: 641–652

Zawdiwski R, Harmon J M, Thompson E B 1983 Glucocorticoid-resistant human acute lymphoblastic leukemic cell line with functional receptors. Cancer Res 43: 3865–3873

2

The clinical use of haemopoietic growth factors

A. P. Haynes   A. E. Hunter   N. H. Russell

A number of growth factors which regulate the proliferation and differentiation of haemopoietic cells have been identified, cloned and three: erythropoietin, granulocyte-colony stimulating factor (G-CSF) and granulocyte-macrophage colony stimulating factor (GM-CSF) are licensed for clinical use. Others including interleukin-3, stem cell factor and interleukin-6 are undergoing clinical trials. Although GM-CSF has more pleiotropic effects in vitro than G-CSF, both agents have been used clinically primarily for their effects in stimulating myelopoiesis. In this respect there have been no randomized large-scale trials to evaluate the relative efficacies of these growth factors.

G-CSF is well tolerated over a wide range of doses with the optimal clinical benefit resulting from doses of 5 µg/kg/day. Recently, however, there have been some studies suggesting that a lower dose of G-CSF such as 50 µg/m^2 may be clinically effective in some situations (Shimazaki et al 1994, Negrin et al 1993). Of necessity owing to the high cost of therapy with these agents, the dose used should be the lowest one to achieve the desired clinical effect. The side effects of a short course of G-CSF are dose related and include myalgia, bone pain and influenza-like symptoms which may be noticed particularly by normal donors undergoing peripheral blood stem cell (PBSC) mobilization. Rarer side effects include exacerbation of psoriasis and Sweet's syndrome of neutrophilic dermatosis. Biochemical abnormalities have included elevations of lactate dehydrogenase (LDH), uric acid and alkaline phosphatase.

GM-CSF stimulates the production of neutrophils, eosinophils and monocytes. It is given at doses of up to 250 µg/m^2 as higher doses cause significant bone pain and occasionally reversible pleural or pericardial effusions. GM-CSF releases interleukin-1 and tumour necrosis factor from monocytes, hence its administration has been associated with fever. Biochemical abnormalities described include elevations of LDH, uric acid or alkaline phosphatase and occasional hypoalbuminaemia. Administration of growth factors by the subcutaneous route may be more effective and associated with less toxicity than after intravenous use. Their degree of glycosylation will also affect their specific activity and receptor binding with possible consequences for efficacy and toxicity.

Both G-CSF and GM-CSF have been evaluated for their role in accelerating myeloid recovery post conventional chemotherapy. Similarly, both have been used to intensify conventional therapy either by reducing the interval between cycles or by increasing the dose of chemotherapy given. However, the major impact of the clinical use of growth factors has not come from their effects on conventional chemotherapy or that on the speed of myeloid engraftment after bone marrow transplantation (BMT), but rather as a result of the observation that these agents can act to mobilize marrow stem and progenitor cells into the peripheral blood. Together with refinements in leucopheresis, this has led to the development and rapid expansion of peripheral blood stem cell transplantation (PBSCT) to support patients undergoing high-dose chemoradiotherapy. Within a few years PBSCT has almost entirely replaced autologous bone marrow transplantation in support of high-dose therapy and is currently being evaluated as an alternative to marrow for allogeneic transplantation.

In this chapter we propose to discuss the use of haemopoietic growth factors in support of patients receiving standard therapy, high-dose therapy and transplantation or in the mobilization of peripheral blood stem cells.

GROWTH FACTORS IN SUPPORT OF CONVENTIONAL THERAPY

Neutropenia and infection are dose limiting side effects of chemotherapy. With the advent of broad spectrum intravenous and prophylactic antibiotics, the mortality from infection is generally low but the economic consequences with attendant hospitalization may be considerable. In haematological patients, trials examining the ability of growth factors to prevent treatment delay, reduce infectious complications and increase dose intensity have largely been restricted to patients with lymphoma. Concern about disease progression has restricted the use of growth factors in patients with acute leukaemia but this experience is now beginning to broaden.

Lymphoma

Pettengell et al have reported a randomized study of G-CSF, 230 $\mu g/m^2$/day subcutaneously in lymphoma patients receiving VAPEC-B, an intensive weekly chemotherapy regimen (Pettengell et al 1992). G-CSF was administered throughout treatment except for the day preceding and the days of chemotherapy. In the patients receiving G-CSF, the incidence of fever and neutropenia was reduced by more than 50%. No differences in antibiotic usage or hospitalization were noted but treatment delay and dose reduction were markedly reduced in the G-CSF treated patients. An approximate increase of 10% in dose intensity was noted in the G-CSF treated patients. A similar magnitude of improvement in dose intensity was reported in lymphoma patients randomized to receive G-CSF or placebo in support of the LNH87 intensive chemotherapy protocol (Gisselbrecht 1993). No beneficial effects on mortality, response rate or survival have been demonstrated in these trials.

Whilst more data from randomized trials is awaited, these limited data indicate that whilst growth factors may reduce the morbidity of chemotherapy, their general use cannot be advocated. Only patients with a high risk of prolonged neutropenia may derive clinical and economic benefit from the use of growth factors. Identifying such patients may be difficult but poor performance status, extensive prior therapy and recent hospitalization may be predictive.

Further increases in dose intensity can be achieved by using growth factors to reduce the interval between courses of chemotherapy. However, other toxicities such as thrombocytopenia or mucositis are significant factors limiting the advantages to be gained from this approach.

The use of growth factors in patients with febrile neutropenia following chemotherapy has been reported (Maher et al 1993). Modest benefits in terms of reduced antibiotic usage or hospitalization have been reported but no clear economic advantage or impact on mortality have been demonstrated. Patients with pneumonia or documented soft tissue infections, particularly involving fungi, may benefit from growth factor support. Such use is likely to remain empirical since randomized trials may be ethically difficult to conduct.

Acute leukaemia

The treatment and support of infection during marrow hypoplasia is a major component in the care of patients with acute leukaemia. Infection remains a major cause of death and morbidity, particularly in older patients.

Pilot studies of the use of growth factors in supportive therapy following induction treatment for acute leukaemia failed to demonstrate disease progression and more randomized studies have now been conducted. The results of trials in acute myeloid leukaemia (AML) have recently been reviewed (Estey 1994). Trials of both G-CSF and GM-CSF given after induction therapy to patients with hypoplastic marrows have demonstrated accelerated neutrophil recovery but no consistent benefit on infection, remission or survival rates. Given the observations that growth factors can enhance the sensitivity of leukaemic cells to cycle-specific agents such as cytarabine, trials have also been conducted with the use of growth factors preceding, during and after induction chemotherapy (Estey 1994). In none of these studies have complete remission rates been improved; indeed one study with GM-CSF showed a lower complete remission and survival rate (Estey et al 1992), which raises the concern that GM-CSF may protect leukaemic cells from apoptosis induced by chemotherapeutic agents (Lotem & Sachs 1992).

More limited data is available concerning the use of growth factors during induction therapy for acute lymphoblastic leukaemia (Kantarjian et al 1993). Accelerated neutrophil recovery has been reported but no significant benefit on clinical outcomes documented.

At present the use of growth factors during induction therapy in acute leukaemia cannot be routinely advocated outside the context of clinical trials or in patients with life-threatening sepsis unresponsive to antibiotic therapy.

Myelodysplasia

Pilot studies have demonstrated the ability of growth factors to elevate neutrophil counts in patients with myelodysplasia. This appears to be a temporary effect lost upon growth factor withdrawal and is more common in patients with a normal karyotype. An increase in blasts was noted in some patients. Two randomized trials have published interim reports. In one, GM-CSF or placebo was administered to patients with all types of myelodysplasia except refractory anaemia with excess blasts (Schuster et al 1990). A rise in neutrophils was recorded with reduction in the incidence of infection. No difference in survival was apparent but the incidence of disease progression was no greater in the GM-CSF group. A second trial using G-CSF was reported in patients with refractory anaemia and excess blasts, or refractory anaemia with excess blasts in transformation (Greenberg et al 1993). No difference was apparent in disease progression but survival was reduced in the G-CSF arm, although G-CSF did increase neutrophil counts. The effect on neutrophil counts has been achieved with low doses of growth factors such as 1 µg/kg G-CSF per day (Negrin et al 1993). The chronic administration of growth factors cannot be recommended on the basis of this information. Growth factors may have a role as an adjunct to antibiotics in patients with severe infection. Trials have also reported the use of growth factors in support of chemotherapy for MDS; the degree of myelosuppression can be ameliorated but no improvement in response rates or survival were documented (Gerhartz et al 1994).

The administration of erythropoietin alone or in combination with other growth factors has generally not resulted in major benefits in terms of transfusion requirements in patients with MDS (Negrin et al 1993).

Miscellaneous

High-dose G-CSF has been reported to improve neutrophil counts in severe aplastic anaemia (Kojima & Matsuyama 1994). Concern has been expressed over the inability to cure the stem cell defect by this therapy and the delay it may bring in such patients receiving potentially curative bone marrow transplantation (Marsh et al 1994). It may be used in the context of severe infection in these patients.

Growth factor administration has been reported to benefit some patients with congenital neutropenia both in resolving acute infection and preventing infection during chronic therapy (Bonilla et al 1994).

Erythropoietin has been reported to improve the anaemia often associated with active myeloma (Barlogie & Beck 1994). Whilst this has benefits for patient morbidity, concerns have been raised about tumour progression and no cost benefit analysis has been presented.

GROWTH FACTORS IN SUPPORT OF HIGH-DOSE THERAPY

As expected from the trial data concerning their use after conventional chemotherapy, phase I/II trials with GM-CSF and G-CSF have demonstrated accelerated neutrophil recovery after high-dose therapy and haemopoietic rescue. Similar data is available from randomized, double-blind, placebo-controlled trials, with additional information documented concerning their benefit in terms of clinical outcomes. Comparison between such trials is complicated by the use of variable dose schedules and administration routes for each growth factor. As our experience of the use of growth factors in this setting has grown, factors which may impact upon the assessment of clinical benefit have become modified. For example, in some trials growth factor was administered for either a standard period of time or until the absolute neutrophil count had exceeded $1 \times 10^9/l$ for 3 days. Such criteria may have masked potential clinical benefits by artificially prolonging hospital stay. High-dose therapy was initially piloted on patients with advanced, heavily pretreated disease but may now be offered to poor-risk patients at an earlier stage in their disease. This may have consequences when comparing the clinical end points of current and older trials. The majority of patients reported in the randomized trials published to date have received high-dose therapy for lymphoid malignancies. Few patients with acute leukaemia were included in the older trials owing to concern that growth factors might stimulate disease progression but as data have accumulated failing to demonstrate this in the setting of myeloablative therapy, the type of patients randomized to growth factor trials have become more heterogeneous. In general, the number of patients randomized to individual trials has been too small to permit statistically valid subgroup analysis and the impact of growth factors on particular patient subgroups may have been missed. Not all trials have reported data detailing the actual or minimum dose and quality of material used for haemopoietic rescue. This may cause difficulties in the comparison and interpretation of trials, particularly those performed on a multicentre basis. Finally, few trials have examined, in a randomized setting, the clinical impact of pharmacological factors such as the degree of glycosylation or the vector from which recombinant growth factors have been obtained.

GROWTH FACTOR SUPPORT AFTER AUTOLOGOUS BONE MARROW TRANSPLANTATION

GM-CSF

The results of published randomized, controlled trials using GM-CSF after high-dose therapy and autologous bone marrow rescue are presented in Table 1. Whilst many of the points raised above are relevant, it is clear that GM-CSF accelerates the rate of myeloid recovery by 4–11 days to achieve a neutrophil count greater than $0.5 \times 10^9/l$ compared to patients not receiving the growth factor. No consistent benefit upon platelet engraftment or blood product support is apparent from this data. The trials indicate that GM-CSF is well tolerated with no impact on procedure related mortality. Given the quality of supportive care with prophylactic and broad spectrum antibiotics

Table 1 Results of randomized trials of the use of GM-CSF in ABMT

Author	No. of patients	Schedule	Duration	PMN > 0.5	Pl > 20	Infection	Antibiotics	In-patient stay
Nemunaitis et al (1991a)	128 2 h IV	250 μg/m²	21/7	19/26*	26/29	17/30%	24/27*	27/33*
Gorin et al (1992)	91	250 μg/m² 24 h IV	PMN > 0.5 x 7/7	14/21*	19/19	27/26%	19/22	23/28*
Advani et al (1992)	69	10 μg/kg 4–6 h IV	PMN > 1.0 x 3/7	12/16*	35/52*	3/18%*	–	27/27
Gulati & Bennett (1992)	24	10 μg/kg 6 h IV	PMN > 1.0 x 3/7	–	13/21*	17/8%	–	37/44
Link et al (1992)	81	250 μg/m² 24 h IV	PMN > 1.0 x 7/7	15/26*	39/31	38/63%	19/19	–
Rabinowe et al (1993)	128	250 μg/m² 2 h IV	21/7	20/27*	–	–	11/19*	23/27*
Khwaja et al (1992a)	61	250 μg/m² SC/IV	PMN > 0.5 x 5/7	14/20*	25/19	28/20%	11/10	24/25

Unless otherwise stated the numbers represent days post marrow infusion.
*Statistically significant difference between treatment and placebo groups.

and the Gram-positive nature of most microbially documented infections, it is perhaps not surprising that patients not receiving growth factor are unlikely to die from infection as a consequence of the delay in their myeloid engraftment. To be of general use, the accelerated myeloid recovery seen with GM-CSF must translate into improved morbidity or reduced resource utilization. In vitro and ex vivo data demonstrate a beneficial effect of GM-CSF on neutrophil function but this has not translated into a clear reduction in the incidence of documented infection, fever or antibiotic usage in the ABMT setting. This may in part relate to the occurrence of fever as a side effect of GM-CSF administration and the relatively small sample size of most trials. Data also indicate that over 90% of infections following ABMT occur during the period of absolute neutropenia (neutrophils $< 0.1 \times 10^9/l$) and GM-CSF has little impact on the duration of this period. A positive benefit is apparent from the data in terms of in-patient stay with a 4–8 day reduction in hospital stay. The reported side effects are those expected after GM-CSF administration. The older trials are now reporting longer term follow-up with no increased risk of death, relapse, acute leukaemia or graft failure in patients who received GM-CSF post ABMT. In vitro and ex vivo data have been published demonstrating improved natural killer cell and cytotoxicity function associated with the use of GM-CSF. The randomized data published to date do not suggest a major clinical impact for such observations in terms of reduced relapse risk after ABMT. Finally, the use of GM-CSF has been described in the context of poor engraftment following ABMT (Brandwein et al 1991). A 14-day course of GM-CSF resulted in improved neutrophil counts in half of the patients reported but this effect was lost after growth factor withdrawal in the majority of these patients.

G-CSF

The results of phase I/II trials suggest accelerated myeloid recovery when using G-CSF post ABMT with a reduction in fever, antibiotic usage, infection and in-patient stay compared to historical controls. Data are available from randomized, controlled trials following ABMT (Table 2).

The multicentre British trial was a placebo-controlled dose finding study with 102 of the 121 randomized patients receiving ABMT (Linch et al 1993). The trial elegantly demonstrated a dose-response effect for recombinant human G-CSF administered by intravenous infusion over 30 minutes. A dose of 5 µg/kg was superior to 2 µg/kg, similar to 10 µg/kg and only marginally worse than 20 µg/kg in terms of the rate of neutrophil recovery. All doses were well tolerated. Hospital stay was reduced by 11–15 days but no benefit was seen in terms of fever, infection, antibiotic usage, platelet engraftment or blood product support.

The multicentre European trial randomized 315 patients to placebo or G-CSF and included 245 patients receiving ABMT (Gisselbrecht et al 1994). In a subanalysis, neutrophil recovery was accelerated in ABMT patients receiving G-CSF compared with those receiving placebo, and the number of

Table 2 Results of randomized trials of G-CSF following ABMT

Author	No. of patients	Schedule	Duration	PMN > 0.5	Pl > 20	Infection	Antibiotics	In-patient stay
Linch et al (1993)	102	2–20 µg/kg 30 min IV	PMN > 1.0 x 3/7	14/19*	–	24/12%	20/23	23/36*
Gisselbrecht et al (1994)	224	5 µg/kg 30 min IV	PMN > 1.0 x 3/7	14/20*	–	10/13%	15/19*	25/29*
Stahel et al (1994)	43	10 µg/kg 24 h IV	PMN > 1.0 x 3/7	10/21*	–	24/29%	8/12	18/21

Unless otherwise stated the numbers represent days post bone marrow infusion.
*Statistically significant difference between treatment and placebo groups.

febrile days, documented infections, days of antibiotic usage and days of hospitalization were reduced by G-CSF. In an open-label randomized trial of G-CSF in patients receiving ABMT for lymphoma, these findings were confirmed although the reduction in antibiotic usage and hospital stay did not reach statistical significance (Stahel et al 1994). These trials reported no effect of G-CSF upon procedure related mortality and no difference in the incidence of side effects compared to placebo.

In general terms, G-CSF may be more effective than GM-CSF following ABMT, and better tolerated, but randomized trial data is not available to confirm this by direct comparison. A single institution non-randomized trial has demonstrated that delaying the onset of G-CSF administration until 8 days following ABMT has no deleterious impact upon myeloid engraftment or clinical end points compared with historical controls receiving growth factor from the day after bone marrow return (Khwaja et al 1993). The dosage schedule of G-CSF following ABMT may therefore be modified with attendant cost savings but this data awaits confirmation in a randomized trial.

M-CSF

M-CSF is a monocyte-macrophage growth factor originally isolated from human urine but now available as a recombinant product. Besides stimulating stem cell differentiation into monocyte and macrophage colonies, M-CSF also increases the in vitro production of other cytokines by monocytes and enhances monocyte function. In a non-randomized dose finding trial, recombinant human M-CSF was administered by intravenous infusion to 20 patients, with refractory lymphoma, receiving ABMT (Khwaja et al 1992a). No adverse clinical side effects were apparent but an acute fall in platelet count at the end of the intravenous infusion was noted. No impact on the speed of myeloid engraftment, incidence of infection or antibiotic usage were noted but the duration of hospital stay was reduced compared with historical controls not receiving growth factor. Platelet engraftment was more rapid in patients receiving a mononuclear cell dose greater than 2×10^8/kg. Therefore the role for M-CSF following ABMT appears limited but these results await confirmation in a randomized setting.

IL-3

IL-3 is a multipotential growth factor which acts on immature progenitor cells and has synergistic activity with a number of other growth factors. In phase I/II trials, IL-3 demonstrated activity in stimulating all lineages in patients with solid tumours, myelodysplasia and bone marrow failure. Randomized trials are currently ongoing, exploring the benefit of IL-3 in support of conventional chemotherapy, but few data have been published concerning its use after high-dose therapy. In a dose finding study, IL-3 was administered as a 2 hour intravenous infusion for 21 days to 30 patients with lymphoid malignancies undergoing ABMT (Nemunaitis et al 1993a). No benefit in terms of haemopoietic recovery or clinical end points was apparent when compared with historical controls receiving GM-CSF. Of note, however, 17 patients did not complete the full schedule of study medication because of side effects, which makes comparison with historical controls difficult. The authors concluded that the maximum tolerated dose of IL-3 was 2 µg/kg/day. Administration of 2–5 µg/kg IL-3 intravenously in patients with poor engraftment following ABMT, who had failed to respond to GM-CSF, demonstrated transient improvement in neutrophil counts particularly if a further course of GM-CSF was administered following IL-3 (Crump et al 1993). The clinical benefit of IL-3 following ABMT remains to be clarified and further studies are awaited.

Erythropoietin

Studies have demonstrated that erythrocyte recovery after ABMT parallels that of the neutrophils and platelets, with erythropoietin levels remaining appropriate for the degree of anaemia (Beguin et al 1993). Randomized trials using recombinant erythropoietin following ABMT are in progress and published interim analyses demonstrate no benefit at doses of 150–200 U/kg/day in terms of speed of erythrocyte recovery or red cell transfusion (Link et al 1994).

Whilst studies exploring the role of combinations of growth factors in concomitant or sequential designs after ABMT are ongoing, with the rapid emergence of peripheral blood stem cell (PBSC) rescue after high-dose therapy and the attendant benefits compared to ABMT the clinical value of the above trials may be less important than that concerning the use of growth factors to optimize PBSC rescue. This will be discussed in the next section.

GROWTH FACTORS FOR PERIPHERAL BLOOD STEM CELL MOBILIZATION AND TRANSPLANTATION

In steady-state normal haemopoiesis, relatively few stem or progenitor cells are circulating in the peripheral blood. The number of such cells can be increased by up to two logs during the recovery from myelosuppressive chemotherapy (Juttner et al 1989, Kessinger et al 1989, Schwartzenberg et al 1993a) or after administration of growth factors (Gianni et al 1989, Sheridan et al 1992, Bensinger et al 1994); the combination of chemotherapy and growth factor being synergistic (Elias et al 1992, Schwartzenberg et al 1993b, Haas et al 1994, Jones et al 1994). With improvements in leucopheresis technology it has become feasible to harvest such peripheral blood stem cells (PBSC) for use in support of high-dose therapy. Doses of growth factor of 5–10 µg/kg/day have been used after chemotherapy and higher doses of up to 16 µg/kg/day when used alone for mobilization.

The results of non-randomized trials using PBSC in this setting indicate accelerated haemopoietic regeneration compared to the use of ABMT with growth factor support (Table 3). Whilst myeloid regeneration is accelerated compared to ABMT, the most striking effect of PBSC rescue has been upon

Table 3 Trials comparing the quality of PBSC harvests and subsequent engraftment following rescue from high-dose therapy after various mobilization regimens.

Author	Mobilisation regimen	CD34 yield x 10^6/kg	PMN > 0.5 x 10^9/l (days)	PL > 20 x 10^9/l (days)	PL > 50 x 10^9/l (days)	In-patient stay (days)
Dreyfus et al (1992)	Various Chemo	–	11–25	–	8–97	–
To et al (1992)	DAT/Cyclo (4–7 g/m^2)	–	9–17	–	9–365	–
Schwartzenberg et al (1993a)	Various Chemo	0.6–17.1	9–26	5–43	–	6–36
Sheridan et al (1992)	G-CSF 12 µg/kg/day SC	–	8–21	–	10–62	11–32
Chao et al (1993)	G-CSF 10 µg/kg/day IV	–	7–14	7–39	–	10–21
Bensinger et al (1994)	G-CSF 16 µg/kg/day SC	0.13–32.6	7–16	7–60	–	–
Haas et al (1993)	Various Chemo plus G-CSF 300 µg/day SC	0.10–31.0	12	11	–	20
Jones et al (1994)	Cyclo (1.5 g/m^2) G-CSF 10 µg/kg/day SC	0.20–46.6	11	13	–	16
Janssen (1993)	Cyclo/Cyclo+VP16 As above plus G-CSF	4.00–39.0 12.00–49.0	20 12	– –	– –	– –
Sutherland et al (1994)	Cyclo (7 g/m^2) Cyclo+GM-CSF G-CSF	1.1 4.2 4.7	8–62 10–31 –	8–62 9–22 –	– – –	– – –

the speed of platelet engraftment (Sheridan et al 1992). Clinical benefit from reduced transfusion requirements, antibiotic usage and in-patient stay have been reported. The use of PBSC mobilized by the combination of growth factors and chemotherapy appears superior to those mobilized by growth factors alone in terms of the yield of CD34 positive cells and speed of engraftment. The speed of engraftment appears to be predicted by the dose of CD34 positive cells infused. In our own work, patients receiving more than 2.5×10^6 CD34 positive cells/kg experienced rapid neutrophil and platelet engraftment whilst those receiving less than 2.0×10^6/kg had delayed platelet engraftment with only 66% achieving a count greater than 50×10^9/l by day 100 post transplant (Haynes et al 1995). Other groups have shown that in order to realise the beneficial effects of PBSC on engraftment CD34 cells have to exceed a certain threshold dose level; however, the figure quoted has varied (Bender et al 1992, Schwartzenberg et al 1993a, Bensinger et al 1994, Haas et al 1994). Randomized comparisons of PBSC versus autologous bone marrow have been completed and their publication is awaited. Published interim results confirm the benefits of PBSC for engraftment, particularly of platelets, together with in-patient stay (Schmitz et al 1994).

Several studies have analysed the cost benefit of ABMT compared with PBSC rescue. Peters et al (1993) demonstrated that rescue with G-CSF or GM-CSF mobilised PBSC was more effective and cheaper than the use of growth factors following ABMT. In this analysis, G-CSF was more effective and cheaper than GM-CSF when used for PBSC mobilisation. The most economical use of growth factors in support of high-dose therapy would therefore appear to be in the mobilisation of PBSC (Russell & Pacey 1992). The impact of PBSC on clinical end points raises the possibility of out-patient or hostel supervised high-dose therapy, which by reducing the cost of in-patient accommodation would be expected to provide further economic advantages in favour of PBSC.

The economic advantages and benefit to patient morbidity of using growth factors to mobilise PBSC rather than support ABMT are clear but their impact on survival remains to be established as trials mature. It is hoped that the use of PBSC rescue will reduce the short-term in-patient procedure-related mortality of high-dose therapy when compared to ABMT. The more mature studies of growth factors in support of ABMT have demonstrated no impact on long-term survival. Given that the major cause of treatment failure following ABMT remains disease relapse, this is perhaps not surprising. At least in theoretical terms, PBSC may be less contaminated with disease than bone marrow but more recent studies with sensitive molecular techniques have demonstrated residual disease contamination in PBSC harvests returned to patients following high-dose therapy (Bird et al 1994). The significance of this for long-term disease-free survival will await the results of gene-marking studies. By mobilising large numbers of CD34 positive cells into the peripheral blood for harvesting, growth factors facilitate the use of in vitro purging techniques such as CD34 positive selection. The impact of such manipulations on survival after high-dose therapy in diseases such as myeloma and lymphoma, where CD34 expression does not occur, remains to be determined. Finally, given the quality and speed of haemopoietic reconstitution after PBSC rescue together with the yield of growth factor mobilised PBSC, pilot studies are currently exploring the use of sequential or 'tandem' high-dose therapy, which may impact on long-term survival in poor prognosis disease.

The optimal use of growth factors in mobilisation schedules has not been defined. Chemotherapy plus growth factors may be appropriate where further disease control or assessment of chemosensitivity are desirable. In some situations, such as in paediatric practice or mobilisation of allogeneic PBSC from normal donors, chemotherapy is undesirable and growth factors may be used alone. To facilitate forward planning, mobilisation schedules must give a predictable recovery in white cell count, with most centres commencing leucopheresis once the count exceeds $1 \times 10^9/l$. Mobilisation post chemotherapy requires the use of up to 15 days of growth factor whereas the use of growth factors alone requires their administration for only 4 or 5 days but at twice or more the dose. Both types of mobilisation schedule can be administered in an out-patient setting. By daily monitoring of the CD34 positive cell content of the PBSC harvests, leucopheresis can be continued until a threshold dose of CD34 positive cells has been attained. Schedules have been described using growth factors alone or after chemotherapy which mobilise sufficient PBSC to permit a single leucopheresis in some patients (Bensinger et al 1994, Jones et al 1994).

Definitive data indicating the best schedule or combination of growth factors are not available. In a recent pilot studies, recombinant human IL-3 mobilised PBSC have been shown to be superior in terms of subsequent engraftment than those mobilised by GM-CSF, with the concurrent administration of IL-3 and G-CSF being synergistic (Haas et al 1993). The combination of G-CSF and stem cell factor is also being evaluated. Such combinations will only be of clinical benefit if they reduce the period of absolute neutropenia, further accelerate engraftment or permit PBSC mobilisation in difficult cases where current protocols would be predicted to fail. Potential factors predicting failure to mobilise sufficient CD34 positive cells using chemotherapy and G/GM-CSF include the number of previous treatment regimens, previous radiotherapy and patients with Hodgkin's disease or myeloma (Bensinger et al 1994, Haas et al 1994).

The role of growth factors following PBSC transplantation is as yet unclear. Spitzer et al (1994) randomized 37 patients with a variety of tumours, including lymphoma, into a study of post PBSC rescue growth factors. All patients were mobilised with a combination of both G-CSF and GM-CSF but 19 were randomized to receive 7.5 µg/kg G-CSF and 2.5 µg/kg GM-CSF by intravenous infusion every 12 hours post high-dose therapy and rescue with marrow and PBSC. Growth factors were continued until a neutrophil count greater than $1.5 \times 10^9/l$ was attained. The duration of absolute neutropenia was decreased by 2 days and the time to a neutrophil count greater than

0.5 x 10⁶/l by 6 days in patients receiving post transplant growth factors. In spite of this, the incidence of fever and documented infection was unchanged with only a 2-day reduction in hospital stay and no impact on blood product requirements. In a non-randomized study, Shimazaki et al (1994) found a 4 day reduction in the time to achieve a neutrophil count of $> 0.5 \times 10^9/l$ in patients receiving low-dose (50 μg/m²) subcutaneous G-CSF after high-dose therapy and PBSC rescue. This small study demonstrated a reduction in antibiotic usage but no benefit for platelet recovery or blood product usage. Finally, in a non-randomized study of patients with lymphoma, G-CSF 10 μg/kg/day post high-dose therapy and PBSC rescue was found to have no effect on myeloid engraftment, fever or antibiotic usage whilst increasing the cost of the high-dose therapy by 50% (Dunlop et al 1994). Larger randomized studies are awaited but at present there is no clear rationale for the routine use of growth factors following PBSC rescue.

GROWTH FACTOR SUPPORT AFTER ALLOGENEIC TRANSPLANTATION

As with autologous rescue after high-dose therapy, the rationale for the use of growth factors postallogeneic transplantation was to accelerate myeloid recovery with consequent reduction in the incidence of infection, number of febrile days and antibiotic usage. Other potential benefits would include an effect upon graft rejection or potentiation of any graft versus leukaemia effect. Concern over the use of growth factors in this setting surrounded potential adverse effects on graft versus host disease (GVHD) or disease progression in patients with acute leukaemia. Haemopoietic recovery after allogeneic transplantation is more complex than that in the autologous setting and is influenced by factors such as the nature of the GVHD prophylaxis employed. The indication for transplant, the age and the remission status of the patient may influence procedure related mortality and relapse risk hence the overall survival of the procedure. Heterogeneity between centres concerning these factors necessitates careful review of the data when comparing trials of the impact of growth factors on the outcome after allogeneic BMT. The demonstration of any benefit of growth factors on overall survival would necessitate a large randomized study, particularly given that less than 10% of allograft recipients die from early infection.

GM-CSF

Two randomized trials have been published which examined the use of GM-CSF post matched sibling allogeneic BMT (Table 4). Powles et al (1990) randomized 40 patients transplanted for acute leukaemia or chronic myeloid leukaemia to a 14-day course of GM-CSF or placebo given by continuous intravenous infusion in a double-blind protocol. No benefit in terms of the time to reach a neutrophil count greater than $0.5 \times 10^9/l$ was apparent; a significant increase in the number of days of antibiotic usage was noted and attributed to the ability of GM-CSF to cause fever. No difference in the length of hospital stay was noted. Similar results were reported by De Witte et al (1993) in a trial of T-cell depleted transplantation for a variety of haematological malignancies, using the same dose and administration schedule as Powles et al (1990). No benefit was seen on myeloid engraftment, the number of infections or duration of hospital stay. The incidence of post-transplant pneumonia was less in the GM-CSF treated group. In neither study was the incidence of acute GVHD affected by the use of GM-CSF but the De Witte study used T-cell depleted grafts. With relatively short median follow up, GM-CSF had no impact on the incidence of relapse. In a randomized dose finding study with historical controls, Nemunaitis et al (1991b) reported the use of a 2-hour intravenous infusion of GM-CSF post-allogeneic BMT. Patients receiving cyclosporin and prednisolone GVHD prophylaxis had accelerated myeloid engraftment and reduced in-patient stay with GM-CSF but these benefits were abrogated in patients receiving cyclosporin and methotrexate GVHD prophylaxis.

Nemunaitis et al (1992) have extended the use of post-transplant GM-CSF to matched unrelated donor allogeneic transplantation where engraftment can be slower than that of sibling transplants and transplant related complications are a major cause of mortality. In a non-randomized study, the use of GM-CSF was associated with a minor impact on neutrophil engraftment but a reduction in the number of febrile days, fewer septicaemic episodes but more importantly a reduction in non-relapse mortality when compared to historical controls. The incidence of GVHD, graft rejection and relapse were unaffected by GM-CSF. These data, if confirmed in a randomized setting, would suggest a role for growth factors post unrelated donor BMT.

G-CSF

Several trials have reported the use of G-CSF post-allogeneic transplant for a variety of haematological malignancies (Table 4). In a randomized, placebo-controlled trial, Masaoka et al (1989) demonstrated accelerated myeloid engraftment but no impact on platelet engraftment. A larger placebo-controlled phase III trial included 70 patients receiving allogeneic BMT for a variety of haematological malignancies and examined the impact of post-transplant G-CSF (Gisselbrecht et al 1994). A 6-day reduction in the time to reach a neutrophil count greater than $0.5 \times 10^9/l$ in favour of G-CSF was reported in the allograft recipients. For the entire study, including a larger number of ABMT recipients, the duration of antibiotic usage and hospital stay were significantly reduced in the G-CSF group but a separate analysis on the allograft patients was not presented. In none of these studies was the incidence of GVHD, graft rejection or disease relapse affected by G-CSF administration.

Overall, these studies suggest a beneficial effect of G-CSF post-allogeneic BMT in terms of accelerating myeloid engraftment, with possible reduction in

Table 4 Results of randomized trials of the use of growth factors in allogeneic BMT

Author	No. of patients	Donor	Schedule	PMN > 0.5	Pl > 20	Infection	Antibiotics	In-patient stay
GM-CSF								
Powles et al (1990)	40	Sibling	5 µg/kg 24 h IV	13/16	–	–	16/13*	24/24
DeWitte et al (1993)	57	Sibling	5 µg/kg 24 h IV	16/20	–	45/54%	–	43/43
Hiraoka et al (1994)	53	Sibling	10 µg/kg 24 h IV	17/21*	–	–	–	21/30*
G-CSF								
Masaoka et al (1989)	71	Sibling	300 µg/m² IV	15/19*	–	–	–	–
Asano et al (1991)	59	Sibling	5 µg/kg IV	16/27*	21/29	–	–	–
Gisselbrecht et al (1994)	70	Sibling	5 µg/kg 30 min IV	14/20*	–	–	–	–

Unless otherwise stated the numbers represent days post marrow infusion.
*Statistically significant difference between treatment and placebo groups.

the incidence of fever, infection and antibiotic usage. The evidence for clinical benefit from the available trials is, however, not conclusive and additional large randomized placebo-controlled trials are required, with careful cost analysis, before the routine use of these expensive drugs post-allogeneic BMT can be recommended. Approximately 10% of patients undergoing autologous or allogeneic BMT have poor graft function or develop late graft failure; this complication is more frequent with unrelated donors. In a study of over 100 patients who had poor engraftment, defined as failure to achieve either a neutrophil count above $0.2 \times 10^9/l$ by day +28 post transplant or greater than $0.1 \times 10^9/l$ by day +21 in the presence of infection or who had suffered late onset neutropenia, over 60% were reported to respond to one or more 14-day courses of GM-CSF (Nemunaitis et al 1990). The platelet recovery of these patients was unaffected but the overall survival was significantly better than historical controls and a randomized study was considered unethical. After allogeneic BMT, response was more likely if donor haemopoiesis was demonstrable compared to those patients with only host type. There seems little doubt that a trial of growth factors should be given to allograft recipients with delayed engraftment or graft rejection.

Although both GM-CSF and G-CSF stimulate the in vitro proliferation of myeloid blast cells, in none of the studies where these growth factors have been administered to patients transplanted for acute myeloid leukaemia has there been any evidence of an increased risk of leukaemic relapse. It would therefore seem that after myeloablative therapy, residual leukaemic cells are incapable of responding to these growth factors whereas normal progenitor cells are. In this respect a novel use of G-CSF has recently been described in patients relapsing after allogeneic transplant for leukaemia (Giralt et al 1993). Three of seven relapsed patients who received G-CSF alone achieved a complete haematological and cytogenetic remission within 3 weeks of starting therapy. If confirmed by randomized studies, stimulating donor haemopoiesis by growth factors to induce remission in relapsed disease, perhaps in tandem with donor leucocytes to induce a graft versus leukaemia effect, may provide a novel therapeutic approach.

M-CSF

M-CSF has been used following allogeneic BMT. During periods of absolute neutropenia, some protection from infection is afforded by the macrophages of the host fixed reticuloendothelial system, which are relatively resistant to transplant conditioning. Part of the rationale for the use of post-transplant M-CSF therefore centred on the stimulation of monocyte function seen in vitro with M-CSF. Masaoka et al (1990) reported a randomized placebo-controlled trial studying the effects of human urinary M-CSF after allogeneic BMT in 119 patients. The rate of myeloid engraftment and survival to 120 days post-transplant were significantly improved with no effect on the incidence of GVHD or relapse. The benefit on myeloid engraftment was less than that reported with the use of G-CSF or GM-CSF. A further potential role for M-CSF has been defined in a study by Nemunaitis et al (1993b). Some 10% of allograft recipients experience fungal infection up to day 100 post-transplant with an attendant mortality of 80–90%. These authors reported 46 consecutive patients with documented fungal infection post-allogeneic BMT who were treated with M-CSF as an adjunct to standard antifungal therapy (Nemunaitis et al 1993b). The overall survival of the 46 patients was 27% compared with 5% in a group of historical controls not receiving M-CSF. On further subanalysis, the 2 year survival of patients with Candida infections was 50% compared to 15% in historical controls and for Aspergillus infection 20% compared to 0%. Prospective randomized trials are clearly indicated to confirm what appears to be a substantial benefit from the use of M-CSF in this setting.

Erythropoietin

Impairment of the erythropoietin response to anaemia is more common after allogeneic than autologous BMT, and red cell transfusion requirements to day 100 post-transplant are higher in allografted patients. This effect is probably multifactorial with conditioning therapy, renal impairment, infection, GVHD and prophylaxis all contributing. In the European multicentre trial, 215 allograft recipients were randomized to receive 150 U/kg/day recombinant human erythropoietin by intravenous infusion or placebo (Link et al 1994). The time to transfusion independence was reduced by erythropoietin but the impact on red cell transfusion was minor, the biggest effect being seen in patients with GVHD. A potential role for erythropoietin exists post-allogeneic BMT, particularly given the recent papers showing evidence of iron overload in these patients, but trials addressing the optimal dosage and scheduling are awaited.

Mobilised peripheral blood stem cells for allogeneic transplantation

The ability of growth factors alone to mobilise large numbers of PBSC has raised the question of whether allogeneic transplantation can be safely performed using PBSC and indeed whether this type of transplant may be advantageous compared to bone marrow. Transplantation of allogeneic PBSC has the same potential benefits as the use of autologous PBSC rescue; accelerated haemopoietic recovery, earlier hospital discharge and reduced costs. For the donor, the discomfort and risks of a general anaesthetic and marrow harvest procedure would be exchanged for a short course of G-CSF followed by leucopheresis, procedures which are performed on an out-patient basis. Among the agents available for mobilisation, G-CSF would appear to be the safest and a number of groups have now established that it can be safely administered to normal donors in doses which mobilise sufficient stem cells to undertake allogeneic or syngeneic transplantation (Russell et al 1993, Weaver et al 1993, Schmitz et al 1995). The ethical problems associated with this have received wide discussion and although the long-term toxicities, if any, have not been established, the procedure seems to be at least as safe for the donor as a bone marrow harvest.

Schmitz et al (1995) have reported on eight patients with leukaemia transplanted with allogeneic G-CSF mobilised PBSC from HLA identical, MLC negative donors. Donors received G-CSF subcutaneously in doses of 5–10 µg/kg/day. This and the leucopheresis procedures were tolerated without major side effects but donors receiving more than 10 µg/kg/day experienced mild bone pain. Circulating CD34 positive cells peaked on day 5 after the start of G-CSF therapy and 1–3 leucophereses gave a sufficient PBSC yield to cause sustained haemopoietic engraftment in the recipients. The 10 µg/kg dose appears to give greater yields of CD34 positive cells, thus minimizing the number of leucopheresis procedures required (Dreger et al 1994, Schmitz et al 1995). The concept of a target dose of CD34 positive cells/kg resulting in rapid haemopoietic reconstitution is established for autologous PBSC rescue and probably exists for the use of allogeneic PBSCT. Based upon our own experience of autologous PBSCT, we have attempted to collect a minimum of 4–5 x 10^6 CD34 positive cells/kg recipient weight for allogeneic PBSCT, which is a significantly greater number than that found in donor marrow harvests. However, satisfactory engraftment has been recorded with 2–3 x 10^6 CD34 positive cells/kg. Following the completion of conditioning therapy we infuse the first and if necessary second harvest, storing the first overnight at 4°C after dilution with autologous plasma. Alternatively, PBSC can be harvested in advance of the transplant and cryopreserved.

Of the potential advantages for allogeneic PBSCT, the most obvious is the possibility of more rapid engraftment but initial data suggest that the kinetics of both platelet and neutrophil engraftment are more variable than might be predicted from the use of autologous PBSC (Schmitz et al 1995). Large randomized studies will therefore be necessary before definite conclusions concerning the kinetics of engraftment following allogeneic PBSCT can be made. The available data do, however, indicate that long-term engraftment follows allogeneic PBSCT, with documentation of totally donor haemopoiesis greater than 1 year post procedure. A major concern over the use of PBSC for allogeneic transplantation was that the incidence and severity of GVHD would be increased by the presence of large numbers of T-cells in the donor leucopheresis products. Analysis of donor harvests shows that the number of T-cells is approximately one log greater than in bone marrow harvests (Dreger et al 1994, Schmitz et al 1995). Despite this increase in the load of infused T-cells, the risk of acute GVHD does not appear to be increased following the use of allogeneic PBSC from HLA, MLC compatible donors when cyclosporin or cyclosporin and methotrexate were used for GVHD prophylaxis although the risk of chronic GVHD may be higher (Russell et al 1993, Schmitz et al 1995). Thus at the present time, at least for matched sibling transplants, the need for T-cell depletion of donor harvests is not established.

A further theoretical advantage of PBSC over bone marrow for allogeneic transplantation is a greater graft versus leukaemia effect (GVL) mediated by the presence of significantly larger numbers of natural killer cells (NK) infused.

NK cells have been implicated in the GVL reaction and there is a reported 20-fold increase in stem cell compared to marrow harvests (Dreger et al 1994). These possible advantages of PBSCT for both donor and recipient in primary allogeneic transplantation are the subject of a randomized study organized by the European Group for Blood and Bone Marrow Transplantation.

A second potential use for allogeneic stem cells is in the treatment of graft failure. Dreger et al (1993) first reported the successful transplantation of unmanipulated G-CSF mobilised PBSC into a patient with failure to engraft with bone marrow (Dreger et al 1993). Others have successfully used CD34 positively selected PBSC for re-engraftment following poor marrow function after BMT (Arseniev et al 1994). The use of G-CSF mobilised PBSC clearly offers a new therapeutic option for the treatment of marrow graft failure.

FUTURE DEVELOPMENTS

Clinical trials defining the appropriate use of the first generation of human haemopoietic growth factors are now reporting their results. As our understanding of the complexity of the basic biology controlling haemopoiesis has improved, new factors such as stem cell factor, interleukins-6/10/11 and thrombopoietin have been discovered. Such agents will only be of additional value to those of the first generation, such as G-CSF or GM-CSF, if the period of absolute neutropenia or speed of platelet engraftment post-transplant can be further reduced. To this end, interleukin-6 and thrombopoietin, which stimulate megakaryocytopoiesis, are potentially very interesting since our ability to pharmacologically manipulate platelet engraftment is at present restricted. The use of concurrent or sequential growth factor combinations is currently under investigation together with agents such as PIXY 321, a genetically engineered fusion protein with the in vivo activity of both GM-CSF and IL-3. Such therapies will be expensive, hence their clinical and cost benefits must be carefully evaluated in randomized trials. At a scientific level, the wider array of growth factors may make in vitro graft expansion, particularly of cord blood stem cells, more accessible, and graft engineering, with the specific modification of subpopulations within a graft, more feasible. In the context of gene therapy, growth factors give access to large numbers of potential target CD34 positive cells and in vivo appear to increase the chances of transfection occurring.

Growth factors occupy a prominent position in the treatment of patients with haematological disorders, and will continue to do so, but we are all charged with ensuring their use for maximum patient benefit whilst containing the costs to health service expenditure. The appropriate planning and conduct of future clinical trials will be essential to meet these aims.

KEY POINTS FOR CLINICAL PRACTICE

- Peripheral blood stem cells have rapidly replaced the use of autologous bone marrow haemopoietic rescue following high-dose therapy. Growth factor mobilised stem cells result in more rapid engraftment than autologous marrow with growth factor support.

- Stem cells collected after mobilisation regimens that include growth factors are superior to those collected after chemotherapy alone in terms of subsequent engraftment.

- A threshold dose of 2.5–5 x 10^6 CD34 positive cells/kg is associated with rapid engraftment after PBSC rescue and is more likely to be attained by regimens including growth factors.

- The routine use of growth factors following allogeneic transplantation cannot be recommended at present. Their use after unrelated donor transplantation, where engraftment can be delayed for longer and infection is a major cause of mortality, appears promising.

- Growth factors are emerging as a treatment of graft failure post-transplantation.

- The use of growth factors as an adjunct to therapy for invasive fungal infection is a promising development.

REFERENCES

Advani R, Chao N J, Horning S J et al 1992 GM-CSF as an adjunct to autologous haemopoietic stem cell transplant for lymphoma. Ann Int Med 116: 83–89

Arseniev L, Tischler H J, Battmer K et al 1994 Treatment of poor marrow graft function with enriched allogeneic CD34 positive immunoselected from G-CSF mobilised peripheral blood progenitor cells of the donor marrow. Bone Marrow Transplant 14: 791–798

Asano S, Masaoka T, Takaku F et al 1991 Beneficial effect of recombinant human G-CSF in marrow transplanted patients: results of multicentre phase I/II studies. Transplant Proc 23: 1701–1703

Beguin Y, Oris R, Fillet G et al 1993 Dynamics of erythropoietic recovery following bone marrow transplantation: role of marrow proliferative capacity and erythropoietin production in autologous versus allogeneic transplants. Bone Marrow Transplant 11(4): 285–292

Barlogie B, Beck T 1994 Recombinant human erythropoietin and the anaemia of multiple myeloma. Stem Cells 11(2): 88–94

Bender J G, Williams S F, Myers S et al 1992 Characterisation of chemotherapy mobilised peripheral blood progenitor cells for use in autologous stem cell transplantation. Bone Marrow Transplant 10: 281–285

Bensinger W I, Longin K, Applebaum F R et al 1994 Peripheral blood stem cells collected after recombinant human G-CSF: an analysis of factors correlating with the tempo of engraftment after transplantation. Br J Haematol 87: 825–831

Bird J, Bloxham D, Samson D et al 1994 Molecular detection of clonally rearranged cells in peripheral blood progenitor cell harvests from multiple myeloma patients. Br J Haematol 88: 110–116

Bonilla M A, Dale D, Ziedler C et al 1994 Long term safety of treatment with recombinant human G-CSF in patients with severe congenital neutropenia. Br J Haematol 88(4): 723–730

Brandwein J M, Nayar R, Baker M A et al 1991 GM-CSF therapy for delayed engraftment after bone marrow transplantation. Exp Haematol 19(3): 191–195

Chao N J, Schriber J R, Grimes K et al 1993 G-CSF mobilised peripheral blood progenitor cells accelerate granulocyte and platelet recovery after high dose therapy. Blood 81(8): 2031–2035

Crump M, Couture F, Kovacs M et al 1993 IL-3 followed by GM-CSF for delayed engraftment after autologous bone marrow transplantation. Exp Haematol 21(3): 405–410

DeWitte T, Vreugdenhil G, Schattenberg A et al 1993 Prolonged administration of GM-CSF after T depleted allogeneic bone marrow transplantation. Transplant Proc 25: 57–60

Dreger P, Suttorp H, Haferlach T et al 1993 Allogeneic G-CSF mobilised peripheral blood progenitor cells for treatment of engraftment failure after allogeneic transplantation. Blood 81: 1404–1405

Dreger P, Haferlach T, Eckstein V et al 1994 G-CSF mobilised peripheral blood progenitor cells for allogeneic transplantation: safety, kinetics of mobilisation and composition of graft. Br J Haematol 87: 609–613

Dreyfus F, Leblond V, Belanger C et al 1992 Peripheral blood stem cells and autografting in high risk lymphoma. Bone Marrow Transplant 10: 409–413

Dunlop D J, Fitzsimons E, McMurray A et al 1994 Filgrastim fails to improve haematopoietic reconstitution following myeloablative chemotherapy and peripheral blood stem cell rescue. Br J Cancer 70: 943–945

Elias A D, Ayash L, Andersen K C et al 1992 Mobilisation of peripheral blood progenitor cells by GM and G-CSF for haematologic support after high dose intensification for breast cancer. Blood 79: 3036–3044

Estey E H, Thall P F, Kantarjian H H et al 1992 Treatment of newly diagnosed acute myeloid leukaemia with GM-CSF before and during continous infusion high dose cytarabine and daunorubicin: comparison to patients treated without GM-CSF. Blood 79: 246–255

Estey E H 1994 Use of colony stimulating factors in acute myeloid leukaemia. Blood 83(8): 2015–2019

Gerhartz H H, Marcus R E, Delmer A et al 1994 A randomised phase II study of low dose cytarabine plus GM-CSF in myelodysplasia with a high risk of developing leukaemia. Leukaemia 8(1): 16–23

Gianni A M, Siena S, Bregni M et al 1989 GM-CSF to harvest circulating haematopoietic cells for autotransplantation. Lancet ii: 580–585

Giralt S, Escudier S, Kantarjian H H et al 1993 Preliminary results of treatment with Filgrastim for relapse of leukaemia and myelodysplasia after allogeneic transplantation. N Engl J Med 329: 757–761

Gisselbrecht C 1993 Critical review II – What do growth factors contribute to dose intensity and outcome in the treatment of non Hodgkin's lymphomas? Proc 5th Int Conf on Malignant Lymphoma. Lugano, Abstract 32

Gisselbrecht C, Prentice H G, Bacigalupo A et al 1994 Placebo controlled phase III trial of Lenograstim in bone marrow transplantation. Lancet 343: 696–700

Gorin N C, Coiffier B, Hayat M et al 1992 Recombinant human GM-CSF after high dose therapy and autologous bone marrow transplantation with unpurged and purged marrow in non Hodgkin's lymphoma: a double blind, placebo controlled trial. Blood 80(5): 1149–1157

Greenberg P, Taylor K, Larson et al 1993 Phase III randomised multicentre trial of G-CSF versus observation for myelodysplasia. Blood 82: 196a

Gulati S C Bennett C L 1992 GM-CSF as an adjunct therapy in Hodgkin's disease. Ann Int Med 116: 177–182

Haas R, Erhardt H, Witt B et al 1993 Autografting with peripheral blood stem cells mobilised by sequential IL-3/GM-CSF following high dose chemotherapy in non Hodgkin's lymphoma. Bone Marrow Transplant 12(6): 643–649

Haas R, Mohle R, Fruhauf S et al 1994 Patient characteristics associated successful mobilisation and autografting of peripheral blood progenitor cells in malignant lymphoma. Blood 83(12): 3787–3794

Haynes A P, Hunter A E, McQuaker G et al 1995 Engratement characteristics of peripheral blood stem cells mobilized with cyclophosphoride and the delayed addition of G-CSF. Bone Marrow Transplantation 16: 359–363

Hiraoka A, Masoaka T, Mizoguchi H et al 1994 Recombinant human non glycosylated GM-CSF in allogeneic bone marrow transplantation: double blind placebo controlled phase III trial. J Clin Oncol 24(4): 205–211

Janssen W E 1993 Peripheral blood and bone marrow haematopoietic stem cells: are they the same? Semin Oncol 20(5) (Suppl. 6): 19–27

Jones H M, Jones S A, Watts M J et al 1994 Development of a simplified single apheresis approach for peripheral blood progenitor cell transplantation in previously treated patients with lymphoma. J Clin Oncol 12(8): 1693–1702

Juttner C A, To L B, Ho J Q K et al 1989 Early lympho-haemopoietic recovery after autografting using peripheral blood stem cells in acute non lymphoblastic leukaemia. Transplant Proc 20: 40–42

Kantarjian H H, Estey E H, O'Brien S et al 1993 Granulocyte colony stimulating factor supportive therapy following intensive chemotherapy in first remission acute lymphoblastic leukaemia. Cancer 72(10): 2950–2955

Kessinger A, Armitage J O, Smither D M et al 1989 High dose therapy and autologous peripheral blood stem cell transplantation for patients with lymphoma. Blood 74: 1260–1265

Khwaja A, Yong K, Jones H M et al 1992a The effect of M-CSF on haemopoietic recovery after bone marrow transplantation. Br J Haematol 81: 288–295

Khwaja A, Linch D C, Goldstone A H et al 1992b Recombinant human GM-CSF after autologous bone marrow transplantation for malignant lymphoma: a BNLI double blind, placebo controlled trial. Br J Haematol 82: 317–323

Khwaja A, Mills W, Leveridge K et al 1993 Efficacy of delayed G-CSF after autologous bone marrow transplantation. Bone Marrow Transplant 11: 479–482

Kojima S, Matsuyama T 1994 Stimulation of granulopoiesis by high dose recombinant human G-CSF in children with aplastic anaemia and very severe neutropenia. Blood 83(6): 1474–1478

Linch D C, Scarffe H, Proctor S et al 1993 A randomised vehicle controlled dose finding study of glycosylated recombinant human G-CSF after bone marrow transplantation. Bone Marrow Transplant 11: 307–311

Link H, Boogaerts M A, Carella M A et al 1992 A controlled trial of recombinant human GM-CSF after total body irradiation, high dose chemotherapy and autologous bone marrow transplantation for acute lymphoblastic leukaemia and lymphoma. Blood 86(9): 2188–2195

Link H, Fauser A, Hubner G et al 1994 Recombinant human erythropoietin after bone marrow transplantation – the European placebo controlled trial. Br J Haematol 87 (Suppl. 1): 39a

Lotem J, Sachs L 1992 Haemopoietic cytokines inhibit apoptosis induced by TGF beta and cancer chemotherapy compounds in myeloid leukaemia cells. Blood 80: 1750–1757

Maher D, Green M, Bishop J et al 1993 Randomised placebo controlled trial of Filgrastim in patients with febrile neutropenia following chemotherapy. Proc Am Soc Clin Oncol 12: 434a

Marsh J C W, Socie G, Schrezenmeir H et al 1994 Haemopoietic growth factors in aplastic anaemia: a cautionary note. Lancet 344: 172–173

Masoaka T, Takaku F, Kato S et al 1989 Recombinant human G-CSF in allogeneic bone marrow transplantation. Exp Haem 17: 1047–1050

Masoaka T, Shibata H, Ohno R et al 1990 Double blind test of human urinary M-CSF for allogeneic and syngeneic bone marrow transplantation: effectiveness of treatment and two year follow up for relapse of leukaemia. Br J Haematol 76(4): 501–505

Negrin R S, Stein R, Vardiman J et al 1993 Treatment of the anaemia of myelodysplastic syndromes using recombinant human granulocyte colony stimulating factor in combination with erythropoietin. Blood 82(3): 737–743

Nemunaitis J, Buckner C D, Singer J W et al 1990 Use of recombinant human GM-CSF in graft failure after bone marrow transplantation. Blood 76: 245–253

Nemunaitis J, Rabinowe S N, Singer J W et al 1991a Recombinant human GM-CSF for lymphoid cancer. N Engl J Med 324(25): 1775–1778

Nemunaitis J, Buckner C D, Applebaum F et al 1991b Phase I/II trial of recombinant human GM-CSF following allogeneic bone marrow transplantation. Blood 77: 2065–2071

Nemunaitis J, Anasetti C, Storb R et al 1992 Phase II trial of recombinant human GM-CSF in patients undergoing allogeneic bone marrow transplantation from unrelated donors. Blood 79(10): 2572–2577

Nemunaitis J, Applebaum F, Singer J W et al 1993a Phase I trial with recombinant human IL-3 in patients with lymphoma undergoing autologous bone marrow transplantation. Blood 82(11): 3273–3278

Nemunaitis J, Shannon Dorcy K, Applebaum F R et al 1993b Long term follow up of patients with invasive fungal disease who received adjunctive therapy with recombinant human M-CSF. Blood 82(5): 1422–1427

Peters W P, Rosner G, Ross M et al 1993 Comparative effects of GM and G-CSF on priming peripheral blood progenitor cells for use with autologous bone marrow after high dose chemotherapy. Blood 81(7): 1709–1719

Pettengell R, Gurney H, Radford J A et al 1992 Granulocyte colony stimulating factor to prevent dose limiting neutropenia in non Hodgkin's lymphoma: a randomised controlled trial. Blood 80(6): 1430–1436

Powles R, Smith C, Milan S et al 1990 Recombinant human GM-CSF in allogeneic bone marrow transplantation for leukaemia: double blind placebo controlled trial. Lancet 336: 1417–1420

Rabinowe S N, Neuberg D, Bierman P J et al 1993 Long term follow up of a phase III study of recombinant human GM-CSF after autologous bone marrow transplantation for lymphoid malignancies. Blood 81(7): 1903–1908

Russell N H, Pacey S 1992 Economic evaluation of peripheral blood stem cell transplantation for lymphoma. Lancet 340: 1280

Russell N H, Hunter A E, Rogers S et al 1993 Peripheral blood stem cells as an alternative to marrow for allogeneic transplantation. Lancet 341: 1482

Schmitz N, Linch D C, Dreger P et al 1994 A randomised phase III study of Filgrastim mobilised peripheral blood progenitor cell transplantation in comparison with autologous bone marrow transplantation in patients with Hodgkin's disease and non Hodgkin's lymphoma. Blood 84(10): 204a

Schmitz N, Dreger P, Suttorp M et al 1995: Primary transplantation of allogeneic peripheral blood progenitor cells mobilised by filgrastim (granulocyte-colony stimulating factor). Blood 85: 1666-72

Schwartzenberg L, Birch R, Blanco R et al 1993a Rapid and sustained haematopoietic reconstitution by peripheral blood stem cell infusion alone following high dose therapy. Bone Marrow Transplant 11: 369–374

Schwartzenberg L, Birch R, Hazleton B et al 1993b Peripheral blood stem cells mobilised by chemotherapy with or without recombinant human G-CSF. J Haematother 1: 317–327

Sheridan W P, Begley C P, Juttner C A et al 1992 Effect of peripheral blood stem cells mobilised by G-CSF on platelet recovery after high dose chemotherapy. Lancet i: 640–644

Shimazaki C, Oku N, Uchiyama H et al 1994 Effect of granulocyte colony stimulating factor on haematopoietic recovery after peripheral blood progenitor cell transplantation. Bone Marrow Transplant 13: 271–275

Shuster M W, Larson R A, Thompson J A et al 1990 GM-CSF for myelodysplasia: results of a multicentre, randomised controlled trial. Blood 76: 318a

Spitzer G, Adkins D R, Spencer V et al 1994 Randomised studies of growth factors post peripheral blood stem cell transplantation: neutrophil recovery is improved with modest clinical benefit. J Clin Oncol 12(4): 661–670

Stahel R A, Jost L M, Cerny T et al 1994 Randomised study of recombinant human G-CSF after high dose chemotherapy and autologous bone marrow transplantation for high risk lymphoid malignancies. J Clin Oncol 12(9): 1931–1938

Sutherland H J, Eaves C J, Lasdorp G L et al 1994 Kinetics of committed and primitive blood progenitor cell mobilisation after chemotherapy and growth factor treatment and their use in autotransplantation. Blood 83(12): 3808–3814

To L B, Roberts M M, Haylock D N et al 1992 Comparison of haematological recovery times and supportive care requirements of autologous recovery phase peripheral blood stem cell transplants, autologous bone marrow transplants and allogeneic bone marrow transplants. Bone Marrow Transplant 9: 277–284

Weaver C H, Buckner C D, Longin K et al 1993 Syngeneic transplantation with peripheral blood mononuclear cells after the administration of recombinant human G-CSF. Blood 82: 1981–1984

3

Treatment of childhood ALL

J. M. Chessells

The treatment of childhood acute lymphoblastic leukaemia (ALL) is one of the success stories of modern haematology. Recent advances in genetics and molecular biology have increased our understanding of leukaemogenesis and have the potential to influence and improve treatment. This exponential increase in knowledge has been accompanied by steady but real improvement in the numbers of children achieving long-term remission and probable cure; most vividly illustrated, not by selected results of recent therapeutic trials, but by population-based survival figures. An example of this survival improvement

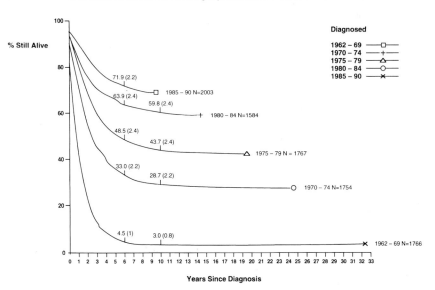

Fig. 1 Survival for consecutive cohorts of children aged 0–15 years in the UK with acute lymphoblastic leukaemia. These are population-based figures derived by the Childhood Cancer Research Group, courtesy of Dr Charles Stiller. Survival percentages with 95% confidence intervals at 6 and 10 years are shown on the graph.

for children in the UK is shown in Fig. 1, which is produced from information obtained by the Oxford Childhood Cancer Research Group.

Despite these encouraging advances problems remain. Treatment is unsuccessful in at least one-third of all children and attempts at retrieval therapy are costly, damaging and frequently do not succeed. Since most children have long first remissions it may take at least 4 to 5 years for any alterations in treatment to prove beneficial. As more children survive, larger numbers of patients are needed to demonstrate any modest improvement in results.

Some of the increasing number of long survivors have late effects of treatment; most commonly problems with memory, learning and growth, but also specific organ toxicities and second neoplasms. Awareness of these issues has led to modifications of treatment, most notably reduction in the use of cranial irradiation.

This review will attempt to summarize recent trends in treatment of ALL and emphasize areas where more work is needed.

PROGNOSTIC FACTORS IN ALL: THE NEED FOR COMMON DEFINITIONS

The concept of risk groups

While the most important factor influencing prognosis in childhood leukaemia is, of course, the treatment, a number of other clinical and biological features influence the chance of cure. This has led to the concept of risk groups and of giving more intensive treatment to children at higher risk of treatment failure or, conversely, avoiding very toxic or dangerous treatment in children who are highly likely to be cured. Almost 10 years have elapsed since the first attempt to define internationally acceptable risk groups in childhood ALL based on age and leukocyte count (Mastrangelo et al 1986); factors which can be measured everywhere and which are known to have a strong prognostic significance. Unfortunately these criteria have not been widely accepted and the various national collaborative groups have very different criteria for risk assignment and, indeed, variable numbers of first line treatment protocols. This is illustrated in Table 1, which has been compiled from published data only and shows how difficult it is for the reader with no inside knowledge to understand the overall treatment strategy in any particular collaborative group, and how the number of protocols varies from group to group, thus hindering international comparisons. The table should also help the reader to interpret the following discussion on recent trial results.

After age and leukocyte count, sex, at least in many reports, appears to have an important influence on outcome, and whenever there are differences girls are always favoured. Recent analysis of results of treatment over 20 years in the MRC UKALL trials (Chessells et al 1995a) has confirmed this finding but has provided no obvious explanation. Boys are not only at risk of testicular relapse but have a higher risk of marrow relapse, particularly after treatment is

Table 1. Definition of Risk Groups in Childhood All (B-All Excluded)

Group and protocols	Years	Risk groups	% Total	Criteria for assignment	Reference
Children's Cancer Group (CCG) 100 Series	1983–1989	Infants Low risk Average risk High risk Lymphoma/leukaemia	2.5 24 43.5 17 13	Age Gender WBC Mass disease Spleen Hb Immunophenotype	Steinherz et al (1991)
MRC UKALL X	1985–1990	Highest risk All other children	12 88	WBC	Chessells et al (1995b)
Paediatric Oncology Group (POG) ALinC; T-Cell3	1986–1991	Infants T-ALL Pre-B ALL	4 15.5 80.5	Age Phenotype	Crist et al (1992)
BFM Group BFM 86	1986–1990	Standard risk Risk group Experimental group	28.6 61.1 10.3	WBC Mass disease Steroid response	Reiter et al (1994)
St Jude Total XI	1984–1988	Lower risk Higher risk	31 69	Age Race WBC Cytogenetics DNA index	Rivera et al (1991)
Dana Farber Institute DFCI 85–01 87–01	1985–1991	Standard risk Higher risk	39 61	Age WBC Phenotype	Sallan (1994)

electively stopped. The theory that the testis acts as a sanctuary site has not been supported by randomized trials of prophylactic testicular irradiation (Eden et al 1990) and it has been postulated that continuing (maintenance) treatment is less effective in boys than girls, possibly because they are more resistant to the mercaptopurine given during continuing treatment in most protocols.

Immunophenotyping

Immunophenotyping is performed with increasing sophistication in ALL using a range of monoclonal antibodies and there have been numerous reviews of the clinical and biological significance of immunophenotype, for example that of Pui et al (1993), which should be consulted for detailed references. Most importantly, immunophenotyping identifies the small group of children (1–2%) with sIg positive B-ALL, previously incurable, who respond to short-term intensive treatment as given for non-Hodgkin's lymphoma. Patients with T-ALL continue to be reported as having a worse prognosis than those with early B-cell disease, but this is largely a result of association with age, mass disease and high leukocyte count (Chessells et al 1995a). There remains some confusion over nomenclature among the early B-cell leukaemias, which comprise the majority; it has been claimed that early pre-B CD10 negative ALL (which is also called null-ALL) has no independent significance once infants, in whom it is common, are excluded from analysis. The majority of children have ALL involving expression of CD10, the common (sometimes called early pre-B) phenotype (CD19+, CD10+) and it now seems clear that the subgroup of these patients with cytoplasmic immunoglobulin expression (confusingly deemed children with pre-B ALL) do not, as previously reported, have a worse prognosis than other subtypes. There is no clear evidence that phenotype-specific treatment is of benefit in ALL other than in sIg positive cases although separate protocols for T-ALL and early B-ALL have been adopted by the Paediatric Oncology Group (POG) (Crist et al 1992) and, to a certain extent, by the American Childrens' Cancer Group (CCG) with their 'Leukaemia Lymphoma' syndrome (Steinherz et al 1991). Unfortunately there have been no randomized trials, on the model of the excellent one performed many years ago in paediatric NHL, and recently updated (Anderson et al 1993) to determine whether phenotype-specific therapy is of benefit other than in B-ALL. Now that monoclonal antibodies are uniformly used in immunophenotyping a number of children with ALL are shown to have myeloid antigen positivity; there are a number of technical problems with the antibodies currently in use for these investigations. Certain subtypes of ALL are more likely to have myeloid lineage features, most notably those occurring in infants with 11q23 cytogenetic abnormalities. However, when these cases are excluded, review of published data on the significance of myeloid antigen positivity shows conflicting results (Drexler et al 1991) and there is, at present, no evidence to recommend that the finding of ALL in association with myeloid antigens should alter the choice of treatment.

Cytogenetics

Conventional cytogenetic analysis, now supplemented by fluorescent in situ hybridization (FISH) and detection of gene rearrangements, also helps to identify another small group of children with a poor prognosis on conventional treatment; there have been many recent reviews of this topic including an excellent one by Raimondi (1993). Some cytogenetic abnormalities such as the t1;19 may lose their previously poor significance with more intensive treatment. However, there are a number of abnormalities associated with a high risk of relapse, most notably near-haploid ALL and the 1–2% of cases with Ph' positive ALL and, perhaps, an additional proportion with BCR/ABL fusion transcript on molecular analysis. Conventional cytogenetic analysis in infants, who have an extremely poor prognosis particularly when under 6 months of age, showed 11q23 rearrangements in 14 of 30, but in an additional 7 on molecular analysis (Chen et al 1993), therefore accounting for the poor prognosis in this age group.

By contrast, high-hyperdiploid ALL, which usually occurs in children with a low leukocyte count and common ALL (Secker Walker et al 1989), has a favourable outcome, and recent studies by the Paediatric Oncology group suggest that ploidy is the single most favourable determinant of outcome (Trueworthy et al 1992). A biological explanation for this is suggested by the finding that cells from patients with high-hyperdiploid ALL accumulate high levels of methotrexate polyglutamates (Whitehead et al 1992).

Cytogenetics in ALL is labour intensive and time consuming, and it has been reported that when patients with a specific abnormality for which the prognostic significance has been well established are removed from analysis the presence of a translocation or other abnormality is of no independent significance (Rubin et al 1991). Perhaps a combination of measurement of ploidy and molecular screening for defined abnormalities with a definite poor prognosis that is Ph' and 11q23 could replace the routine analysis of cytogenetics in all cases of lymphoblastic leukaemia.

Drug sensitivity

There have been a number of recent reports relating in vitro drug sensitivity to long-term outcome and it has been claimed that these findings may be independent of other prognostic features (Pieters et al 1991) but confirmation in large prospective studies is awaited. Meanwhile several groups, most notably the BFM, have adopted response to single agent prednisone as an in vivo prognostic factor (Reiter et al 1994). Therefore, as shown in Table 1, widely different clinical and biological measures are used to identify the 10% or so of patients with a worse prognosis.

TREATMENT STRATEGY

Induction and intensification

It has become apparent in the last 15 years that while prednisolone, vincristine and *l*-asparaginase will achieve remission in over 90% of children with ALL the use of additional drugs during induction and/or a period of further intensification therapy is essential to optimize the chance of event-free survival. There is, however, no evidence that any particular form of intensification therapy is of particular benefit, or whether, if such intensification is given, it is necessary to use additionally toxic drugs in the first days of treatment. For example, the use of daunorubicin in MRC UKALL VIII on days 1 and 2 produced quicker blast regression and less bone marrow relapses, but more toxicity and no overall benefit in event-free survival (Eden et al 1991).

Many schedules in Europe and elsewhere have been based on those of the German BFM group. The group have for many years given an 8-week induction/intensification protocol and showed in unrandomized studies that children who received a further 6-week reinduction intensification did better than historical controls (Riehm et al 1990). The original BFM protocols included moderate-dose combination chemotherapy, which produced myelosuppression over several weeks; its various components were subsequently examined in a large randomized trial by the CCG in protocol 105 with patients receiving either the early intensive 8 week component, the later 6-week component, both or neither (Tubergen et al 1993a). The trial, open to average-risk patients (see Table 1) showed a significant benefit for late intensification in children under 10 years and an apparent although non-significant benefit for early and late intensification in older children. A parallel trial conducted by the Group has shown that similar early and late intensive treatment was superior to standard therapy in high-risk patients (Gaynon et al 1993).

MRC UKALL X was a randomized trial addressing the benefits of 5-day blocks of intensification in all children save for the 10% at highest risk of treatment failure; the results show that double intensification at both 5 and 20 weeks produced a 14% improvement in disease-free survival, but most importantly that this intensification was of benefit to all children including those at lower risk of treatment failure. (Chessells et al 1995b). These results confirm the earlier findings of a small randomized trial conducted by the BFM group, when omission of late intensification in low-risk children was associated with a higher rate of late relapses (Riehm et al 1990).

Single centre protocols for ALL have often used more complicated regimens; in the St Jude study XI all patients received an intensive 6-week induction, but for lower risk children a simple continuing treatment regimen was as effective as a more complex one; higher risk patients all received more intensive treatment throughout (Rivera et al 1991). The Boston Dana-Farber protocols comprised 6 months of pulsed chemotherapy with repeated doses of doxorubicin and high-dose asparaginase; results obtained from this approach appear to be directly comparable with those of the BFM group (Niemeyer et al 1991).

How much intensification is needed and for how long should this type of treatment continue? Some schedules are reaching the limits of tolerance, even when supported by treatment with cytokines. While there is clear evidence that some form of intensification is beneficial during the first 6 months or so of treatment, the need for continued reintensification rather than continuing (maintenance) therapy is uncertain; in MRC UKALL XI we are investigating the benefit of a third intensification course at 8 months from diagnosis. The BFM 86 protocol, recently reported (Reiter et al 1994), included a randomization in the Middle Risk group to receive late intensification at 1 year from diagnosis; the results showed no benefit for this additional treatment but unfortunately only one-quarter of the eligible patients were randomized.

The Paediatric Oncology Group, who use phenotype specific therapy, have attempted to develop protocols largely based on antimetabolite therapy for children with B-lineage ALL. They have investigated the use of intravenous mercaptopurine with methotrexate (Camitta et al 1994) and of intermediate doses of methotrexate and cytarabine as intensification therapy. Repeated courses of methotrexate and cytarabine given during the first 6 months of therapy were as effective as intermittent reintensification given 12 weekly for 18 months (Land et al 1994).

Continuing (maintenance) therapy

Early treatment protocols for ALL, which involved combination chemotherapy for 12–15 months, were associated with a high relapse rate and for many years prolonged outpatient treatment, usually with relatively low doses of mercaptopurine and methotrexate, has become a traditional part of therapy in ALL. Is this phase of treatment necessary in the era of more intensive therapy? In view of the poor outcome after relapse of ALL and the medical costs of retrieval therapy it would be a brave or rather foolhardy move to abandon continuing treatment forthwith and it seems more likely that reduction will be gradual via a series of cautious trials of duration of therapy. Alternatively, the answer may come from investigation of minimal residual disease (see below).

Acute lymphoblastic leukaemia is the only type of cancer where this continuing or maintenance therapy seems beneficial and the possible reasons for this have been the subject of speculation (Gale & Butturini 1991). It seems inherently unlikely that the low dose of drugs given during this phase would kill the leukaemic cells which have survived intensive early treatment, nor, since maintenance is profoundly immunosuppressive, does it seem probable that therapy would be an immunostimulant. An alternative hypothesis is that maintenance therapy controls growth of the leukaemic clone thus facilitating its programmed cell death.

Whatever the role of continuing treatment, current evidence suggests that longer rather than shorter treatment is beneficial in ALL. In MRC UKALL VIII where the duration of therapy was randomized between 2 and 3 years a third year may have decreased the relapse rate but has not, to date, improved overall survival (Eden et al 1991). The BFM group conducted a randomized trial of duration of therapy and found that even after intensive treatment there is a benefit for 2 years rather than 18 months (Riehm et al 1990).

Traditional continuing (maintenance) treatment consists of daily oral mercaptopurine and weekly methotrexate by mouth or injection; additional prednisolone and vincristine given every 4 weeks is not myelosuppressive and may be of benefit (Bleyer et al 1991).

There is no evidence that any more complicated schedule is superior to this combination. More complicated continuing treatment was of no benefit after intensive initial treatment in high-risk children with ALL treated by the CCG (Gaynon et al 1993). It seems probable that drug doses during continuing treatment should be given to the limits of tolerance as determined by the absolute neutrophil count; children who receive larger doses of mercaptopurine and methotrexate and who sustain treatment-induced neutropenia are at less risk of subsequent relapse (Hale & Lilleyman 1991, Pearson et al 1991).

There have been a number of recent investigations of absorption and pharmacology of mercaptopurine and methotrexate and these have shown wide inter- and intrapatient variation (Pearson et al 1991, Lilleyman & Lennard 1994). Preliminary suggestions that rapid clearance of methotrexate is associated with a higher risk of leukaemic relapse have not been confirmed (Pearson et al 1991) but it has been shown that children with low intracellular concentrations of mercaptopurine metabolites are at increased risk of relapse (Lilleyman & Lennard 1994). Variability in concentration of metabolites may be caused by genetic factors (Lennard et al 1990) but may also be related to compliance (Davies et al 1993). It has recently been suggested that thioguanine may be a more appropriate drug than mercaptopurine in continuing therapy (Lennard et al 1993) and several collaborative groups are attempting to examine this issue.

Minimal residual disease

Minimal residual disease (MRD), that is disease occurring at a subclinical level which is not detectable by conventional techniques, can now be detected by the use of the polymerase chain reaction (PCR) to amplify chromosomal translocations or clone specific immunoglobulin heavy chain or T-cell receptor gene rearrangements (Morgan et al 1994). These have the capacity to detect one leukaemic cell in $10^4/10^6$ normal marrow cells. There have now been a number of studies, usually based on retrospective analysis of stored marrow samples, which have shown that in patients who remain in remission the proportion of leukaemic cells detected by PCR declines during therapy and none are usually detectable at the end of treatment. By contrast, patients relapsing during therapy may have a rising proportion of cells of a high level of disease after completion of induction therapy. Patients who subsequently relapse off treatment may have detectable disease in their end-of-treatment bone marrow

(Wasserman et al 1992) and, remarkably, MRD was detected retrospectively in end-of-treatment samples in two children relapsing more than 8 years off treatment (Potter et al 1993). There are, however, a number of technical pitfalls in assessment of MRD, such as false positive findings and the lack of a true method of quantitation, while clonal evolution may produce false negative results (Steward et al 1994). Such problems are less likely to arise when both IgH and T-cell receptor gene rearrangements are investigated. It is not clear whether the presence of MRD at the end of treatment necessarily heralds subsequent relapse, or whether some long-term survivors may have evidence of MRD. Large prospective studies of molecular monitoring are needed to confirm the significance and clinical value of these retrospective studies. If these preliminary findings are validated they offer hope for individual tailoring of duration of therapy and late intensification.

An alternative approach to detection of minimal residual disease is the use of double marker immunofluorescence that can be used to detect blast cells which are absent from normal blood and marrow, for example, in cases of T-cell leukaemia (Campana et al 1990). However, extreme caution should be exercised in reliance on immunological techniques to diagnose relapse in childhood ALL. Lymphocytes that are CD19, CD10 terminal-transferase positive are, of course, present in normal bone marrow and this phenotype may be expressed by reactive cells in cerebrospinal fluid.

CNS directed therapy

Treatment to prevent overt leukaemic infiltration of the central nervous system is essential for all children with ALL, but it has become apparent that this treatment should be tailored for the age and risk group of the patient. Results of recent clinical trials have shown that for many children the previous standard therapy, comprising a short-term course of intrathecal methotrexate injections and cranial irradiation in a dose order of 18 to 24 Gy, can be effectively replaced by regular intrathecal chemotherapy with or without high-dose systemic methotrexate. It is important to recognize the interaction between systemic and CNS directed treatment, illustrated over 10 years ago in a randomized comparison of cranial irradiation plus short-term intrathecal MTX and intermediate dose MTX. In children with leukocyte counts under $20 \times 10^9/l$ the former provided better CNS protection and the latter better bone marrow and testicular protection, but overall event-free survival was similar in the two groups of patients (Freeman et al 1983).

A course of short-term intrathecal methotrexate alone will not prevent CNS relapse (Ortega et al 1987), but the combination of such a course with regular intrathecal methotrexate has been shown by CCG to provide adequate treatment for children with low-risk ALL (Littman et al 1987). CCG protocol 105, in addition to investigating the benefits of intensification therapy, contained a randomized comparison of long-term intrathecal MTX and short-term intrathecal MTX plus cranial irradiation. Intrathecal MTX alone afforded adequate CNS protection in younger children who had also received intensified systemic therapy, while children over 10 appeared to have a better event-free survival if they received cranial irradiation (Tubergen et al 1993b). Children with lymphoma-leukaemia syndrome treated by CCG with the LSA_2L_2 protocol had superior event-free survival and a lower CNS relapse rate when treated with cranial irradiation as well as regular intrathecal chemotherapy; the benefit was not apparent in patients with leukocyte counts below $50 \times 10^9/l$ (Cherlow et al 1993).

There have been no direct comparisons of intrathecal methotrexate with triple intrathecal chemotherapy, a combination favoured by the POG for all children, irrespective of leukocyte count save those with T-ALL (Crist et al 1992). The group have recently shown in a randomized trial that this combination is superior to short-term triple intrathecal chemotherapy and regular intermediate-dose intravenous methotrexate (Pullen et al 1993). High-dose intravenous methotrexate in any dose from 500 mg to 34 G has been used with apparent effect in a number of unrandomized studies, and in a randomized comparison from St Jude hospital, lower risk patients who received regular intravenous methotrexate every 6 weeks had a better event-free survival, albeit a higher CNS relapse rate, than children who received cranial irradiation (Pui et al 1992).

Therefore it appears that regular intrathecal chemotherapy affords adequate protection for children with low or average-risk leukaemia defined variously on the basis of leukocyte count or immunophenotype. For children at higher risk additional treatment is needed, either cranial irradiation or high-dose intravenous methotrexate. The present MRC UKALL XI involves a randomized comparison of regular intrathecal MTX and intrathecal plus intravenous MTX in children with initial leukocyte counts below $50 \times 10^9/l$ and of intrathecal and intravenous MTX with cranial irradiation in the remainder.

The confounding effects of systemic chemotherapy must always be considered as shown in the previous examples. Long-term follow-up of an early trial from the Cancer and Leukaemia Group B (ancestor of the POG) suggests that dexamethasone is superior to prednisolone for prevention of CNS disease, a finding which warrants further appraisal (Jones et al 1991).

The interpretation of CSF findings can be difficult during regular intrathecal chemotherapy and there is contradictory evidence about the significance of low numbers of blast cells in the CSF. Children on protocol 105 whose CSF showed blast cells without pleocytosis (> 5 WBC/ml) on one or two occasions were not necessarily at increased risk of CNS relapse and the yield of routine CSF examinations was low (Tubergen et al 1994). These findings emphasize the need for caution in diagnosis of CNS relapse (thus subjecting patients to more toxic treatment) during regular intrathecal chemotherapy, and perhaps question the value of routine cytological examinations in patients with a low CSF leukocyte count.

ALTERNATIVE TREATMENTS

B-ALL

The conventional approach to treatment reviewed above is not appropriate for a small minority of children with ALL. The group for whom it is most clearly inappropriate is the 1–2% with surface membrane immunoglobulin positive B-ALL. These children, previously incurable, have responded to treatment with various combinations of short-term high-dose chemotherapy as used in paediatric non-Hodgkin lymphoma of mature B-cell phenotype, which includes high-dose cyclophosphamide, methotrexate and cytarabine. Such patients are at high risk of CNS relapse but prevention can be obtained in the majority of patients with the use of high-dose intravenous and intrathecal chemotherapy without cranial irradiation. There are a number of similar protocols reported with excellent results, most notably perhaps those of the French LMB group (Patte et al 1994) who in their latest series of protocols have reported event-free survival of over 80% for children with B-ALL. The main adverse prognostic factor at diagnosis is CNS involvement, although the group have claimed improved survival with the use of intensified systemic treatment and subsequent cranial irradiation.

Infants

Infants under 1 year, and particularly under 6 months of age, are at high risk of both marrow and CNS relapse; a recent analysis of prognostic factors showed that the strongest predictor of treatment failure was 11q23/MLL involvement of blast cells (Pui et al 1994). The probability of continuous complete remission in the intensive protocol developed by the CCG was 31% (Heerema et al 1994) and recent attempts to intensify treatment by the MRC were associated with a high incidence of toxicity and a number of relapses after high-dose chemotherapy and autologous BMT in first remission (Chessells et al 1994a). Clearly, innovative therapy is needed in this age group, at least in those children with 11q23 abnormalities.

Bone marrow transplant in first remission ALL

There is continued debate about the role of high-dose chemotherapy and bone marrow transplantation in first remission of ALL. This form of treatment would seem appropriate, at least for the small number of children with an extremely poor prognosis who have a histocompatible sibling donor. These would include the rare children who fail to respond to intensive induction therapy, those with Ph positive ALL and perhaps t4;11 and near-haploid ALL and others selected on the basis of leukocyte count and/or additional criteria. This higher risk group would not comprise more than, at most, one-tenth of children with ALL. In MRC UKALL X children with a leukocyte count greater than $100 \times 10^9/l$ and a histocompatible sibling donor were eligible for BMT at the discretion of family and physician. Only 34 of 198 children with high counts received BMT, which significantly reduced the relapse rate but, since it was associated with more toxic deaths than chemotherapy, had no overall effect on disease-free survival (Chessells et al 1992). These results suggest that, with reduced toxicity, BMT might play a role in first remission ALL in selected children. We continue to explore BMT in UKALL XI but patients are now selected on the basis of a risk score derived from age and sex as well as leukocyte count (Chessells et al 1995a).

Adolescents

Adolescents and young adults are frequently eligible for both paediatric and adult trials of therapy. Recent analysis of adults aged 16–21 treated on CCG protocols in the 100 series showed a creditable 6 year event-free survival of 60%, similar to the results in the 10–15+ age group, and better than reports from most adult trials (Nachman et al 1993). Similarly, a steady improvement has been shown in the outcome of 10–18-year-olds treated at St Jude hospital (Rivera et al 1993). These results suggest that paediatric protocols may be optimal for the treatment of adolescents and young adults.

Treatment after relapse

Despite the success of modern treatment, one-third to one-quarter of children still experience a relapse, most often in the bone marrow. The outlook for such patients, as illustrated in Figures 2 and 3 remains poor, the duration of second remission depending on the type of relapse (Fig. 2) and the length of first remission (Fig. 3).

It has been accepted for some time that chemotherapy is rarely successful in treatment of early marrow relapse (occurring up to at least 6 months after treatment has been electively stopped) and that for children who have a histocompatible sibling donor BMT is the most effective treatment despite the instability of second remissions and the high risk of post-transplant relapse (Dopfer et al 1991). The BFM group have reported that children with later marrow relapses may respond to further intensive chemotherapy (Henze et al 1991); our own experience is that, while such children may achieve long second remissions they remain at risk of a second relapse (Chessells et al 1994b). A recent comparison of data from the International Bone Marrow Transplant Registry with the results of children receiving chemotherapy on POG protocols has shown that BMT carries a significantly lower probability of relapse and a greater chance of leukaemia-free survival than chemotherapy, which is independent of time of relapse, age, leukocyte count or immunophenotype (Barrett et al 1994). For children who do not have a histocompatible sibling donor the alternatives are intensive chemotherapy, autologous transplantation (Billett et al 1993), reputedly successful in later relapses, or

TREATMENT OF CHILDHOOD ALL   57

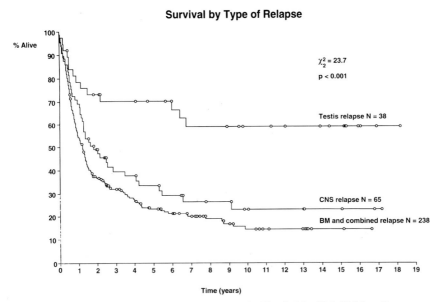

Fig. 2 Survival in all children with ALL treated at the Hospital for Sick Children from 1972–1990 who have relapsed and received further treatment. Survival is shown according to site of relapse; all relapses with bone marrow involvement are analysed together.

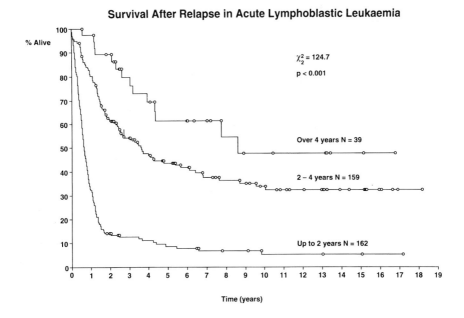

Fig. 3 Survival in the same population of children as Fig. 2 according to length of the first remission.

use of a matched unrelated donor. As the probability of obtaining HLA-matched donors improves there will be the potential for critical evaluation of MUD transplants in second remission and we are currently trying to organize such a study in relapsed ALL.

For children with late extramedullary relapses, particularly in the testis, intensified chemotherapy and local irradiation continues to afford a good chance of prolonged second remission; the recent BFM study showed two-thirds of patients alive in remission at 6 years (Henze et al 1991). There are few large studies of treatment of CNS relapse in children who have received modern protocols; in a recent report from POG, 120 children with an isolated CNS relapse received further induction, cranial irradiation and monthly triple intrathecal chemotherapy; the event-free survival at 4 years was 46% but children with earlier relapses (less than 3 years from diagnosis) had a significantly worse prognosis (Winick et al 1993). These results suggest that, for most children who will not have received cranial irradiation, it may be possible to dispense with the spinal component of radiotherapy after CNS relapse. These results would also justify trials of cranial irradiation and long-term regular intrathecal chemotherapy as a substitute for craniospinal irradiation in the 1–2% of children who present with overt CNS disease at diagnosis. Early CNS relapse in 12–18 months from diagnosis has a poor prognosis and it may be reasonable to consider BMT in these patients.

Potential new approaches to treatment

It is salutary to recognize that the majority of drugs effective in ALL have been available for at least 20 years. The resurrection of interest in thioguanine (Evans & Relling 1994) and in intravenous mercaptopurine (Pinkel 1993) are timely reminders that all is not known yet about these old reliables. Conjugated immunotoxins, usually linked to monoclonal antibodies, have undergone preliminary studies in lymphohaemopoetic neoplasms (Vallera 1994) and have the potential to deliver targeted therapy. Modern developments in molecular biology have allowed development of antisense sequences, which have the potential to downregulate products of a target gene, thus acting as therapy for minimal residual disease or perhaps altering drug resistance (Kirkland et al 1994). The increasing interest in programmed cell death and its role, particularly in B-cell precursors has led to the study of agents inducing apoptosis in experimental conditions; an interesting preliminary report suggests that IL-4 may have the potential to induce apoptosis in cells from patients with high-risk leukaemia (Manabe et al 1994). No doubt by the time of the next review of this topic the clinical relevance of these approaches will have become more apparent.

LATE EFFECTS OF TREATMENT

No review of treatment of childhood ALL would be complete without mention of the late effects of treatment, which may take years to become apparent and which have led to many of the recent modifications of therapy. It is now accepted that children who received cranial irradiation at a young age are at risk of cognitive impairment (Cousens et al 1988) and recent evidence supports the concept that previous reductions in the dose of cranial irradiation to 18 Gy have not eliminated that risk (Jankovic et al 1994); it remains unclear whether alternative CNS directed treatment will prove less damaging, and in one prospective study children who did not receive cranial irradiation also developed cognitive defects and changes on computerized tomography of the brain (Ochs et al 1991). There are as yet no detailed studies of growth and puberty in children treated without cranial irradiation but it seems unlikely that they will develop the growth failure or precocious puberty encountered after previous protocols. While there have been as yet no large-scale studies of fertility in long-term survivors there is no evidence of impaired fertility in patients who have not received spinal or total body irradiation, or drugs with recognized impairment of fertility such as cyclophosphamide.

Perhaps the most worrying late effect of treatment reported in recent years is anthracycline-induced cardiac toxicity; in a recent detailed study of this complication, while age and total dose of drug were the only two independent predictors of toxicity, no safe cumulative dose could be determined (Lipshultz et al 1991). Toxicity may cause late cardiac decompensation as a result of pregnancy or weight training. Many groups are now attempting to develop guidelines for prevention of this serious complication by dose limitation, serial monitoring, scheduling and the use of cardioprotectants (Hale & Lewis, 1994).

The risk of second cancers after ALL has been reported as increased sevenfold over the normal age-adjusted population, that is with an incidence of 2.53% at 15 years after diagnosis. The most common second cancer is a primary CNS tumour, but these have only been reported in children who have received cranial irradiation and the under 5s are at highest risk (Neglia et al 1991). The risk of secondary myeloid leukaemia is low except after intensive epipodophyllotoxin therapy (Pui et al 1991). These reports emphasize the need for both individual and population based follow-up of all long-term survivors of childhood leukaemia. Many collaborative groups are now developing guidelines for follow-up, which are tailored to the individual treatment protocol.

KEY POINTS FOR CLINICAL PRACTICE

- Despite the steady improvement in outlook for children with acute lymphoblastic leukaemia, treatment is unsuccessful in perhaps one-third of patients.

- There is no internationally accepted definition of risk groups, but age, gender and leukocyte count are the most important clinical features influencing prognosis. Cytogenetic analysis and measurement of ploidy help to define low- and high-risk patients.

- A standard approach to treatment is indicated for 90% of children. The exceptions are those with B-ALL, infants and a small number who fail induction and/or have other very adverse prognostic features.

- Bone marrow transplantation may be of benefit in highest risk children in first remission, but in all others is only indicated after relapse.

- There is good evidence that one or more additional periods of post remission intensification treatment improves the chance of disease-free survival in all patients.

- All children require CNS directed therapy but the type of treatment should be determined by the age and risk group of the patients.

- Intrathecal chemotherapy alone affords adequate CNS protection for low-risk children, but those at higher risk of CNS relapse require additional treatment with cranial irradiation or possibly high-dose intravenous methotrexate.

- Despite the introduction of more intensification treatment most children require at least 2 years of treatment; the latter part as continuing (maintenance) therapy.

- Modern techniques of molecular biology enable detection of low levels of minimal residual disease but prospective studies are needed to confirm the clinical feasibility and value of detection of MRD.

- All children who have completed treatment require long-term follow-up to detect and minimize potential late effects of therapy.

REFERENCES

Anderson J R, Jenkin D T, Wilson J F et al 1993 Long-term follow-up of patients treated with COMP of LSA2L2 therapy for childhood non-Hodgkin's lymphoma: A report of CCG-551 from the children's Cancer Group. J Clin Oncol 11: 1024–1032

Barrett A J, Horowitz M M, Pollock B H et al 1994 Bone marrow transplants from HLA-identical siblings as compared with chemotherapy for children with acute lymphoblastic leukaemia in a second remission. N Engl J Med 331: 1253–1258

Billett A L, Kornmehl E, Tarbell N J et al 1993 Autologous bone marrow transplantation after a long first remission for children with recurrent acute lymphoblastic leukemia. Blood 81: 1651–1657

Bleyer W A, Sather H N, Nickerson H J et al 1991 Monthly pulses of vincristine and prednisone prevent bone marrow and testicular relapse in low-risk childhood acute lymphoblastic leukemia: A report of the CCG-161 study by the Childrens Cancer Study Group. J Clin Oncol 9: 1012–1021

Camitta B, Mahoney D, Leventhalt B et al 1994 Intensive intravenous methotrexate and mercaptopurine treatment of higher-risk non-T, non-B acute lymphocytic leukemia: a pediatric oncology group study. J Clin Oncol 12: 1383–1389

Campana D, Coustan-Smith E, Janossy G 1990 The immunologic detection of minimal residual disease in acute leukemia. Blood 76: 163–171

Chen C-S, Sorensen P H B, Domer P H et al 1993 Molecular rearrangements on chromosome 11q23 predominate in infant acute lymphoblastic leukemia and are associated with specific biologic variables and poor outcome. Blood 81: 2386–2393

Cherlow J M, Steinherz P G, Sather H N et al 1993 The role of radiation therapy in the treatment of acute lymphoblastic leukemia with lymphomatous presentation: A report from the childrens cancer group. Int J Rad Oncol Biol Phys 27: 1001–1009

Chessells J M, Bailey C, Wheeler K et al 1992 Bone marrow transplantation for high-risk childhood lymphoblastic leukaemia in first remission: experience in MRC UKALL X. Lancet 340 (ii): 565–568

Chessells J M, Eden O B, Bailey C C et al 1994a Acute lymphoblastic leukaemia in infancy: experience in MRC UKALL trials. Report from the Medical Research Council Working Party on childhood leukaemia. Leukemia 8: 1275–1279

Chessells J M, Leiper A D, Richards S M 1994b A second course of treatment for childhood acute lymphoblastic leukaemia: Long-term follow-up is needed to assess results. Br J Haematol 86: 48–54

Chessells J M, Richards S M, Bailey et al 1995a Gender and treatment outcome in childhood lymphoblastic leukaemia: Report from the MRC UKALL trials. Br J Haematol 89: 364–372

Chessells J M, Bailey C, Richards S M 1995b Intensification of treatment improves survival for all children with lymphoblastic leukaemia: results of MRC UKALL X. Lancet: 345: 143–148

Cousens P, Waters B, Said J et al 1988 Cognitive effects of cranial irradiation in leukaemia: A survey and meta-analysis. J Clin Psychol Psychiat 29: 839–852

Crist W, Shuster J, Look T et al 1992 Current results of studies of immunophenotype-, age- and leukocyte-based therapy for children with acute lymphoblastic leukemia. Leukaemia 6 (Suppl 2): 162–166

Davies H A, Lennard L, Lilleyman J S 1993 Variable mercaptopurine metabolism in children with leukaemia: A problem of non-compliance? Br Med J 306: 1239–1240

Dopfer R, Henze G, Bender-Götze C et al 1991 Allogeneic bone marrow transplantation for childhood acute lymphoblastic leukemia in second remission after intensive primary and relapse therapy according to the BFM- and CoALL-protocols: Results of the German Cooperative Study. Blood 78: 2780–2784

Drexler H G, Thiel E, Ludwig W-D 1991 Review of the incidence and clinical relevance of myeloid antigen-positive acute lymphoblastic leukemia. Leukemia 5: 637–645

Eden O B, Lilleyman J S, Richards S 1990 Testicular irradiation in childhood lymphoblastic leukaemia. Br J Haematol 75: 496–498

Eden O B, Lilleyman J S, Richards et al 1991 Results of medical research council childhood leukaemia trial UKALL VIII (Report to the Medical Research Council on behalf of the Working Party on Leukaemia in Childhood). Br J Haematol 78: 187–196

Evans W E, Relling M V 1994 Mercaptopurine vs thioguanine for the treatment of acute lymphoblastic leukemia. Leuk Res 18: 811–814

Freeman A I, Weinberg V, Brecher M L et al 1983 Comparison of intermediate-dose methotrexate with cranial irradiation for the post-induction treatment of acute lymphocytic leukemia in children. N Engl J Med 308: 477–484

Gale R P, Butturini A 1991 Maintenance chemotherapy and cure of childhood acute lymphoblastic leukaemia. Lancet 338: 1315–1318

Gaynon P S, Steinherz P G, Bleyer W A et al 1993 Improved therapy for children with acute lymphoblastic leukemia and unfavourable presenting features: A follow-up report on the Childrens Cancer Group Study CCG-106. J Clin Oncol 11: 2234–2242

Hale J P, Lilleyman J S 1991 Importance of 6-mercaptopurine dose in lymphoblastic leukaemia. Arch Dis Child 66: 462–466

Hale J P, Lewis I J 1994 Anthracyclines: cardiotoxicity and its prevention. Arch Dis Child 71: 457–462

Heerema N A, Arthur D C, Sather H et al 1994 Cytogenetic features of infants less than 12 months of age at diagnosis of acute lymphoblastic leukemia: Impact of the 11q23 breakpoint on outcome: A report of the Childrens Cancer Group. Blood 83: 2274–2284

Henze G, Fengler R, Hartmann R et al 1991 Six-year experience with a comprehensive approach to the treatment of recurrent childhood acute lymphoblastic leukemia (ALL-REZ BFM 85). A relapse study of the BFM group. Blood 78: 1166–1172

Jankovic M, Brouwers P, Valsecchi M G et al 1994 Association of 1800 cGy cranial irradiation with intellectual function in children with acute lymphoblastic leukaemia. Lancet 344: 224

Jones B, Freeman A I, Shuster J J et al 1991 Lower incidence of meningeal leukaemia when prednisolone is replaced by dexamethasone in the treatment of acute lymphocytic leukaemia. Med Pediatr Oncol 19: 269–275

Kirkland M A, O'Brien S G, Goldman J M 1994 Antisense therapeutics in haematological malignancies. Br J Haematol 87: 447–452

Land V J, Shuster J J, Crist W M et al 1994 Comparison of two schedules of intermediate-dose methotrexate and cytarabine consolidation therapy for childhood B-precursor cell acute lymphoblastic leukaemia: a pediatric oncology group study. J Clin Oncol 12: 1939–1945

Lennard L, Lilleyman J S, Van Loon J et al 1990 Genetic variation in response to 6-mercaptopurine for childhood acute lymphoblastic leukaemia. Lancet 336: 225–229

Lennard L, Davies H A, Lilleyman J S 1993 Is 6-thioguanine more appropriate than 6-mercaptopurine for children with acute lymphoblastic leukaemia? Br J Cancer 68: 186–190

Lilleyman J S, Lennard L 1994 Mercaptopurine metabolism and risk of relapse in childhood lymphoblastic leukaemia. Lancet 343: 1188–1190

Lipshultz S E, Colan S D, Gelber R D et al 1991 Late cardiac effects of doxorubicin therapy for acute lymphoblastic leukemia in childhood. N Engl J Med 324: 808–815

Littman P, Coccia P, Bleyer W A et al 1987 Central nervous system (CNS) prophylaxis in children with low risk acute lymphoblastic leukemia (ALL). Int J Rad Oncol Biol Phys 13: 1443–1449

Manabe A, Coustan-Smith E, Kumagai M-A et al 1994 Interleukin-4 induces programmed cell death (apoptosis) in cases of high-risk acute lymphoblastic leukaemia. Blood 83: 1731–1737

Mastrangelo R, Poplack D G, Bleyer W A et al 1986 Report and recommendations of the Rome workshop concerning poor-prognosis acute lymphoblastic leukemia in children: Biologic bases for staging, stratification, and treatment. Med Pediatr Oncol 14: 191–194

Morgan G J, Shiach C, Potter M 1994 The clinical value of detecting gene rearrangements in acute leukaemias. Br J Haematol 88: 459–464

Nachman J, Sather H N, Buckley, J D et al 1993 Young adults 16–21 years of age at diagnosis entered on children's cancer group acute lymphoblastic leukemia and acute myeloblastic leukemia protocols. Cancer 71: 3377–3385

Neglia J P, Meadows A T, Robison L L et al 1991 Second neoplasms after acute lymphoblastic leukemia in childhood. N Engl J Med 325: 1330–1336

Niemeyer C M, Reiter A, Riehm et al 1991 Comparative results of two intensive treatment programs for childhood acute lymphoblastic leukemia: The Berlin-Frankfurt-Munster and Dana-Farber Cancer Institute protocols. Ann Oncol 2: 745–749

Ochs J, Mulhern R, Fairclough D et al 1991 Comparison of neuropsychologic functioning and clinical indicators of neurotoxicity in long-term survivors of childhood leukemia given cranial radiation or parenteral methotrexate: A prospective study. J Clin Oncol 9: 145–151

Ortega J A, Nesbit M E, Sather H N et al 1987 Long-term evaluation of a CNS prophylaxis trial-treatment comparisons and outcome after CNS relapse in childhood ALL: A report from the children's cancer study group. J Clin Oncol 5: 1646–1654

Patte C, Michon J, Frappaz D et al 1994 Therapy of Burkitt and other B-cell acute lymphoblastic leukaemia and lymphoma: Experience with the LMB protocols of the SFOP (French Paediatric Oncology Society) in children and adults. Ballieres Clin Haematol 7: 339–348

Pearson A D J, Amineddine H A, Yule M et al 1991 The influence of serum methotrexate concentrations and drug dosage on outcome in childhood acute lymphoblastic leukaemia. Br J Cancer 64: 169–173

Pieters R, Huismans, D R, Loonen A H et al 1991 Relation of cellular drug resistance to long-term clinical outcome in childhood acute lymphoblastic leukaemia. Lancet 338: 399–403

Pinkel D 1993 Intravenous mercaptopurine: Life begins at 40. J Clin Oncol 11: 1826–1831

Potter M N, Steward C G, Oakhill A 1993 The significance of detection of minimal residual disease in childhood acute lymphoblastic leukaemia. Br Haematol 83: 412–418

Pui C-H, Ribeiro R C, Hancock M L et al 1991 Acute myeloid leukemia in children treated with epipodophyllotoxins for acute lymphoblastic leukemia. N Engl J Med 325: 1682–1687

Pui, C-H, Simone J V, Hancock M L et al 1992 Impact of three methods of treatment intensification on acute lymphoblastic leukaemia in children: Long-term results of St Jude total therapy study X. Leukemia 6: 150–157

Pui C-H, Behm F G, Crist W M 1993 Clinical and biologic relevance of immunologic marker studies in childhood acute lymphoblastic leukemia. Blood 82: 343–362

Pui C-H, Behm F G, Downing J R et al 1994 11q23/MLL rearrangement confers a poor prognosis in infants with acute lymphoblastic leukemia. J Clin Oncol 12: 909–915

Pullen J, Boyett J, Shuster J et al 1993 Extended triple intrathecal chemotherapy trial for prevention of CNS relapse in good-risk and poor-risk patients with B-progenitor acute lymphoblastic leukemia: A Pediatric Oncology Group Study. J Clin Oncol 11: 839–849

Raimondi S C 1993 Current status of cytogenetic research in childhood acute lymphoblastic leukemia. Blood 81: 2237–2251

Reiter A, Schrappe M, Ludwig W-D et al 1994 Chemotherapy in 998 unselected childhood acute lymphoblastic leukemia patients, results and conclusions of the multicenter trial ALL-BFM 86. Blood 84: 3122–3133

Riehm H, Gadner H, Henze G et al 1990 Results and significance of six randomized trials in four consecutive ALL-BFM studies. Haematol Blood Trans 33: 439–450

Rivera G K, Raimondi S C, Hancock M L et al 1991 Improved outcome in childhood acute lymphoblastic leukaemia with reinforced early treatment and rotational combination chemotherapy. Lancet 337: 61–66

Rivera G K, Pui C-H, Santana V M et al 1993 Progress in the treatment of adolescents with acute lymphoblastic leukemia. Cancer 71: 3400–3405

Rubin C M, Le Beau M M, Mick R et al 1991 Impact of chromosomal translocations on prognosis in childhood acute lymphoblastic leukemia. J Clin Oncol 9: 2183–2192

Sallon SE 1994 Overview of Dana Karber Cancer Institute – Consortium Childhood Acute Lymphoblastic Leukemia Protocols: 1973-1992 in Acute Leukemias IV Buchmer et al, eds. Springer-Verlag, Berlin, Heidelberg, pp 322-329

Secker Walker L M, Chessells J M, Stewart E L et al 1989 Chromosomes and other prognostic factors in acute lymphoblastic leukaemia: a long term follow-up. Br J Haematol 72: 336–342

Steinherz P G, Siegel S E, Bleyer W A et al 1991 Lymphomatous presentation of childhood acute lymphoblastic leukemia: A subgroup at high risk of early treatment failure. Cancer 68: 751–758

Steward C G, Goulden N J, Katz F et al 1994 A polymerase chain reaction study of the stability of Ig heavy-chain and T-cell receptor delta gene rearrangements between presentation and relapse of childhood B-lineage acute lymphoblastic leukemia. Blood 83: 1355–1362

Trueworthy R, Shuster J, Look T et al 1992 Ploidy of lymphoblasts is the strongest predictor of treatment outcome in B-progenitor cell acute lymphoblastic leukemia of childhood: A Pediatric Oncology Group Study. J Clin Oncol 10: 606–613

Tubergen D G, Gilchrist G S, O'Brien R T et al 1993a Improved outcome with delayed intensification for children with acute lymphoblastic leukemia and intermediate presenting features: A Children's Cancer Group Phase III trial. J Clin Oncol 11: 527–537

Tubergen D G, Gilchrist G S, O'Brien R T et al 1993b Prevention of CNS disease in intermediate-risk acute lymphoblastic leukemia: Comparison of cranial radiation and intrathecal methotrexate and the importance of systemic therapy: A Children's Cancer Group Report. J Clin Oncol 11: 520–526

Tubergen D G, Cullen J W, Boyett J M et al 1994 Blasts in the CSF with a normal cell count do not justify alteration of therapy for acute lymphoblastic leukemia in remission: A Children's Cancer Group Study. J Clin Oncol 12: 273–278

Vallera D A 1994 Immunotoxins: will their clinical promise be fulfilled? Blood 2: 309–317

Wasserman R, Galili N, Ito Y et al 1992 Residual disease at the end of induction therapy as a predictor of relapse during therapy in childhood B-lineage acute lymphoblastic leukemia. J Clin Oncol 10: 1879–1888

Whitehead V M, Vuchich M J, Lauer S J et al 1992 Accumulation of high levels of methotrexate polyglutamates in lymphoblasts from children with hyperdiploid (>50 chromosomes) B-lineage acute lymphoblastic leukemia: A Pediatric Oncology Group Study. Blood 80: 1316–1323

Winick N J, Smith S D, Shuster J et al 1993 Treatment of CNS relapse in children with acute lymphoblastic leukemia: A Pediatric Oncology Group Study. J Clin Oncol 11: 271–278

4

New therapies for chronic lymphocytic leukemia

C. A. Koller   M. J. Keating

Chronic lymphocytic leukemia (CLL) is a clonal expansion of B-lymphocytes with a low proliferative index but prolonged cell survival. It is the most common adult leukemia in the USA; its incidence increases with age. Progress in understanding and treating CLL has been slow since the original clinical description by Minot and Isaacs (1924). However, new insights into the biology of this disease, better diagnostic and staging criteria (Binet et al 1981, Rai & Han 1990), and the development of more potent therapeutic agents are changing the outlook for CLL patients. Indeed, recent gains in remission rates and survival (Dillman et al 1989, Juliusson et al 1993, Keating et al 1993) and the potential role of bone marrow transplantation (Bandini et al 1991) and of biotherapy in the adjuvant setting have raised expectations for the eventual cure of this disease. Cases of chronic lymphocytosis with a T-cell phenotype are rare and account for less than 5% of cases of chronic lymphocytic leukemia. Based on the immunologic, biologic, and clinical differences from B-cell CLL, most investigators recommend that unless specifically mentioned otherwise, T-cell CLL should not be included in a discussion of CLL.

TREATMENT CONSIDERATIONS

Biology and staging

It is beyond the scope of this review to discuss in depth the newest insights into the biology and staging of CLL and the reader is referred to several recent reviews (O'Brien et al 1995, Faguet 1994, Cheson 1993). It must be noted, however, that the link between tumor burden and survival is so strong that disease staging has become the basis for therapy. Of the many staging systems proposed (Rai & Han 1990, Binet et al 1981, Jaksic & Vitale 1981), the modified Rai and the Binet approaches are widely accepted.

The modified Rai staging system stratifies patients into low, intermediate, and high-risk categories based on their clinical picture: monoclonal B-cell lymphocytosis of blood and marrow, lymphocytosis plus lymphadenopathy with or without splenomegaly, and lymphocytosis plus anemia (hemoglobin level < 11 g/dl) or thrombocytopenia (platelet count < 100 000/µl), respectively. These categories, which correspond to Rai's initial stages 0, I plus II, and III plus IV (Rai et al 1975), represent 30%, 60%, and 10% of newly diagnosed CLL patients and are associated with 10-, 6-, and 3-year survival rates, respectively.

The Binet staging system is based on the number of lymph node areas involved and the presence of anemia or thrombocytopenia. Less than three node bearing areas are classified as stage A; three or more node bearing areas are classified as stage B. Patients with anemia (hemoglobin level < 10 g/dl) or thrombocytopenia (platelet count < 100 000/µl) are classified as stage C. In contrast to Rai's categories, Binet's stages A, B, and C account for 60%, 30%, and 10% of newly diagnosed cases, but exhibit comparable median survival rates (9, 5, and 2 years, respectively).

Therefore, the staging workup should include a thorough physical examination and a complete blood cell count. Bone marrow aspiration and biopsy with cell surface marker analysis is indicated to confirm the B-cell phenotype and the pattern of infiltration. In certain cases, computed tomographic scanning of the chest and abdomen may be indicated to assess intracavity lymphadenopathy and organomegaly that are not clinically detectable.

Response criteria

The National Cancer Institute (NCI) (Cheson et al 1988) and the International Workshop on Chronic Lymphocytic Leukemia (IWCLL) (1989) proposed uniform guidelines for response criteria (Table 1). A subset of patients with complete response (CR) may have residual lymphoid nodules, which are sometimes seen in normal marrow. Disappearance of the malignant clone by immunophenotypic parameters and gene rearrangement studies are not requirements for CR. Therefore, patients achieving CR may be heterogeneous, and include hematologic and clonal CRs. Furthermore, the impact of achieving a clonal CR on the natural history of this disease is not clear. Robertson et al (1992) evaluated patients who achieved CR with fludarabine and prednisone therapy, based on whether CD5-positive B cells were present in remission. For complete responders having no residual disease, the 2-year progression-free survival rate was 84% compared to 39% in patients having residual disease detected by two-color flow cytometry ($p < 0.001$).

When should treatment be initiated?

The heterogeneity of outcome in CLL has generated a variety of opinions as to when treatment should be initiated in patients with chronic lymphocytic leukemia. Treatments which were available in the past had a low probability of achieving a complete remission and there were no data to suggest that treatment changed the natural history of the disease. Thus, clinicians used clinical judgment as to when to initiate treatment. When the staging systems identified that anemia and/or thrombocytopenia were associated with a poor prognosis, clinicians decided to initiate treatment when these complications

Table 1 Response criteria in chronic lymphocytic leukemia (CLL) CLL

A. NCI criteria for response in CLL (Cheson et al 1988)

Site	Complete response	Partial response
Physical exam		
Nodes	None	≥50% decrease
Liver/spleen	Not palpable	≥50% decrease
Symptoms	None	not applicable
Peripheral blood		
Neutrophils	≥1500/µl	≥1500/µl or >50% improvement from baseline
Platelets	>100 000/µl	>100 000/µl or >50% improvement from baseline
Hemoglobin (untransfused)	>11.0 g/dl	>11.0 g/dl or >50% improvement from baseline
Lymphocytes	≤4000/µl	≥50% decrease
Bone marrow	<30% lymphocytes	not applicable

B. International Workshop on Chronic Lymphocytic Leukemia (1989) Response Criteria

Complete remission	Resolution of lymphadenopathy and hepatosplenomegaly
	Resolution of constitutional symptoms
	Normalization of complete blood count
	  Neutrophils > 1500/µl
	  Platelets >100 000/µl
	  Lymphocytes <4000/µl
	Normalization of bone marrow
	  Nodular or focal lymphoid infiltrates are compatible with complete response

Partial remission	Change from stage C to A or B, or from stage B to A
Stable disease	No change in the stage of the disease

developed. In addition, if patients were having symptoms related to the leukemia which were interfering with their quality of life, or if there was evidence of progressive enlargement of liver, spleen, or lymph nodes, massive lymph node enlargement, or massive splenomegaly, treatment was usually commenced on treatment. However, these decisions remained arbitrary.

Definition of 'active' disease

The National Cancer Institute (NCI) sponsored Working Group has developed a series of guidelines for chronic lymphocytic leukemia protocols (Cheson et al 1988). A definition of 'active' disease was developed, which included the presence of weight loss of ≥ 10% of body weight during the previous 6 months, extreme fatigue, fever, unrelated to infection, of > 100.5°F for more than 2 weeks, night sweats, development of anemia, thrombocytopenia, and autoimmune anemia, and/or thrombocytopenia that was not responding to corticosteroid therapy. In addition, massive splenomegaly or lymphadenopathy, progressive lymphocytosis with an increase of > 50% over a 2 month period, or lymphocyte doubling time of less than 6 months were indications to start treatment. Marked hypogammaglobulinemia or development of a monoclonal protein were not considered sufficient causes for initiation of treatment. In addition, there was no evidence that inducing a patient into a remission necessarily improved the gammaglobulin production. The NCI guidelines were set up for entry on clinical trials to try to establish homogeneity of patients entering clinical trials in a variety of environments.

Definition of 'smoldering' disease

Following the report from the French Cooperative Group on Chronic Lymphocytic Leukemia (1990a) that a subgroup of Binet Stage A patients have a survival that is equivalent to an age and sex-matched population, Montserrat et al (1988) developed a term called 'smoldering' chronic lymphocytic leukemia. They classified Binet A into smoldering disease or active disease. The criteria for smoldering disease were similar to the French study with a hemoglobin level of ≥ 12 g/dl, lymphocyte count < 30 000/µl, and a platelet count > 150 000/µl. A non-diffuse pattern in the biopsy with < 80% lymphocytes in the bone marrow aspirate and a prolonged doubling time of > 12 months were also parameters that were found to be associated with a good life expectancy. The disease progression rate in the smoldering leukemia group is approximately 15% at 5 years, and survival rate is no different than in age and sex-matched controls. Montserrat et al (1988) considered that 25–30% of all CLL patients fulfilled the criteria of smoldering CLL at the time of diagnosis. One emerging feature is that an increasing number of patients are being diagnosed as having CLL, coincidentally, as a result of increased complete blood count examinations for evaluation of other conditions. Therefore, in the future, more patients are likely to be diagnosed at the time that they fulfill the criteria of smoldering CLL. It is obvious from the studies that are being conducted that nothing is lost from observing these patients to establish whether they develop symptoms related to their disease, show progressive disease in blood marrow or other organs, or evidence of marrow compromise.

Immediate versus delayed treatment

A trial initiated by the French Cooperative Group on CLL (1990a) was one of the few clinical trials to address the issue of timing of treatment. In 1980, a randomized clinical trial was initiated in which 612 good prognosis patients (Binet stage A) received either no treatment ($n=309$) initially or (for an indefinite period) treatment with chlorambucil at a daily dose of 0.1 mg/kg ($n=303$). The 'no treatment' group of patients had treatment delayed until clinical progression. Patients who progressed from stage A to stage B then received chlorambucil, and patients who evolved to stage C were treated with a COP (cyclophosphamide, vincristine, and prednisone) regimen. In the chlorambucil-treated patients, those who evolved to stage B or directly to stage C received COP. Patients who had progressed to stage B and then developed stage C in the chlorambucil treatment group were given a CHOP (COP plus doxorubicin) regimen.

Overall survival of the patients was the major endpoint in this clinical trial. Survival was slightly superior in the 309 patients randomized to 'no treatment', with 50 patients dying compared to 62 patients on the immediate-treatment group. The survival was not significantly different even after adjusting for a variety of prognostic factors. Five-year survival rates were compared for the two groups and were 82% for the untreated group and 75% for the immediate chlorambucil group. Immediate chlorambucil treatment demonstrated the ability to delay progression to stage B or stage C. After 9 months of follow-up treatment the immediate chlorambucil group had a 40% clinical and hematologic remission rate with disappearance of adenopathy, splenomegaly, or hepatomegaly, and a lymphocyte count $< 4000/\mu l$ with a hemoglobin level of > 12 g/dl and a platelet count of $> 150\,000/\mu l$. In addition, another 28% of patients achieved a partial remission. The 5-year survival rate was 89% for patients who achieved clinical remission, 76% for those who achieved a partial remission, 82% for patients with stable disease, and 55% for patients with progressive disease. Survival after disease progression to stage B or stage C was significantly worse for patients with immediate chlorambucil versus those with no initial treatment.

An additional contribution of that study was to demonstrate that stage A patients with a hemoglobin level of > 12 g/dl, and a lymphocyte count $< 30\,000/\mu l$ had a survival rate that was not significantly different from that of an age and sex-matched French population. The recommendation from that study was that no treatment should be given to Binet stage A patients until disease progression was observed. One of the issues of concern in the study was that chlorambucil, a known mutagenic agent, may have increased the rate of development of the epithelial cancers. In the 'no treatment' group only 3 of the 50 deaths were associated with the development of an epithelial cancer, whereas 13 of 62 deaths in the chlorambucil treatment arm were associated with an epithelial cancer.

A similar outcome was reported from a summary of the Medical Research Council CLL trials in the UK (Catovsky et al 1991). In those studies, the effect of early treatment versus delayed therapy in stage A patients was investigated and showed no advantage for the earlier treatment. Six hundred patients with stage A CLL were randomized. No difference in the incidence of second cancers was noted between the two groups. The conclusion from these studies is that there appears to be a subset of patients that do not have progressive disease and should not receive treatment. However, a number of patients do develop progressive disease and the exact timing of intervention is, so far, not established. The recommendation for patients with Binet A and B disease and Rai 0–II disease is to delay treatment unless the patient has massive lymphadenopathy or hepatosplenomegaly, or has symptoms of weight loss and fever related to the leukemia and not associated with infection. Most investigators would initiate treatment immediately for patients who present with Rai stage III and IV disease.

TREATMENT OF CLL

Conventional treatment

The most commonly used chemotherapeutic regimen in CLL is the combination of chlorambucil and prednisone. The evidence supporting the use of the combination instead of either drug alone is based on two small, randomized studies in which no significant difference in survival was evident for the different treatment groups (Sawitsky et al 1977, Han et al 1973). Responses with this combination ranged from 38–87%. This wide variation in response is a result of several factors, including differences in response criteria and in drug dose schedules. The issue of dose intensity for chlorambucil is evident in the trial conducted by Jaksic & Brugiatelli (1988). In their study, 181 patients with CLL were randomized to treatment with continuous daily chlorambucil (15 mg daily to CR or toxicity) or with weekly doses of chlorambucil (75 mg weekly for 6 weeks) plus prednisone. The total dose of chlorambucil was six times higher with the daily chlorambucil regimen, which resulted in a CR rate of 70% compared to 31% with the weekly schedule. Survival of patients randomized to the high-dose regimen was also significantly superior.

Various other drug combinations have been investigated. COP (cyclophosphamide, vincristine, and prednisone) was associated with a response rate range of 44–82% (French Cooperative Group on CLL 1990b, Raphael et al 1991), with much of the outcome diversity accounted for by different patient characteristics, response criteria, and drug dose schedules. In randomized trials, COP results were no better (Montserrat et al 1985) or inferior to those obtained with chlorambucil and prednisone. The addition of doxorubicin to the COP regimen (CHOP) yielded superior survival results than COP alone, and higher response rates than chlorambucil plus prednisone. A recent update from the French randomized study of CHOP versus chlorambucil plus prednisone for stage B CLL patients failed to show a significant survival difference between the two groups (Chevret et al 1992). When CHOP was compared to high-dose chlorambucil, no significant differences in overall response rates were seen between regimens. Other combination chemotherapy regimens have included M2 (vincristine, BCNU, cyclophosphamide, melphalan and prednisone) (Kempin et al 1982), CMP (cyclophosphamide, melphalan, and prednisone), CAP (cyclophosphamide, doxorubicin, and prednisone) and POACH (cyclophosphamide, doxorubicin, cytosine arabinoside, vincristine, and prednisone) (Keating et al 1988). Although these regimens induce higher CR rates, they are more toxic, and not clearly superior to chlorambucil plus prednisone.

Nucleoside analogs

Nucleoside analogs are a major new group of structurally similar drugs with activity in slow growing lymphoid maligancies (Fig. 1). Fludarabine phosphate has documented activity in CLL, indolent lymphoma, Waldenstrom's macroglobulinemia, and hairy cell leukemia (Kantarjian et al 1990). Cladribine has marked activity in hairy cell leukemia and substantial activity in CLL and indolent lymphoma (Carson et al 1984). Pentostatin has marked activity in hairy cell leukemia, some activity in CLL, and also in indolent lymphoma and mycosis fungoides (O'Dwyer et al 1988). Pentostatin is a potent inhibitor of adenosine deaminase, whereas this is not noted for the other two analogs. The common interaction in areas of purine, DNA, and RNA metabolism suggests that there is some, as yet undefined, common mechanism of action.

Fludarabine phosphate

Fludarabine (2-fluoro-araAMP; FAMP; Fludara®) was first evaluated in a Southwestern Oncology Group phase II CLL protocol by Grever et al (1988). The characteristics of the patient population were as expected in the phase II trial with a median age of 63 years, and a median performance status of one.

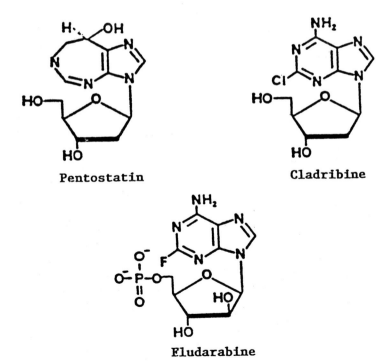

Fig. 1. Structure of nucleoside analogs useful in chronic lymphocytic leukemia.

Three patients were Rai stage 0, five stage I, six stage II, four stage III, and four stage IV. Myelosuppression was noted to be the most frequent toxicity indicator with 13 patients having a decline in platelets and some declining in granulocytes. All patients had received prior therapy. One patient achieved a complete remission, three an excellent partial remission, and 15 patients had additional evidence of improvement. A study of fludarabine in 68 patients with previously treated CLL was reported from the University of Texas MD Anderson Cancer Center (Keating et al 1989). Ten patients achieved a complete remission and 30 (44%) a partial response. Response rates for Rai stages 0–II, III, and IV were 64%, 58%, and 50% respectively. Using the NCI criteria for complete remission, which allows the persistence of residual nodules in the bone marrow, the CR rate was 29%. Twenty-eight percent of patients fulfilled the NCI criteria for a partial response. The conclusion from this study was that the cytoreductive potency of fludarabine was substantial. Ten patients died during the study, seven during the first three courses of treatment. Survival was correlated with response to treatment; those with a complete remission had a superior survival rate to the partial remission patients. Median survival of the patients on the study was 16 months. In addition to stage, other factors associated with high response rates were a low white blood cell count, a decreased number of lymph nodes, normal hemoglobin and platelet levels, and normal serum albumin and alkaline phosphatase levels. Factors significantly associated with survival were the serum albumin level, serum alkaline phosphatase level and the platelet count. While some association of survival with Rai and Binet stage was noted, it was not significant.

Episodes of fever or infection were the major toxic reactions associated with fludarabine. Three hundred and thirty-seven courses of treatment were evaluated for toxic reactions, with 25 episodes of pneumonia noted. In addition, 28 episodes of fever of unknown origin were noted. Septicemia was uncommon being found in only four patients, and 16 patients developed minor documented infections. Myelosuppression was the most common morbidity. Fifty-six percent of courses were associated with a low neutrophil count of $<500/\mu l$ and 25% with a low platelet count of $<50\,000/\mu l$. Myelosuppression was significantly more common in patients with advanced pretreatment Rai and Binet stages. Nausea, vomiting, stomatitis, and diarrhea were noted in <5% of courses. Three patients had some symptoms suggestive of a peripheral neuropathy but these were transient in nature.

Fludarabine was then used at the same dose (30 /mg/m^2 per day for 5 days intravenously every 4 weeks) to treat 33 patients with previously untreated CLL (Keating et al 1991). Patients had advanced Rai stage III or IV disease or progressive Rai stage 0–II disease. The complete remission rate using the NCI Working Group guidelines was 75%. Fourteen out of the 25 CR patients had residual lymphoid nodules in the bone marrow as their only evidence of disease. Six of the 33 patients failed to respond. Three patients, all of whom were older than 75 years and had a pretreatment Rai stage of III–IV, died of infection during the first three cycles of treatment. Two of the patients had

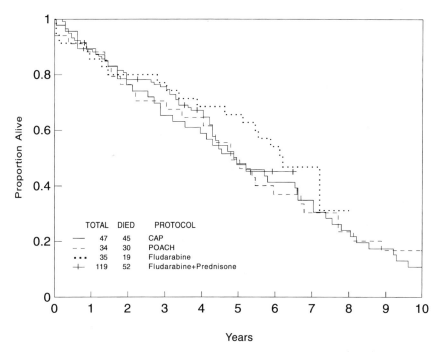

Fig. 2. Survival of previously untreated chronic lymphocytic leukemia patients by treatment regimen.

pneumonia (one Nocardia), and the third patient had disseminated candidiasis. This initial study did not demonstrate any substantial difference in survival with the fludarabine regimen compared to the CAP and POACH regimens (Fig. 2).

A second generation study performed at the M D Anderson Cancer Center studied the addition of prednisone to fludarabine for previously treated patients with CLL. One hundred and sixty nine patients were analyzed (O'Brien et al 1993). Thirty-seven percent of patients obtained a complete remission with two-thirds of patients having persistent lymphoid nodules in the bone marrow. An additional 15% of patients obtained a partial remission, giving a total response rate of 52%. There was no evidence of an improvement in response rate with the addition of prednisone to fludarabine. As with the single agent study, the major toxicity was febrile episodes and documented infection. It is interesting that in the more recent study with prednisone, *Pneumocystis carinii* and Listeria infections were noted whereas they were not seen in the fludarabine single agent study. Patients with Rai stage III and IV disease and those that failed to respond had a higher probability of developing infections with fludarabine. The survival of previously treated patients using fludarabine as a single agent or combined with prednisone as compared with POACH is illustrated in Figure 3.

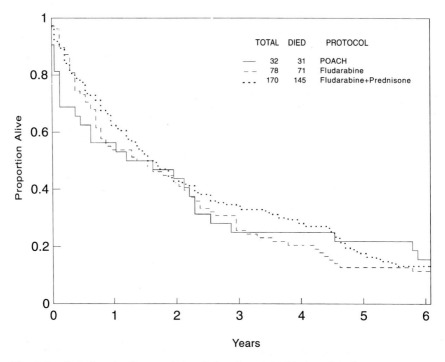

Fig. 3. Survival of previously treated chronic lymphocytic leukemia patients by treatment regimen.

Careful immunophenotypic and molecular studies were conducted by these same investigators to assess the completeness of response to fludarabine (Robertson et al 1992). No residual disease could be detected by two-color flow cytometry or surface light-chain expression in 72% of CRs, 45% of nodular CRs, or 16% of partial remissions. In addition, studies of immunoglobulin gene rearrangements revealed a return to germline configuration in 83% of CRs and 20% of nodular CRs. Of note was a reversal of the CD4:CD8 ratio, which appeared to correlate with the incidence of viral infections, but eventually resolved following postfludarabine therapy.

A different schedule of fludarabine, utilizing a loading dose followed by a continuous infusion, was studied by Puccio et al (1991). Fludarabine was administered as a single bolus injection of 20 mg/m^2 intravenously on day 1 followed by a continuous infusion of 30 mg/m^2 per day for 2 days. This regimen was repeated at 4-week intervals. Forty-two patients were evaluable for response. Twenty-two obtained a partial response, with 12% having stable disease. No complete remissions were noted. Improvement in Rai stage was noted with 6 patients achieving Rai stage 0. As with the other studies, myelosuppression was the main toxicity. Non-hematologic toxicity was mild.

Fludarabine appears to be a major new agent in the management of patients with chronic lymphocytic leukemia. Fludarabine is bioavailable orally and oral formulations of fludarabine are in development.

Cladribine

Cladribine (2-chlorodeoxyadenosine; 2-CDA; Leustatin®) is structurally similar to fludarabine. The initial report from the Scripps clinic of cladribine in CLL demonstrated that 10 (55%) of 18 patients 'responded' to cladribine (Beutler et al 1988). The median number of courses was two and overall 4/18 patients achieved a partial response and 6/18 patients achieved clinical improvement. Almost all of the patients in this study had anemia or thrombocytopenia. Patients were not maintained on study and duration of remission was short (range, 2–15 months). Three of four patients with autoimmune hemolytic anemia had resolution of the hemolytic state. While acute toxicity was mild, the major problem was infection. One patient developed disseminated herpes zoster, two patients had pneumonia of unknown etiology, and this was noted to be associated with aspergillus infection. Twenty-eight percent of patients experienced a reduction in the platelet count during treatment. An association between failure of response and the development of progressive thrombocytopenia was noted in this study.

A follow-up study of 94 patients with refractory CLL treated with cladribine has been reported by the Scripps investigators (Saven et al 1991). The dose given was 0.1 mg/kg per day by continuous infusion for 7 days. Patients were treated at 4-week intervals until maximum response or toxicity intervened. The median number of cycles received was two. All patients had failed prior therapy but whether they were resistant or not was not noted. Eighty-seven patients had stage C disease. Four percent obtained a complete remission, and 44% a partial response. The median duration of response was 4 months. Thrombocytopenia was noted to be dose limiting. Pulmonary infiltrates were developed by 10% of patients, 4% with documented infection. Six patients developed herpes zoster (three dermatomal, and three disseminated). In addition, three patients also developed meningitis. As with fludarabine and pentostatin, clardribine appears to be a drug with marked activity in CLL. Dose limiting marrow toxicity and opportunistic infections appear to be associated with the administration of this agent. Unlike fludarabine, cladribine should probably be given by a central venous line because of the incidence of phlebitis when given by peripheral line.

Pentostatin

Pentostatin (2'-deoxycoformycin; 2'-DCF; Nipent®) is an adenosine deaminase inhibitor. Toxicity was noted when pentostatin had been administered at high doses in the past (Koller & Mitchell 1983). Grever and colleagues treated 25 patients with refractory CLL (Grever et al 1985) with a dose of 4 mg/m^2 of pentostatin every 2 weeks. In this study one CR and four partial remissions were noted in an overall response rate of 20%. Seventeen of the patients had Rai stage IV disease. In addition to the five patients who responded, four had clinical improvement in their disease. No significant difference was noted in the pretreatment activity of adenosine deaminase between responding patients and patients who failed to respond. The patients entered on this study had failed standard alkylating agents and the investigator suggested that pentostatin would not be cross resistant with current agents used to treat CLL. Dillman et al (1989) reported on a phase II trial of pentostatin in CLL conducted by Cancer and Leukemia Group B. The pentostatin dose was 4 mg/m^2 IV weekly for 3 weeks and then every 2 weeks. Of 39 eligible patients who were evaluable 31% were stage B and 33% had no prior treatment. Three percent of patients obtained a complete remission, 23% a partial response, 28% clinical improvement, and 38% had stable disease. Forty-six percent obtained a remission in the 'no prior treatment' group versus 15% for the prior-treated group of patients. The major toxicity noted was infection. Severe, life-threatening, or lethal bacterial infection occurred in 34% of patients. Opportunistic infections developed in 26% including six patients with herpes simplex, three with herpes zoster, two with candidiasis, and one with *Pneumocystis carinii* pneumonia. Mostly all of these complications occurred within 6 weeks of the initiation of pentostatin therapy. Riddell and colleagues (1985) used a similar regimen in 16 patients; seven showed improvement in peripheral blood findings, but no criteria for objective responses were reported in that study. Pentostatin appears to be active in refractory CLL patients. Based on initial reports, the infectious morbidity of pentostatin makes it less suitable than fludarabine.

Biologic response modifiers

Biologic response modifier agents are conceptually attractive given their non-cytotoxic mechanisms of action and because their side effects are different and for the most part milder than those associated with chemotherapy. Of the many biologic response modifier agents available, relatively few, notably interleukin-2 and interferon alfa-2β, have reached clinical trials and their effectiveness in CLL has been largely disappointing. Indeed, interleukin-2 appears to have little activity against CLL (Kay et al 1988). Likewise, overall response rates to interferon alfa-2β were less than 50% in CLL patients with Binet stages A and B, and less than 10% in those with advanced-stage disease, indicating that interferon alfa-2β might prolong chemotherapy-induced responses (Ferrara et al 1992).

Bone marrow transplantation

Experience with allogeneic bone marrow transplantation in CLL patients younger than 50 years of age is slowly accumulating (Michallet et al 1991, Bandini et al 1991). The combined international experience was summarized for 47 CLL patients who received allogeneic transplants between 1984 and

1992 (Michallet et al 1993). Conditioning usually consisted of cyclophosphamide and total body irradiation; the most common graft-versus-host disease (GVHD) prophylaxis consisted of methotrexate and cyclosporin. The median age was 42 years (range, 21–58) and 56% of patients were Rai stage III–IV at the time of bone marrow transplantation. GVHD was a significant problem and the most common cause of death post-bone marrow transplantation; 38% of patients experienced greater than grade I acute GVHD and 47% had chronic GVHD (extensive in 17%). The projected leukemia-free survival rate was 40% ± 18% at 5 years with stage of disease being the most important factor influencing survival.

Rabinowe et al (1993) treated eight patients with CLL with a T-cell depleted allogeneic bone marrow transplant, using cytoxan and total body irradiation for conditioning. Patients were treated at a minor disease stage with chemotherapy, including fludarabine in six patients. Only one patient had severe acute GVHD and eventually died of *Pneumocystis carinii* pneumonia. With a median follow-up of 11.7 months, six patients remain in CR and one patient has bone marrow involvement as the only sign of residual disease.

The results from a study at MD Anderson (Khouri et al 1994) are similar to that of Rabinowe et al (1993). Ten patients were treated with allogeneic and one with syngeneic bone marrow transplantation using T-cell depletion and the same preparative regimen. However, all patients were refractory or relapsing after a median of three regimens, and nine patients were staged Rai III–IV. All patients had received fludarabine. Eight patients achieved CR and one achieved PR. No patient developed greater than grade 1 acute GVHD; one patient developed chronic extensive GVHD. Ten patients are alive with a median follow-up of 10 months.

In contrast to the European study, the incidence of severe GVHD, with consequent early death, is lower in the American studies. All but two patients in the American studies received therapy with fludarabine, a potent immunosuppressive agent, while none of the European patients were treated with this drug. T-cell suppression, seen with fludarabine, may interfere with antigen presentation to the donor cells, resulting in a decrease in the incidence of GVHD. Because of age constraints and donor availability, only a minority of CLL patients can be considered for allogeneic bone marrow transplantation. Its application in CLL is investigational, and patients should be treated in the setting of clinical trials.

Autologous bone marrow transplantation may be an alternative investigational option for this older group of patients. Purged autologous marrow has been used as consolidation remission in low-grade lymphoma, and analogous disease entity. Patients rendered negative for *bcl*-2 rearrangement at the polymerase chain reaction (PCR) level had prolonged disease-free survival (Gribben et al 1991). Rabinowe et al (1993) used monoclonal antibody purged autologous bone marrow to treat 12 patients with CLL, using cyclophosphamide and total body irradiation as the preparative regimen. Like the allogeneic bone marrow transplantation patients, all 12 achieved a minimal disease state with chemotherapy prior to bone marrow transplantation. One patient died with pulmonary hemorrhage; all but one of the other patients remain in CR with a median follow-up of 5 months.

Khouri et al (1994) treated 11 CLL patients with purged autologous bone marrow transplantation. All patients had relapsed after fludarabine therapy and the median number of prior regimens was three. There was one death from cytomegalovirus infection and one death from complications of liver biopsy; 3 patients remain in CR with a median follow-up of 10 months.

Monoclonal antibodies, immunotoxins and radioimmunoconjugates

Monoclonal antibodies directed against cell-surface antigens are potentially useful as therapeutic agents. Target cells can be lysed by triggering complement or by antibody-dependent cell-mediated cytotoxicity, or the antibody molecule can carry radioisotopes or cytotoxic agents to the target cell surface or interior. Until tumor-specific antigens are identified in humans, targeted immunotherapy must be directed against differentiation antigens, particularly those preferentially expressed by maligant cells. Unfortunately, tumor-associated antigens are also expressed to some degree by normal cells, including cells of markedly different lineages. Non-specific antigen expression contributes to non-specific cytotoxicity and has the effect of diluting antibody interaction with the targeted malignant cell population. Nonetheless, several CLL-associated antigens, including CD5, CD19, CD20, CD25, cCLLa, Lym–1, Lym–2, surface IgM, surface IgD, surface idiotype, and the CAMPATH-binding glycoprotein, (Dyer et al 1989, Dillman et al 1984) have been selected for immunotherapy of CLL. Early trials using CD5 as the target antigen established the safety of unconjugated monoclonal anti-CD5, but only modest and transient reductions in circulating CLL were seen and no significant effect on the size of involved lymph nodes was noted (Dyer et al 1989, Dillman et al 1984). A few CLL patients have been treated with the CAMPATH-1 monoclonal antibody, including one refractory patient who achieved a CR. Monoclonal antibodies can also be used as carriers of cytotoxic agents, particularly plant or bacterial toxins, such as ricin, pokeweed antiviral protein, saporin, and pseudomonas exotoxin (Pastan et al 1986) or radioactive isotopes, such as iodine 131 (Kaminsky et al 1993). Most CLL patients have been treated with ricin chain-A-based immunotoxin directed against the CD5 (Frankel 1993), or with blocked ricin conjugated to an anti-CD19 monoclonal antibody (Grossbard et al 1992). In one study, the carrier was ligand (interleukin-2) conjugated to modified (DAB_{486}) diphtheria toxin (LeMaistre et al 1992). To date, conjugated immunoreagents have proved ineffective for treating CLL. Current attempts are directed toward developing more efficacious, second-generation immunotoxins and maximizing their effect.(Jaffrezou et al 1992).

KEY POINTS FOR CLINICAL PRACTICE

- Not all patients with CLL require intervention.

- Most patients will benefit from a period of observation which will help define the activity of the disease, including the lymphocyte doubling time.

- Non-diffuse (nodular or interstitial) infiltration of the bone marrow biopsy plus prolonged (> 12 months) lymphocyte doubling time predicts an indolent course.

- The gold standard of chlorambucil ± prednisone remains unchallenged by any other alkylating agent regimen.

- There are very little data to support that corticosteroids, vincristine or anthracyclines add to response rate or survival.

- Nucleoside analogs such as fludarabine, cladribine, and pentostatin have shown dramatic cytoreductive activity in CLL; fludarabine is obviously the most active single agent studied to date.

- The ability to achieve complete marrow remission with nucleoside analogs has raised the possibility of autologous bone marrow transplantations.

- Preliminary results with cyclophosphamide and total body irradiation are encouraging in a small group of allogeneic transplant patients, and should be considered for select patients.

- Continued progress will hopefully lead to curative approaches for CLL.

REFERENCES

Bandini G, Michallet M, Rossi G et al 1991 Bone marrow transplantation for chronic lymphocytic leukemia. Bone Marrow Transpl 7: 251–253

Beutler E, Piro L D, Saven A et al 1988 2-Chlorodeoxyadenosine (2-CDA): A potent chemotherapeutic and immunosuppressive nucleoside. Leuk Lymphoma 5: 1–8

Binet J L, Auquier A, Dighiero G et al 1981 A new prognostic classification of CLL derived from multivariate survival analysis. Cancer 48: 198–206

Carson D A, Wasson D B, Beutler E 1984 Anti-leukemic and immunosuppressive activity of 2-chloro-2′-deoxyadenosine. Proc Natl Acad Sci USA 81: 2232–2236

Catovsky D, Richards S, Fooks J et al 1991 CLL trials in the United Kingdom–The medical research council CLL trials 1, 2 and 3. Leuk Lymphoma 5 (Suppl): 105–111

Cheson B D (ed.) 1993 Chronic lymphocytic leukemia. Scientific advances and clinical developments. Marcel Dekker, New York

Cheson B D, Bennett J M, Rai K R et al 1988 Guidelines for clinical protocols for chronic lymphocytic leukemia: recommendations of the National Cancer Institute sponsored Working Group. Am J Hematol 29: 152–163

Chevret S, Travade P, Chastang C et al 1992 The CHOP polychemotherapy in stage B-chronic lymphocytic leukemia (CLL): interim results of a controlled clinical trial on 287 patients. Proc Am Soc Clin Oncol 11: 267

Dillman R O, Shawler D L, Dillman J B et al 1984 Therapy of chronic lymphocytic leukemia and cutaneous T-cell lymphoma with T101 monoclonal antibody. J Clin Oncol 2: 881–891

Dillman R O, Mick R, McIntyre O R 1989 Pentostatin in chronic lymphocytic leukemia: A phase II trial of cancer and leukemia group B. J Clin Oncol 7: 433–438

Dyer M J, Hale G, Hayhoe F G et al 1989 Effects of CAMPATH-1 antibodies in vivo in patients with lymphoid malignancies: Influence of antibody isotype. Blood 73: 1431–1439

Faguet G B 1994 Chronic lymphocytic leukemia: An updated review. J Clin Oncol 12: 1974–1990

Ferrara F, Rametta V, Mele G et al 1992 Recombinant interferon-alpha 2A as maintenance treatment for patients with advanced stage chronic lymphocytic leukemia responding to chemotherapy. Am J Hematol 41: 45–49

Frankel A E 1993 Immunotoxin therapy of cancer. Oncology 7: 69–78

French Cooperative Group on Chronic Lymphocytic Leukemia 1990a Effects of chlorambucil and therapeutic decision in initial forms of chronic lymphocytic leukemia (stage A): Results of a randomized clinical trial on 612 patients. Blood 75: 1414–1421

French Cooperative Group On Chronic Lymphocytic Leukemia 1990b A randomized clinical trial of chlorambucil *vs* COP in stage B chronic lymphocytic leukemia. Blood 75: 1422–1425

Grever M R, Leiby J M, Kraut E H et al 1985 Low-dose deoxycoformycin in lymphoid malignancy. J Clin Oncol 3: 1196–1201

Grever M R, Kopecky K J, Coltman C A et al 1988 Fludarabine monophosphate: A potentially useful agent in chronic lymphocytic leukemia. Nouv Rev Fr Hematol 30: 457–459

Gribben J G, Freedman A S, Neuberg D et al 1991 Immunologic purging of marrow assessed by PCR before autologous bone marrow transplantation for B-cell lymphoma. N Engl J Med 325: 1525–1533

Grossbard M I, Freedman S A, Ritz J et al 1992 Serotherapy of B-CLL neoplasms with anti-B4-blocked ricin: A phase I trial of daily bolus infusion. Blood 79: 576–588

Han T, Ezdinli E Z, Shimaoka K et al 1973 Chlorambucil vs. combined chlorambucil-corticosteroid therapy in chronic lymphocytic leukemia. Cancer 31: 502–8

International Workshop on Chronic Lymphocytic Leukemia 1989 Recommendations for diagnosis, staging, and response criteria. Ann Int Med 110: 236–238

Jaffrezou J P, Levade T, Thurneyssen O et al 1992 In vitro and in vivo enhancement of ricin-A chain immunotoxin activity by novel indolizine calcium channel blockers: Delayed intracellular degradation linked to lipodosis induction. Cancer Res 52: 1352–1359

Jaksic B, Vitale B 1981 Total tumor mass score (TTM): A new parameter in chronic lymphocytic leukaemia. Br J Haematol 49: 405–413

Jaksic B, Brugiatelli M 1988 High dose continuous chlorambucil *vs* intermittent chlorambucil plus prednisone for treatment of B-CLL. IGCI CLL-01 trial. Nouv Rev Fr Hematol 30: 437–442

Juliusson G, Liliemark J 1993 High complete remission rate from 2-chloro-2'-deoxyadenosine in previously treated patients with B-cell chronic lymphocytic leukemia: Response predicted by rapid decrease of blood lymphocytic count. J Clin Oncol 11: 679–689

Kaminsky M S, Zasadny K R, Francis I R et al 1993 Radioimmunotherapy of B-cell lymphoma with ^{131}I-anti-B1 (antiCD20) antibody. N Engl J Med 329: 459–465

Kantarjian H M, Redman J R, Keating M J 1990 Fludarabine phosphate therapy in other lymphoid malignancies. Semin Oncol 17 (Suppl. 8): 66–70

Kay N E, Oken M M, Mazza J J et al 1988 Evidence for tumor reduction in refractory or relapsed B-CLL patients treated with infusional interleukin-2. Nouv Rev Fr Hematol 30: 475–478

Keating M J, Scouros M, Murphy S et al 1988 Multiple agent chemotherapy (POACH) in previously treated and untreated patients with chronic lymphocytic leukemia. Leukemia 2: 157–164

Keating M J, Kantarjian H, Talpaz M et al 1989 Fludarabine: A new agent with major activity against chronic lymphocytic leukemia. Blood 74: 19–25

Keating M J, Kantarjian H, O'Brien S et al 1991 Fludarabine: A new agent with marked cytoreductive activity in untreated chronic lymphocytic leukemia. J Clin Oncol 9: 44–49

Keating M J, O'Brien S, Kantarjian H et al 1993 Nucleoside analogs in the treatment of chronic lymphocytic leukemia. Leuk Lymphoma 10: 139–145

Kempin S, Lee B J, Thaler H T et al 1982 Combination chemotherapy of advanced chronic lymphocytic leukemia: the M-2 protocol (vincristine, BCNU, cyclophosphamide, melphalan, and prednisone). Blood 60: 1110–1121

Khouri I F, Keating M J, Vriesendorp H M et al 1994 Autologous and allogeneic bone marrow transplantation for chronic lymphocytic leukemia: preliminary results. J Clin Oncol 12: 748–758

Koller C A, Mitchell B S 1983 Alterations in erythrocyte adenine nucleotide pools resulting from 2'-deoxycoformycin therapy. Cancer Res 43: 1409–1414

LeMaistre C F, Meneghetti C, Rosenblum M et al 1992 Phase I trial of an interleukin-2 (IL-2) fusion toxin (DAB_{486}IL-2) in hematologic malignancies expressing the IL-2 receptor. Blood 79: 2547–2554

Michallet M, Corront B, Hollard D et al 1991 Allogeneic bone marrow transplantation in chronic lymphocytic leukemia: 17 cases. Report from the EB-MTG. Bone Marrow Transplant 7: 275–279

Michallet M, Archimbaud E, Bandini G et al 1993 HLA-identical sibling bone marrow transplants for chronic lymphocytic leukemia (CLL) – A collaborative study of the European Bone Marrow Transplantation Group (EBMTG) and International Bone Marrow Transplantation Registry (IBMTR). Blood 82 (Suppl. 1): 345a

Minot G P, Isaacs R 1924 Lymphatic leukemia. Age, incidence, duration and benefit derived from irradiation. Boston Med J 191: 1–9

Montserrat E, Alcala A, Parody R et al 1985 Treatment of chronic lymphocytic leukemia in advanced stages: A randomized trial comparing chlorambucil plus prednisone versus cyclophosphamide, vincristine, and prednisone. Cancer 56: 2369–2375

Montserrat E, Vinolas N, Reverter J C et al 1988 Natural history of chronic lymphocytic leukemia: On the progression and prognosis of early clinical stages. Nouv Rev Fr Haematol 30: 359–361

O'Brien S, Kantarjian H, Beran M et al 1993 Results of fludarabine and prednisone therapy in 264 patients with chronic lymphocytic leukemia with multivariate analysis-derived prognostic model for response to treatment. Blood 82: 1695–1700

O'Brien S, del Giglio A, Keating M 1995 Advances in the biology and treatment of B-cell chronic lymphocytic leukemia. Blood 85: 307–318

O'Dwyer P J, Wagner B, Leyland-Jones B et al 1988 2'-Deoxycoformycin (Pentostatin) for lymphoid malignancies. Ann Intern Med 108: 733–743

Pastan I, Willingham M C, Fitzgerald D J 1986 Immunotoxins. Cell 47: 641–648

Puccio C A, Mittelman A, Lichtman S M et al 1991 A loading dose continuous infusion schedule of fludarabine phosphate in chronic lymphocytic leukemia. J Clin Oncol 9: 1562–1569

Rabinowe S N, Soiffer R J, Gribben J G et al 1993 Autologous and allogeneic bone marrow transplant for poor prognosis patients with B-cell chronic lymphocytic leukemia. Blood 82: 1366–1376

Rai K R, Han T 1990 Prognostic factors and clinical staging in chronic lymphocytic leukemia. Hematol Oncol Clin North Am 4: 447–456

Rai K R, Sawitsky A, Cronkite E P et al 1975 Clinical staging of chronic lymphocytic leukemia. Blood 46: 219–234

Raphael B, Andersen J W, Silber R et al 1991 Comparison of chlorambucil and prednisone versus cyclophosphamide, vincristine, and prednisone as initial treatment for chronic lymphocytic leukemia: long-term follow-up of an Eastern Cooperative Oncology Group randomized clinical trial. J Clin Oncol 9: 770–776

Riddell S, Johnston J B, Bowman D et al 1985 2'-Deoxycoformycin (DCF) in chronic lymphatic leukemia (CLL) and Waldenstrom's macroglobulinemia (WM). Proc Am Soc Clin Oncol 4: 167

Robertson L E, Huh Y O, Butler J J et al 1992 Response assessment in chronic lymphocytic leukemia after fludarabine plus prednisone: clinical, pathologic, immunophenotypic, and molecular analysis. Blood 80: 29–36

Saven A, Carrera C J, Carson D A et al 1991 2-Chlorodeoxyadenosine treatment of refractory chronic lymphocytic leukemia. Leuk Lymphoma 5: 133–138

Sawitsky A, Rai K R, Glidewell O et al 1977 Comparison of daily versus intermittent chlorambucil and prednisone therapy in the treatment of patients with chronic lymphocytic leukemia. Blood 50: 1049–1059

5

Gaucher disease

A. Zimran   E. Beutler

During the late 19th century the French medical student Phillipe C E Gaucher was stimulated by an unusual clinical presentation in one of his patients to write a descriptive case report as his thesis for the degree of medicine (Gaucher 1882). He regarded the large splenic cells that today bear his name as a manifestation of a primary neoplasm of the spleen. In 1906 Marchand proposed that the disease was caused by storage of material in the reticuloendothelial cells, and in 1924 Epstein demonstrated an alcohol-soluble substance in the spleens of Gaucher patients that was shown by Lieb to be a cerebroside and then, by Aghion, to be a glucosyl ceramide. In 1965, Brady et al in the USA and Patrick in Britain, using different methodologies, both demonstrated that Gaucher disease is a result of a deficiency in the enzyme glucocerebrosidase. This made possible diagnosis of the disease by enzyme assays carried out on small numbers of peripheral blood leukocytes using a convenient, soluble artificial substrate, and heterozygote detection became possible for the first time (for references see Beutler & Grabowski 1994).

The partial purification of this enzyme from human placental tissue was first achieved by Pentchev et al. In 1985, Sorge et al were able to clone and sequence the glucocerebrosidase cDNA, and the cDNA was cloned independently by Tsjui et al. Enzyme replacement therapy for Gaucher disease was first investigated in the 1970s, and a commercially available preparation was licensed in the US in 1991.

CLINICAL MANIFESTATIONS

In attempting to portray the 'typical' Gaucher patient with type I disease, one is confronted with the truism that nothing is more common than the lack of commonalty. Descriptive statistics are bound to overestimate the severity of a disease such as Gaucher disease where many of the patients have subclinicial disease; it is only those Gaucher patients who are symptomatic or have a positive family history who come to attention.

Table 1. Age of symptom onset in surveys of type I Gaucher disease, expressed as percentages

	Matoth & Fried (1965)	Chang-Lo et al (1967)	Kolodny et al (1993)	Zimran et al (1992a)	Zevin et al (1993)*	Sibille et al (1993)**	Beutler (1994) unpublished	Beutler (1994) unpublished**
No. cases	32	12	48	53	34	59	231	79
<10 years	69	25	31	51	91	12	98	11
>50 years	2	50	15	14	NA	NA	18	14

*all children
**all genotype 1226G/1226G

Age of onset of symptoms

Type I Gaucher disease

The age of symptom onset has considerable prognostic value in that the earlier the onset of symptoms the less mild the predicted disease course. Today, as clinicians more accurately diagnose Gaucher disease in its incipient stages, the age of onset of symptoms is more closely concomitant with the age of diagnosis.

Although the term 'adult' Gaucher disease has persisted as a synonym for type I disease, this form has been long recognized even in infants (Bernstein & Sheldon 1959). In fact, in most series of symptomatic patients the age of onset in childhood or adolescence occurs in approximately one-third of cases (Table 1). Therefore, in an early report of 34 patients by Matoth and Fried in Israel (1965), two-thirds of the patients presented before the age of 18 years; 7 of 17 cases (41%), where exact information was available, showed manifestations of the disease before the age of 5 years. In a report from New York, nearly one-third of 48 patients (15 patients) had been diagnosed before the age of 10 years (Kolodny et al 1982). In a larger series from California (Zimran et al 1992a), the mean age at diagnosis was 21 years; however, 26 of the 53 type I patients (51%) presented before the age of 12 years. Of the last 111 patients seen personally by one of the authors (E Beutler) the median age of diagnosis or first symptoms was 17.

However, the oldest patient reported in the literature, at 86 years of age (Brinn & Glabman 1962), had no history of Gaucher-related symptoms. Similarly, surveys of family members of Gaucher patients for unrelated diseases have revealed other elderly asymptomatic patients (Beutler 1977a).

The age of onset differs strikingly in patients with different genotypes: patients diagnosed late in life almost always have the 1226G/1226G genotype, while onset in early childhood is characteristic of those with the 1226G/84GG and 1226G/IVS2(+1) genotypes. In a series of 100 Ashkenazi Jewish patients we found that the median (mean) age of symptom onset of the four most common genotypes were as follows: 1226G/1226G, 26 (28.9); 1226G/84GG, 5 (12.8); 1226G/1448C, 15 (16.5); and 1226G/IVS2(+1) 4 (9.4). One-quarter of patients with the 1226G/1226G genotype became symptomatic or were diagnosed after the age of 45 (Beutler 1992). Our most recent analysis of 78 patients with the 1226G/1226G genotype showed a median age of onset of 27 years of age; of 31 patients with the 1226G/84GG genotype a median onset age of 6 years; of 27 patients with the 1226G/1448C genotype a median onset age of 10 years and of 8 patients with the 1226G/IVS2(+1) genotype, a median onset age of 4 years. These results have been confirmed in a large series of patients from New York and Cincinnati (Sibille et al 1993).

Type II Gaucher disease

The age distribution in type II disease is *per force* restricted. Most children succumb to rapidly progressive neurologic disease before the second year of life. Neurologic complications are invariably evident by 6 months of age (Brady et al 1993). It has been suggested that there is a late onset form of type II disease wherein most developmental markers are normal during the first year or into the second year (Kolodny et al 1982), and only then does the neurological component become evident. Sidransky et al (1992a) have documented a subset of type II patients in whom death occurs prenatally, or at the latest by age 4.5 months.

Type III Gaucher disease

Type III disease has been studied most intensively in the Norbottnian population in northern Sweden, where there is a high prevalence of the 1448C mutation. Here, despite the genetic homogeneity of the disease, there is considerable variation in age of onset (Svennerholm et al 1982). Onset of symptoms varied between 1 month and 3 years of age (with a median of 1 year), and one patient who was diagnosed at 14.2 years of age. Subclassification of this form of the disease into type IIIa and type IIIIb has been proposed (Patterson et al 1993). Of 18 children who were classified as type IIIa, the mean age of onset of the slowly progressive neurologic component comparable to that seen in type II disease was 7.4 years of age. Thirteen children who were classified type IIIb, i.e. had isolated horizontal supranuclear gaze palsy but no other neurologic sign, had a mean age of onset of 4 years. Of 16 type III patients studied by Sidransky et al (1992b), the mean age at diagnosis was 1.9 years.

Spleen

The earliest sign of Gaucher disease is generally splenomegaly, which may not be visible or palpable, but will nonetheless be demonstrable by ultrasound (Hill et al 1986). The rate of splenic enlargement is apparently correlated with the rate of disease progression and when an abrupt change in that rate is noted in adulthood (after the initial, expected growth of childhood), a second process, possibly an infection or hematological malignancy, should be suspected. Splenomegaly often leads to functional hyperactivity, i.e. hypersplenism. In a series of 53 patients (Zimran et al 1992a), the most common presenting symptoms were bleeding manifestations including epistaxis, bruising and prolonged bleeding after superficial trauma; splenomegaly was seen in 24 of the 29 non-splenectomized patients.

The second consequence of splenomegaly is mechanical obstruction and/or displacement of the neighbouring tissues and organs owing to the often massive enlargement. This can result in overt discomfort or pain. In a report of the abdominal findings of 44 type I Gaucher patients, all of whom had splenomegaly on examination, using MRI, the average splenic enlargement was 2200% (range: 103–6293%) (Hill et al 1992). Of these patients, 14 had nodules and 15 patients had infarcts seen as subcapsular, wedge-shaped areas, more common in larger spleens and often accompanied by pain. Owing to attempts to minimize imaging exposure time, the finding of approximately 30% occurrence of nodules and infarcts is probably an underestimate. Indeed, we found in ultrasound evaluation of 85 Gaucher patients with splenomegaly that 25 patients (29.4%) had focal lesions, consisted of hypo-echogenic (11 of these 25), hyper-echogenic (9) or of mixed echogeneity (5). Enlarged accessory spleens were also noted among 17 (20%) of these 85 patients, some of which reached a few cm in size. These accessory spleens tend to be larger in splenectomized patients, who also present with enlarged periportal and retroperitoneal lymph nodes.

In one study (Sibille et al 1993), the average splenic enlargement in 33 patients homozygous for the 1226G mutation was 8.6-fold normal, versus 33.7-fold normal in 9 patients with the 1226G/84GG genotype. Therefore it appears that patients with the more severe genotypes have a greater degree of splenomegaly.

A third consequence of splenomegaly is growth retardation in children (see the section on Growth and Height, below)

Liver

In most symptomatic Gaucher patients there is some degree of liver involvement (Lee 1982). In patients with massively enlarged spleens, hepatomegaly is often greater than in patients with lesser degrees of splenomegaly; in patients in whom a splenectomy had been performed, the hepatomegaly tends to be greater than in those patients who have intact spleens. In one study (Hill et al 1992), the liver was enlarged in all 46 patients (44 with type I disease and 2 patients with type III disease). The average increase in volume was 85% (range 16–236%). These results confirm the findings by others of liver enlargement in 67% of 48 patients (Kolodny et al 1982), 77% of 53 patients (Zimran et al 1992a), 96% of 25 patients (James et al 1982), 100% of 161 patients (Sibille et al 1993), and 100% of 34 children (Zevin et al 1993). Nine of the 46 patients in one MRI based study (Hill et al 1992) had focal abnormalities; three of these underwent liver biopsies that revealed portal and sinusoidal infiltration by Gaucher cells and some degree of fibrosis. Several types of abnormalities were documented: inflammation and fibrosis, and/or ischemia. The accumulation of lipid in the cells of the reticuloendothelial system may also interfere with their inherent functions. The severity of liver involvement appears to be a marker of severe complications in other organs (James et al 1982). Although liver failure is rare (James et al 1981), cirrhosis that may be defined as regenerating nodules infiltrated by Gaucher cells has been described (James et al 1982) in 12% of 25 cases. Portal hypertension is also relatively uncommon (James et al 1982, Kolodny et al 1982). Bleeding from esophogeal varices has been reported (Fellows et al 1975, James et al 1982). Hepatocytes do not appear to be affected in that they are not a depot for lipid storage.

Generally, liver function tests are normal or slightly abnormal. SGOT and

SGPT were elevated in 64% and 32% of patients, respectively, in one series (James et al 1982); 18 of 53 patients (34%) had elevated SGOT values in another (Zimran et al 1992a).

Bone

Perhaps the most variable of all the symptoms attributed to Gaucher disease is that of bone involvement, particularly the pain that it engenders. This comment applies to both type I and type III disease. Beighton et al (1982) found significant orthopedic problems in 83% (29 of 35) of patients over the age of 16 years. This is a higher percentage than found in most other surveys: 21% of patients (10 of 48) (Kolodny et al 1982); 44% of patients (15 of 34) (Matoth & Fried 1965); 81% of patients (43 of 53) (Zimran et al 1992a); and 100% in the Norbottnian type III population (Svennerholm et al 1982). In a study of children, 80% of patients (30 of 34) were found to have some bone involvement (Zevin et al 1993). Beighton et al (1982) categorized eight types of orthopedic complications:

1. Non-specific bone pain, that may be episodic and last for a few days but which will resolve without major medical intervention;

2. Pseudo-osteomyelitis, which is accompanied by pain, tenderness, redness, swelling, warmth and has a variable duration of days to weeks with consequent fever, elevated erythrocyte sedimentation rate and leucocytosis;

3. Pyogenic osteomyelitis;

4. Chronic pain associated with stiffness of the large joints and relieved by rest and analgesics;

5. Aseptic necrosis of the head of femur;

6. Pathological fractures;

7. Spinal malalignment; and

8. Growth and stature reduction owing to spinal deformity.

Involvement of the hip is the most common (Amstutz 1973), although the shoulder, knee and vertebral joints are also known to be affected (Beighton et al 1982). The mechanism by which these pathological changes occur are as yet unexplained (Mankin et al 1990). The most prevalent, and probably pathognomonic abnormality (Beighton et al 1982) is failure of bone remodeling that is seen in approximately 80% of adults and, hence, is often used as a screening tool (Kolodny et al 1982). Bones have a wide metaphyseal-diaphyseal region that has become known as the 'Erlenmeyer flask' deformity; it is generally bilateral and rather symmetrical. Bone density, as seen on X-ray or CT scan is often reduced either in a non-homogeneous, diffuse pattern or a localized one (Kolodny et al 1982). It has been suggested that diffuse bone loss may correlate with more severe manifestations in other organ systems and/or with age per se (Beighton et al 1982, Stowens et al 1985). The epiphyses are generally spared. Clinical symptoms of active bouts of bone pain are correlated with altered marrow signal patterns on MRI (Hermann et al 1993). These areas of increased intensity on T2-weighted images correspond to increased water, i.e. edema, associated with acute infarcts, or with hemorrhage-associated marrow displacement (Horev et al 1991). Compression and collapse of vertebral bodies are not uncommon and spinal cord/nerve involvement have been reported (Markin & Skultety 1984). The extent of the bone pathology that can be directly attributed to Gaucher cell accumulation is uncertain. However, it is generally conceded that the intraosseous pressure caused by the burden of the lipid-laden cells is a major factor in achieving cortical erosion.

Another poorly understood aspect of bone involvement is that of bone crises. The pain during a crisis may develop suddenly or insidiously, and the consequence after the crisis passes may be unremarkable or may result in alterations in bone integrity. Although most truly septic cases of osteomyelitis are probably secondary to intervention (Stowens et al 1985), these crises often mimic periostosis or aseptic osteomyelitis; infarction of bone is the probable underlying pathology. The patient intially complains of intense, localized pain that is often accompanied during the acute phase by fever, leucocytosis and the classic signs of inflammation, hence the description, pseudo-osteomyelitis (see classification by Beighton et al 1982). A crisis may subside after 1 to 3 days or may linger for weeks with only gradual abatement of symptoms. Although there is no predictable criterion for occurrence, these crises often appear, in prone patients including young children and adolescents post-splenectomy, on a schedule of up to several times a year.

Lung

There appears to be a paucity of studies on the extent of lung involvement in symptomatic type I Gaucher patients. More than one-third of autopsied Gaucher patients had significant abnormalities in the lung (Lee & Yousem 1988). The pathological findings were grouped into three categories:

1. Interstitial infiltration of Gaucher cells;

2. Capillary plugging resulting in pulmonary hypertension;

3. Alveolar consolidation reminiscent of the pneumonia seen in type II Gaucher disease.

These descriptions are consistent with other reports of diffuse reticulonodular infiltrate or miliary pattern on X-ray in several Gaucher patients with diverse clinical pictures. However, significant lung abnormalities on autopsy, including overt Gaucher cell infiltration, are not always indicative of a clinically significant process in life; and similarly, as indicated by Thiese & Ursell (1990), marked pulmonary hypertension need not necessarily be accompanied by Gaucher cell infiltration.

Of the several large series of type I Gaucher patients only two deal, albeit tangentially, with the manifestations in the lung (Kolodny et al 1982, Zimran et al 1992a). In a study of the effects of enzyme replacement therapy on two type I Gaucher patients with frank pulmonary disease, pulmonary function tests, among others, were evaluated by Beutler et al (1991a): one patient who had a normal transbronchial biopsy had been on continuous nasal oxygen because of severe dyspnea, and a second patient who had developed shortness of breath over a 1-year period showed Gaucher cell infiltration on transbronchial biopsy. In both of these women, steady-state diffusing capacity was reduced (30% and 43% of predicted values, respectively) and FEV1/FVC (forced expiratory volume in 1 second relative to forced vital capacity) was moderately reduced, probably indicative of (small) airway obstruction. Similar results were obtained by Pelini et al (1994).

In a recent study of pulmonary fuction tests in 81 patients over the age of 6 years with type I Gaucher disease (Kerem et al, unpublished) nearly half showed abnormal Kco, a measure of diffusion capacity, and approximately one-fifth had various abnormal pulmonary function tests that were indicative of small airway obstruction. Interestingly, less than 10% of these patients had clinical signs and symptoms of lung involvement.

Pulmonary involvement has been noted in type II and type III Gaucher disease in conjuction with hepatic decompensation; and pneumonia (often aspiration) and/or apnea are ultimately the most common causes of death in the neuronopathic forms (Beutler & Grabowski 1994). Anecdotal reports of lung failure in children with type II and type III Gaucher disease (Bernard et al 1961) are described almost exclusively in patients with severe hepatic disease. In cases of liver transplantation in a Gaucher patient, pulmonary oxygen supply was immediately improved (Carlson et al 1990, DuCerf et al 1992, Smanik et al 1993).

Kidney

Kidney involvement is uncommon in Gaucher disease although Gaucher cells have been found in glomeruli, cortex, medulla, and interstitum (Ross 1969, Smith et al 1978, Groen & Garrer 1948) without significant renal complications. In a series of 48 patients one patient presented with nephrotic syndrome and one with glomerulonephritis (Kolodny et al 1982).

Heart

Anecdotal reports of cardiac involvement include constrictive pericarditis (Groen & Garrer 1948), rheumatic aortic valve disease (Tamari et al 1983), infiltration of myocardial interstitium by Gaucher cells (Smith et al 1978, Edwards et al 1983), as well as a familial occurrence of non-rheumatic heart disease in a presentation of a new syndrome of Gaucher disease with several unusual features (Uyama et al 1992). There have also been two case reports of type III patients, one of whom died with fibrosis of the aorta and coronary artery (Wilson et al 1985), and the other who died of aortic and mitral valve involvement (Tsutsumi 1982).

Recently, a new range of symptoms seen in Gaucher disease, each with a cardiac component and a neurological manifestation, has been presented (Chabas et al 1993). Three siblings with enzymatically proven Gaucher disease died of calcified aortic and mitral valves and ascending aorta; two of these patients had hyporeflexia, saccadic eye movements and ophthalmoplegia. The index patient did not carry either the 1448C or 1504T mutations. Twelve Arab patients have been reported with enzymatically proven Gaucher disease, all under the age of 20 years, and all with overt horizontal supranuclear gaze palsy and, except for the very youngest children, echocardiographic evidence of heart valve sclerosis. Molecular diagnosis revealed that all 12 patients were homozygous for the 1342C mutation (Zimran et al 1993a).

Skin

The unusual finding of ichthyoses in the subset of very early onset type II patients (Sidransky et al 1992a) is as yet unexplained but may be a result of enzyme deficiency, since the mouse model of glucocerebrosidase deficiency shows comparable symptoms. The pterygium and pingueculae in the conjuctiva of the eyes of many Gaucher patients may not be attributable to this disease (Kolodny et al 1982).

Growth and height

Matoth & Fried (1965) concluded that stunted growth is not apparent in their adult patients, whereas in their pediatric population deviation from the normal growth patterns began with the advent of the disease process, and the magnitude of deviation was correlated with the severity of the disease. In this study, of 14 children under the age of 16 years, 3 (21%) showed growth retardation. In the survey by Kolodny et al (1982), of 13 children under the age of 16 years, 5 (39%) are described as being of 'very short stature'. Of the 9 children under the age of 16 years in the series by Zimran et al (1992a), only one (11%) was noted to be growth retarded. In the series of 34 children studied by Zevin et al (1993), 10 children (29%) were evaluated as showing growth retardation, i.e. below the 10th percentile for age, and that in children with the more severe genotypes 1448C/1448C (L444P/L444P) and 1226G/84GG (N370S/84GG) the deviation was more pronounced. In this study, height discrepancies were more common than weight retardation; in two adolescents sexual maturation was delayed. This latter finding of delayed sexual maturation or sexual infantilism was also noted by others (Matoth & Fried 1965). In the Norbottnian variant, body growth was retarded and height retardation was between one and five standard deviations below the normal for age value (Svennerholm et al 1982).

Central nervous system

By definition, type I Gaucher disease does not have a neurological component. Nonetheless, in routine autopsies of type I patients, Gaucher cell infiltration has been noted (Soffer et al 1980) in several areas in the brain, without evidence of central nervous system (CNS) involvement during life. Conversely, CNS complications in type I patients, such as seizures and intellectual deterioration may not be related to the primary processes of Gaucher disease. A Parkinson-like syndrome, which developed between the fourth and fifth decades of life, has been noted in patients with enzymatically proven Gaucher disease and no other neurological manifestation (Turpin et al 1987).

In type II disease signs of cranial nerve nuclei and extrapyramidal tract involvement are common, as is the 'classical triad' of trismus, strabismus and retroflexion of the head (Brady et al 1993). Spasticity, hyperreflexia, positive Babinski as well as seizures (myoclonic and grand mal) are seen in most of these children within the first year of life (Brady et al 1993). Patients with type III disease are reported to manifest horizontal supranuclear gaze palsy, myoclonic epilepsy, dementia and spasticity (Nishimura & Barranger 1980, Svennerholm et al 1982, Winkelman et al 1983, Patterson et al 1993) although onset and progression of these signs are variable. Oculomotor apraxia has been described in both type II and type III Gaucher disease (Tripp et al 1977) and as an unique presentation without other neurological complications (Patterson et al 1993).

Hematological manifestations

Anemia and thrombocytopenia are among the main features of Gaucher disease, and are frequently responsible for the presenting symptoms. These are typically caused by the hypersplenism and by infiltration of the marrow by Gaucher cells. In one study of 53 patients (Zimran et al 1992a) thrombocytopenia was seen in 28 patients (52%), 22 patients had (mostly mild) anemia (42%), and 3 patients (6%) had pancytopenia; splenic status in these patients varied so that anemia appeared more often than thrombocytopenia in splenectomized patients whereas non-splenectomized patients manifested thrombocytopenia more often. In children (Zevin et al 1993), anemia was present in 80% and thrombocytopenia in 60% of patients, with anemia being most severe in the 2–5 year olds. In addition to the well-recognized thrombocytopenia and anemia associated with hypersplenism and/or infiltration of bone marrow with Gaucher cells, other hematological abnormalities may occur in Gaucher disease. Iron deficiency anemia may result from bleeding. The association of Gaucher disease with autoimmune disorders, such as autoimmune hemolytic anemia or with hematologic malignancies, should be considered when confronted with a patient whose condition has been stable and who suddenly presents with severe cytopenia.

Interference with the normal blood clotting mechanisms may be a clinically significant feature in some patients. The partial thromboplastin time and prothrombin time may be prolonged. Factor IX deficiency is probably an artifact and does not lead to bleeding (Boklan & Sawitsky 1976). The frequency of factor XI deficiencies in patients with Gaucher disease is probably a result of the high prevalence of this genetic disorder in the Ashkenazi Jewish population and it segregates independently from Gaucher disease (Seligsohn et al 1976). Nonetheless, it is of clinical importance in terms of excessive bleeding following trauma and in particular during dental procedures and surgery. Very mild Gaucher disease patients have often been discovered following excessive bleeding after tooth extraction or similar mild surgical interventions, when, in fact, factor XI deficiency is the underlying disorder.

Immune system

While there are no compelling data regarding the susceptibility of Gaucher disease patients to infection impaired chemotaxis of neutrophils (Aker et al 1993) as well as in the suppression of superoxide generation, staphylococcal killing and phagocytosis by monocytes (Liel et al 1994) have been documented in many Gaucher patients. The defect in the neutrophils was correctable by low-dose high-frequency enzyme replacement therapy (Zimran et al 1993b), which also reduced the incidence of infections within 1 year.

T-lymphocyte deficiencies in both spleen and blood, as gauged by impaired skin-test response (Burns et al 1977) and decreased natural killer T-cells (Burstein et al 1987) have been reported. In addition, there have been reports of increased immune activity (Shoenfeld et al 1980) in Gaucher disease. Hypergammaglobulinemia, diffuse immunoglobulin elevations and monoclonal gammopathies have all been documented. Apparently there is an increase in the predicted level of immunoglobulins with age (Pratt et al 1968) and there is a change in isotype from IgM to IgG and IgA as the disease progresses (Shoenfeld et al 1982). Numerous individual cases of progression of these immunopathologies to multiple myeloma have been reported. According to one survey (Shiran et al 1993), hematologic cancers are more prevalent in Gaucher patients, with up to a 14.7-fold increase. There have been case histories of other malignancies concomitant with Gaucher disease: Hodgkin's disease, chronic lymphocytic leukemia, chronic granulocytic leukemia and acute leukemias. Solid tumors and carcinomas have also been documented in association with Gaucher disease. (Literature references may be found in recent reviews: Beutler & Grabowski 1994; Beutler 1988a,b.)

Gynecological and obstetric aspects

Several of the most common signs of (type I) Gaucher disease, including thrombocytopenia, anemia, hepatosplenomegaly, tendency to bleed and susceptibility to infections, may pose special problems for women in their reproductive years. The obstetric histories of women with Gaucher disease have suggested that pregnancy is not contraindicated (Goldblatt & Beighton 1985, Young 1985, Mazor et al 1986, Zlotogora et al 1989). Nonetheless, the rate of spontaneous abortions in Gaucher disease patients may be higher than in other women (Teton & Treadwell 1957) as may be the rate of stillbirths and neonatal death (Hsia et al 1962). This apparent finding is probably not because of the mechanical compression caused by organomegaly (Goldblatt & Beighton 1985). However, a recent study (Granovsky-Grisaru et al 1994) of 53 women of childbearing age shows several dysfunctional features in their gynecological/obstetric profiles. Delay of puberty was seen in nearly two-thirds of women, but there was no consequent infertility. Heavy menstrual bleeding was a major problem in most women. Of the 102 pregnancies recorded in these women, 25 (24.5%) terminated in spontaneous abortion in the first trimester. Aggravation of thrombocytopenia and anemia was prominent in most women during pregnancy. The incidence of early postpartum hemorrhage and fevers was also increased, regardless of the type of delivery.

Other associated findings

Although there is no clear correlation between the level of acid phosphatase and the clinical severity of the disease, monitoring of this enzyme has been useful in following the response to enzyme therapy. Acid phosphatase levels were elevated in all or nearly all patients in some series (James et al 1982, Pastores et al 1993) and 63% in another study (Zimran et al 1992a); in children (Zevin et al 1993) this parameter was elevated in 82% of the 28 patients tested.

The activity of angiotensin converting enzyme in the serum of Gaucher patients is very commonly elevated (Lieberman & Beutler 1976) and hence is often used as a marker by clinicians. The mechanism by which this enzyme is related to the abnormal lipid accumulation is unknown. Chititriosidase activity was recently found (Hollak et al 1994) to be elevated in type I Gaucher disease to approximately 600 times the normal level. The usefulness of this method to detect Gaucher disease is impaired by the fact that a deficiency of this enzyme apparently occurs independently; 2 of the 32 Gaucher disease patients (6%) had undetectable levels, a finding that apparently is also seen in the population at large.

Hypocholesterolemia, possibly caused by increased catabolism of both low- and high-density lipoproteins, has been demonstrated (Ginsberg et al 1984) and may also be attributed to macrophage dysfunction resulting from lipid accumulation (Le et al 1988).

Other serum abnormalities include increased macrophage colony-stimulating factor, increased soluble CD 14, increased ferritin, increased transcobalamin II, increased β-hexosaminidase activity and increased lysozyme activity.

THE MOLECULAR BIOLOGY OF GAUCHER DISEASE

The glucocerebrosidase genes and cDNA

The glucocerebrosidase gene is located on chromosome 1 at band q21 (Barneveld et al 1983); its total length is nearly 7 kilobases (Horowitz et al 1989). Downstream from the glucocerebrosidase gene is a highly homologous pseudogene; both the active gene and the pseudogene have been cloned and sequenced (Horowitz et al 1989, Beutler et al 1992a). The availability of the complete sequences of both the active glucocerebrosidase gene and the pseudogene has been crucial to the development of strategies for molecular diagnosis of Gaucher disease. The pseudogene is shorter than the active gene; its length is only 5769 base pairs, yet is nearly 96% homologous to the functional gene (Horowitz et al 1989). The pseudogene is actively transcribed (Sorge et al 1990), but no functional product is formed. There are two ATG initiating codons (Sorge et al 1987, Beutler et al 1988), each of which can be translated into a discrete, functional product.

Mutations

More than 50 mutations in the active glucocerebrosidase gene have been discovered to date (Table 2). Most of these are point mutations; however, other mechanisms are also known to give rise to mutations in the glucocerebrosidase gene including insertions, deletions, splicing, gene conversion and crossing-over between the functional gene and the pseudogene. When an allele cannot produce an active product, i.e. cannot synthesize a functional enzyme, such a mutation in the homozygote state is probably incompatible with life. Mice lacking a glucocerebrosidase gene do not survive longer than a few hours after birth (Tybulewicz et al 1992). The following are among the most common and/or important mutations.

Mutation 1226: A→G (Asn370→Ser). The most frequent mutation in Gaucher disease is a point mutation in exon 9 (Tsuji et al 1988). It is the prototype of what has been designated the mild type of mutation (Beutler 1992, 1994) that is found exclusively in patients with type I disease and accounts for more than 75% of Gaucher alleles in Ashkenazi Jews and 36% of alleles among non-Jews (Beutler 1992). Studies correlating the mutations with the severity of the clinical manifestations have shown an apparent association of the 1226G mutation with mild phenotypic expression of the disorder, as well as rather late age of onset of symptoms (Zimran et al 1989, Sibille et al 1993, Beutler 1991, 1992, 1993a,b, Beutler & Gelbart 1993, Beutler et al 1992b). The clinical course of compound heterozygotes is influenced by the severity of the mutation on the other allele. However, it is generally conceded that the 1226G

Table 2A Point mutations in the glucocerebrosidase gene that cause Gaucher disease

	Amino Acid mature protein	cDNA 1st ATG	Genomic	Exon	Base substitution *PseudoGC	Amino acid substitution	Rapid detection method	Disease type	Class	Other allele	Reference
1	43	245	1749	3	C→T	Thr→Ile	+AccI	I	Unknown		Graves et al (1988)
2	48	259	1763	3	C→T	Arg→Trp	(+StyI)	I	Unknown	1448G	Beutler et al (1993b)
3	120	476	3060	5	G→A	Arg→Gln	+BstNI EcoRII	I	Unknown		Eyal et al (1991)
4	122	481	3065	5	C→T	Pro→Ser	−KpnI	I	Mild		Eyal et al (1991)
5	140	535+	3119	5	G→C	Asp→His	+BspHI+NlaIII+MnlI	I	Unknown	586C	
6	157	586		5	A→C	Lys→Gln	+ScrFI	I,II	Severe	535C, 1093A, and with 1448C in II	
7	176	644	3438	6	C→A	Ala→Asp	−PflMI	I	Unknown	1226G	Beutler et al (1994b)
8	182	661	3455	6	C→A	Pro→Thr	−HphI	I	Unknown	1226G	Beutler et al (1994b)
9	202	721	3515	6	G→A*	Gly→Arg	−NciI	I, II	Severe	12261448	Beutler et al (1994b)
10	212	751	3545	6	T→C	Tyr→His	+DraIII	I	Unknown	1226G	Beutler et al (1993b)
11	213	754	3548	6	T→A*	Phe→Ile	(+NsiI)	I,III	Severe		Kawame & Eto (1991)
12	216	764	4113	7	T→A	Phe→Tyr	+KpnI	I	Mild	XOVR, IVS2	Beutler & Gelbart (1990)
13	257	887	4236	7	G→A	Arg→Gln	−BsmAI	I	Unknown	1226G	Beutler et al (1994b)
14	285	970	4319	7	C→T	Arg→Cys	(+NsiI)	I	Unknown	1226G	Beutler et al (1994b)
15	289	983	4332	7	C→T	Pro→Leu	(−BglI)	I	Mild	754A	He et al (1992)
16	309	1043	5259	8	C→T	Ala→Val	−BanI+MaeIII	I	Mild	1226G	Latham et al (1991)
17	312	1053	5269	8	G→T	Trp→Cys	−KpnI, −BanI-NlaIV	I	Mild	1448C	Latham et al (1991)
18	323	1085	5301	8	C→T	Thr→Ile	+FokI	I	Unknown	1504T	He et al (1992)
19	325	1090	5306	8	G→A*	Gly→Arg	+Bsu36I	II	Severe		Eyal et al (1990)
20	326	1093+	5309	8	G→A	Glu→Lys	−BsmaI, +BbvII+MboII	I	Unknown	586C	Eyal et al (1991)
21	342	1141	5357	8	T→G	Cys→Gly	−StuI	II	Severe		Eyal et al (1990)
22	359	1192	5408	8	C→T	Arg→Stop	−TaqI-Sau3AI	I,II	Severe	1448C	Beutler & Gelbart (1994a)
23	359	1193	5409	8	G→A	Arg→Gln	−TaqI	I	Mild	1448C	Kawame et al (1992)
24	364	1208	5424	8	G→C	Ser→Thr	(+AlwNI)	I	Mild	1448C	Latham et al (1991)
25	370	1226	5841	9	A→G	Asn→Ser	(+XhoI)	I	Mild		Tsuji et al (1988)
26	377	1246	5861	9	G→A	Gly→Ser	+PvuII	I	Mild	1448C	Laubscher et al (1993)
27	378	1249	5864	9	T→G	Trp→Gly	ASOH	I	Unknown	764A	Beutler et al (1994b)
28	380	1255	5870	9	G→A	Asp→Asn	(+XcmI)	I	Unknown	1226G	Beutler et al (1994b)
29	380	1256	5871	9	A→C	Asp→Ala	+ScrFI	I	Unknown		Walley & Harris (1993)

Table 2A (continued)

30	394	1297	5912	9	G→T	Val→Leu	(−BanI)	I, III	Severe		Theophilus et al (1989)
31	399	1312	5927	9	G→A	Asp→Asn	−TaqI	II	Severe	1448C	Beutler & Gelbart (1994a)
32	409	1342	5957	9	G→C*	Asp→His	−StyI	I, III	Severe		Theophilus et al (1989)
33	409	1343	5958	9	A→T	Asp→Val	−AflII+MaeIII	III	Severe	1448C	Theophilus et al (1989)
34	415	1361	5976	9	C→G	Pro→Arg	+HhaI	II	Severe		Wigderson et al (1989)
35	417	1366	5981	9	T→G	Phe→Val	+NcoI	I	Unknown	1226G	Choy et al (1994)
36	418	1370	5985	9	A→G	Tyr→Cys	+BglI	I	Unknown	1226G	Tuteja et al (1994)
37	425	1390	6375	10	A→G	Lys→Glu	(+SacI)	III	Severe		Kawame et al (1992)
38	444	1448	6433	10	T→G	Leu→Arg	+BstEI	II	Severe	1447del	Uchiyama et al (1994)
39	444	1448	6433	10	T→C*	Leu→Pro	+NciI	I, II, III	Severe		Tsuji et al (1987)
40	463	1504	6489	10	C→T	Arg→Cys	+BsrI–MspI	I	Unknown	?	Hong et al (1990)
41	463	1505	6490	10	G→A	Splice	+BsrI	III	Severe	1342C	Ohshima et al (1993)
42	478	1549	6628	11	G→A	Gly→Ser	+AluI	I	Unknown	1226G	Beutler et al (1993b)
43	496	1603	6682	11	C→T	Arg→Cys	−BsaHI	I	Mild	1603T homozy	Kawame et al (1992)
44	496	1604	6683	11	G→A	Arg→His	+HphI	I	Mild		Beutler et al (1993b)

Table 2B Insertions and deletions in the glucocerebrosidase gene that cause Gaucher disease

	Amino Acid mature protein	cDNA 1st ATG	Genomic	Exon	Base substitution *PseudoGC	Amino acid substitution	Rapid detection Method	Disease type	Class	Other allele	Reference
1	NA(-15)	72	1023	2	C→>DEL	Frameshift	+AluI	I	Lethal	?	Beutler et al (1993b)
2	NA(-11)	84	1035	2	G→>GG	Frameshift	(+BsaBI)	I	Lethal	1226G	Beutler et al (1991b)
3	IVS2+1	IVS2+1	1067	IVS2+1	G-A	Splice	-HphI	I	Lethal	1226G	Beutler et al (1992b)
4	NA(29)	203	1707	3	C>DEL	Frameshift	ASOH	I	Lethal	1226G	Beutler et al (1994b)
5	NA(382)	1263–1317 Del	5879–5932	9	55DEL	Frameshift	-SalI	I	Lethal	1226G	Beutler et al (1993b)
6	NA(444)	1447–1466 Del	6432–6451	10	20 bp del, TG insertion	Frameshift	Size difference	II	Lethal	1448G	Uchiyama et al (1994)
7	NA	Total gene del.	All	All	NA	NA	PCR gene quantitation	I	Lethal	1226G	Beutler & Gelbart (1994b)

Table 2C Complex mutations in the glucocerebrosidase gene that cause Gaucher disease

	Crossover Event	Crossover location					Exons affected	Genomic number	cDNA number	Amino acid substitution	Detection method	Type	Other allele	Reference
		cDNA		Genomic										
		5'limit	3'limit	5'limit	3'limit									
1	GC to PseudoGC	455	475	3039	3059	5	3059	475 C-T	Arg 120 Trp	-NciI	I	1226G	Latham et al (1991)
	PseudoGC to GC	754	812	3548	4161	6	3461	667 T-C	Trp 184 Arg	ASOH			
						6	3475	681 T-G	Asn 188 Lys	+StyI			
						6	3483	689 T-G	Val 191 Gly	ASOH			
						6	3497	703 T-C	Ser 196 Pro	+HaeIII			
						6	3515	721 G-A	Gly 202 Arg	-NciI			
						6	3548	754 T-A	Phe 213 Ile	(+NsiI)			
2	GC to PseudoGC	1317	1343	5932	5958	9	5957	1342 G-C	Asp 409 His	-StyI	I	1226G	Eyal et al (1990)
						10	6433	1448 T-C	Leu 444 Pro	+NciI	I	1226G	Latham et al (1990)
						10	6468	1483 G-C	Ala 456 Pro	+BcgI	III	1297T	Latham et al (1990)
						10	6482	1497 G-C	Val 460 Val	ASOH			
						int 9	6272 c-t			-PstI			
						int 9	6309 t-c						
3	GC to PseudoGC	1342	1388	5957	6272	10	6433	1448 T-C	Leu 444 Pro	+NciI	II	1448C	Eyal et al (1990)
						10	6468	1483 G-C	Ala 456 Pro	+BcgI	I	?	Eyal et al (1990)
						10	6482	1497 G-C	Val 460 Val	ASOH	I	1226G	Hong et al (1990)
											II	1448C	Lathem et al (1990)
													Zimran et al (1990a)

mutation on one allele is protective against the development of central nervous system involvement, an important consideration in prenatal diagnosis.

Mutation 1448: T→C (444Leu→Pro). This point mutation, the first to be discovered in the glucocerebrosidase gene (Tsuji et al 1987), is in exon 10. It is the prototype of the *severe* type of mutation (Beutler 1992, 1994) and has therefore been identified in all three phenotypic forms of the disease. It is the most frequent mutation in patients with types II and III Gaucher disease, including the Norbottnian variant. Most patients with this mutation are not Jewish and in this group it is also the most common mutation found in type I disease. The normal sequence of the pseudogene matches the sequence of the active gene with this mutation, implying that the occurrence of this mutation may be the result of recombination events between the active gene and the pseudogene, such as gene conversion or unequal crossing-over. This situation also underscores the need for separation of active gene from pseudogene during molecular diagnosis.

Mutation 84GG. This is a mutation wherein an extra guanine is inserted into the cDNA at position 84 (Beutler et al 1991b); no enzyme is produced, and it is the prototype of what has been designated the *lethal* type of mutation (Beutler 1992, 1994). It is the second most common mutation in the Ashkenazi Jewish population, accounting for 10–13% of mutated alleles (Beutler 1992).

Mutation IVS2(+1). This is a splice site mutation where an adenine is substituted for a guanine between exon 2 and intron 2, resulting in loss of exon 2; a non-functional enzyme is produced (Beutler et al 1992b, He & Grabowski 1992). It is another *lethal* Gaucher disease mutation that has never been seen in the homozygous form or in combination with the 84GG mutation. In the heterozygous form with the 1226G on the other allele, it represents 1–5% of genotypes in type I Gaucher disease in Jewish patients.

Mutation 1604: G→A (496Arg→His). This point mutation in exon 11 (Beutler 1992) has been identified only in a few compound heterozygotes. We have seen three patients in whom the 1604A mutation was inherited together with the 84GG mutation, one with the IVS2+1 mutation, and only once with the 1226G mutation. None of these patients developed neuronopathic disease, establishing this mutation as a mild mutation. Moreover, it is of significance that in patients with Gaucher disease the 1604A mutation is found predominantly with the less common, lethal mutations. This is best interpreted as indicating that individuals of the 1604A/1226G genotype, who should be more common in the Jewish population, do not come to notice because they are not clinically affected. This implies that the 1604A mutation is not only mild, but is even milder than the 1226G mutation.

Fusion genes and recombinations

In a number of Gaucher patients cDNA has been found to represent a transcript from a fusion gene in which the 5' end is the active gene and the 3' end is the pseudogene (Zimran et al 1990a). Although rare, these types of fusion genes provide information regarding the molecular anatomy of both the active gene and the pseudogene, and have significant implications with respect to the molecular pathogenesis and diagnosis of Gaucher disease.

Two different mechanisms appear to operate to form such a gene. One of these mechanisms is fusion of the functional gene and pseudogene into a single gene, analogous to the βδ hemoglobin fusion gene found in hemoglobin Lepore. As a result the gene/pseudogene complex is shortened, and this can be appreciated on Southern blotting (Zimran et al 1990a). This type of mutation was originally designated XOVR. The other type of recombinant gene is produced when the pseudogene sequence is imprinted on the 3' end of the functional gene, without loss of the pseudogene. When this occurs the size of the gene/pseudogene complex remains unaltered. The mechanism by which this type of change occurs is not well understood, but has been designated *gene conversion*. XOVR and one of these latter mutations designated variously as complex A (Latham et al 1990) or recNci (Horowitz et al 1989) includes three discrete point mutations: 1448C, 1483G, and 1497C. This complex allele is generally associated with moderate to severe type I disease and, when appearing with mutation 1448, can cause type II disease.

The second complex allele, designated as recTL (Firon et al 1990) or complex B (Latham et al 1990) includes a fourth G→C transversion at nucleotide 1342 in addition to the above three point mutations of the recNci/complex A mutation.

Interestingly, in the homozygous state, the point mutation 1342C can cause type III Gaucher disease: a unique variant with some unusual features including oculomotor apraxia and a progressive heart valve defect but only minimal other organ involvement (Zimran et al 1993a). The recTL allele has only been seen in the compound heterozygous state in conjunction with the 1226G mutation, and in spite of its similarity to the recNci complex allele, it is apparently associated with asymptomatic to mild Gaucher disease (Zimran & Horowitz 1994).

Saposin C and A

The glucocerebrosidase enzyme has an activator, saposin C, of 80 amino acids, which enhances substrate degradation. A prosaposin product is translated and processed into four discrete activators of four related lysosomal enzymes. Mutations in the area of the saposin C activator of the prosaposin molecule resulted in Gaucher disease in two known cases (Christomanou et al 1987, 1989, Schnabel et al 1991). A second protein activator, saposin A, has been described (Morimoto et al 1989) but has not been as extensively characterized.

Polymorphisms in the glucocerebrosidase gene

Early in the study of the glucocerebrosidase gene a DNA restriction polymorphism of the glucocerebrosidase gene complex, the *Pvu*II polymorphism, was found. It provided the first evidence at molecular level of the existence of genetic heterogeneity in Gaucher disease (Sorge et al 1985), that had heretofore only been suspected on the basis of clinical observations and family studies. Subsequent studies showed the existence of a complex of 12 polymorphic sites in the introns of the glucocerebrosidase gene (Beutler et al 1992a), but these were all found to be in strong linkage dysequilibrium, and therefore the *Pvu*II polymorphism serves as a surrogate for all of the polymorphic sites within the gene. This polymorphism is characterized by the presence or absence of a 1.1 kilobase fragment (Pv1.1$^+$ and Pv1.1$^-$ respectively) following digestion with the restriction enzyme *Pvu*II. With the complete sequence of both Pv1.1$^+$ and Pv1.1$^-$ human glucocerebrosidase available, the site of the *Pvu*II polymorphism was localized in intron 6, constituting a G→A single base substitution at position 3931 of the genomic sequence (Zimran et al 1990b). DNA analysis of unrelated Gaucher patients showed complete linkage dysequilibrium between the Pv1.1$^-$ genotype and the 'common Jewish' mutation 1226G (Zimran et al 1990b, Beutler et al 1992b), suggesting that the 1226G mutation arose only once in a Pv1.1$^-$ allele. Similarly, the 84GG is always in the Pv1.1$^+$ context (Beutler et al 1991b, 1992b) and IVS2(+1) in the Pv1.1$^-$ context (Beutler et al 1992b, Beutler 1993a). In contrast, it appears that the 1448C mutation arose more than once since there was no linkage dysequilibrium between either Pv1.1 allele and the 1448C mutation. Therefore, the Gaucher mutations are more recent in origin than the *Pvu*II polymorphism. A more extended and somewhat more diverse haplotype is provided by the nearby gene for the liver/red cell pyruvate kinase, designated *PKLR*. Here a silent polymorphism at cDNA nucleotide 1705, an A→C transition that destroys a *Bsph*I restriction site, is also in marked linkage dysequilibrium with all of the polymorphic Gaucher disease mutations (Glenn et al 1994). A microsatellite in the *PKLR* gene (Lezner et al 1994) increases the number of haplotypes and thus the diagnostic power of this linkage group.

The fact that the 1226G mutation and the IVS (2+1) mutation are always associated with the Pv1.1$^-$ haplotype, and the 84GG mutation is associated with the Pv1.1$^+$ haplotype, supports the concept of a single origin for each of these mutations, which are most common in the Ashkenazi Jewish community (Beutler 1992). The premise that the evolutionary process allowed an increase in the frequency of these mutations, despite the obvious deficiencies in the homozygote state, argues for a selective advantage within this ethnic community (Diamond 1994, Beutler 1991). To date, we have examined the role of resistance to infection, e.g. tuberculosis, increased fertility, and enhanced intellectual capacity as possible explanations for the selective advantage in carriers of the defective allele, but no evidence that any of these factors is operative has been found.

CLINICAL MANAGEMENT

Until recently therapy for Gaucher disease was very unsatisfactory, being directed at providing symptomatic relief. Only in the past few years, with the advent of enzyme replacement therapy, has management of Gaucher patients had an impact on the underlying mechanism of the disease. Treatment modalities were either supportive, e.g. control of infections, psychological, analgesics, nutrition, or surgical, such as splenectomy and corrective orthopedic procedures. While the need for such measures has been decreased by the advent of enzyme replacement and may be obviated by gene therapy, there is still an important place for symptomatic management of Gaucher disease.

Surgical

Splenectomy will generally correct the hematologic complications, relieve the symptoms of mechanical compression, engender a compensatory growth spurt in children and improve the nutritional status of adults. However, although it has been suggested that the progression of the disease was not related to the splenectomy (Lee 1982), some investigators have suggested that there was significant acceleration in liver and bone involvement following total splenectomy in patients with type I disease (Rose et al 1982, Ashkenazi et al 1986). In the Norbottnian patients (type III disease), a similar acceleration was seen (Conradi et al 1984, Nilsson et al 1985) and was attributed to increased lipid accumulation in other tissues and organs (Beutler 1988b) since the spleen was not available as a storage depot. In 1977, one of us (Beutler 1977b) introduced the use of partial splenectomy to reverse the hematologic and mechanical complications without sacrificing liver or bone integrity. Although early reports were encouraging (Guzzetta et al 1990, Fleshner et al 1991, Cohen et al 1992), the long-term clinical outcome in 24 patients with partial splenectomy has been rapid regrowth of the splenic remnant, recurrence of hypersplenism and development of new, bone-related complications in many patients (Zimran et al 1995).

Today, performance of splenectomy is restricted to a few specific situations: when enzyme replacement therapy is not available; when the thrombocytopenia is life-threatening or there is the need for major surgery when the thrombocyte count is low, since in these cases the platelet response may be too slow; when the spleen is massively enlarged (Zimran et al 1994, Pastores et al 1993); for vena cava syndrome; for abdominal pain caused by (recurrent) splenic infarction; and when there is severe pulmonary involvement and concern for respiratory failure (Zimran & Horowitz 1994).

Total hip replacement is appropriate treatment for aseptic necrosis of the femoral head; prolonged benefit has been documented (Goldblatt et al 1988). A similar case can be made for the shoulder joint in those patients whose primary bone-related focus is in the humeral head. Today, total joint replacement should be considered in those whose avascular necrosis is both painful and restricts the range of limb mobility, compromising the quality of life.

Spinal cord compression may occur as a result of the collapse of one or more adjacent vertebral bodies. In the case of compression, conservative management and surgical decompression have both been employed to reduce the consequent pain as well as correct the neurologic deficit and (local) gibbus formation.

Pathologic fractures, most commonly in the long bones and the ribs, are manifestations of the loss of normal bone integrity which cause concern. Management of these fractures is specific to the site wherein they occur and to the patient, although preference is for non-surgical treatment whenever possible. Relatively slow healing of the fracture is common and there is difficulty in applying internal fixation devices. It has been suggested that the occurrence of fractures can be correlated with the incidence of bone crises in the previous 2 to 12 months (Yosipovitch & Katz 1990) wherein the processes of repair post-crisis are retarded by internal porosity caused by ischemia. Because of possible increased susceptibility to infection in Gaucher patients, scrupulous attention to adequate antibiotic coverage, and to hematological stability, is advisable in all cases of surgical intervention.

Organ transplantation

In an attempt to provide enzyme to Gaucher patients, both renal and splenic allografts have been investigated (Groth et al 1971, 1979). In these cases engraftment was incomplete and therefore these modes have been abandoned. Liver transplantation has been performed in a few cases; while engraftment did occur (Carlson et al 1990, DuCerf et al 1992, Smanik et al 1993, Starzl et al 1993) one cannot expect response of a hemopoietic stem cell disease to hepatic transplantation, although it has been claimed that microchimerism occurs and may produce a generalized benefit (Starzl et al 1993).

Bone marrow transplantation (BMT) has been used to replace the patient's (recipient) genetically defective macrophages with those of the donor, thereby curing those aspects of the disease that are the consequence of macrophage engorgement with glycolipid, i.e. the manifestations of Type I Gaucher disease. Transplantation of the first such patient showed regression of storage cells, but the patient died of infectious complications (Rappeport & Ginns 1984). In the 5-year follow-up report of the first successful BMT in Gaucher disease, Ringdén et al (1988) document in a 9-year-old type III girl who had previously undergone splenectomy, normalization of liver size by 2 years post-transplant, complete disappearance of Gaucher cells from the bone marrow by 3 years and a growth spurt in both height and weight. However, despite normal plasma and erythrocyte glucosylccramide levels, she has manifested a gradual but progressive intellectual deterioration in the latter 3 years since BMT. In a series of six children under the age of 16 years who underwent BMT, only one death was noted, and was attributable to hypersplenism. The other five patients were doing well, with regression of some of their Gaucher symptoms and considerable improvement in their quality of life, approximately 1–4 years post-BMT (Hobbs et al 1987).

ENZYME REPLACEMENT THERAPY

The concept of enzyme replacement therapy as a means of treatment for patients suffering from lysosomal storage diseases was first suggested by DeDuve in 1964. Gaucher disease was regarded a prime candidate for this therapeutic modality because of the sparing of the central nervous system and the suitability of the macrophages to take up the exogenously administered enzyme. Brady suggested this form of treatment for Gaucher disease in 1966, 1 year after his discovery of the inherited deficiency of glucocerebrosidase as the etiology of this disorder. Brady et al (1974) infused partially purified enzyme intravenously into patients with Gaucher disease. Although their results were encouraging in that biochemical changes in red cell and liver glucocerebroside levels could be demonstrated, no clinically significant effect were achieved in their early trials (Brady & Barton 1994). Beutler and his group improved the delivery of the enzyme to the macrophage-monocyte system by incorporating the enzyme into resealed red blood cells either with or without coating them with IgG, and was the first to report clinical improvement in a patient so treated (Beutler et al 1977, Beutler 1981, Dale & Beutler 1982). Belchetz et al (1977) attempted to use liposomes as the delivery vehicles with disappointing results.

A major common obstacle to all early attempts to induce a clinical response in Gaucher patients by infusion of the native glucocerebrosidase was the lack of sufficient quantities of the placental enzyme. This problem was overcome in the 1980s when, with the introduction of commercial production, large quantities of placental glucocerebrosidase became available. In addition, the native enzyme has been modified to expose increased numbers of mannose residues as a means of targeting the enzyme to the macrophages. Although this has also been considered to be an important contribution to the success of the present enzyme replacement therapy (Brady et al 1994, Barton et al 1990), it is now apparent that the enzyme preparation is not selectively taken up only by macrophages (Beutler 1994, Sato & Beutler 1993).

An objective clinical response to infusions of 'mannose-terminated-glucocerebrosidase' was reported in 1990 in a 4-year-old child with type I Gaucher disease over a 20 week period. This child demonstrated an increase in hemoglobin level from a mean level of 6.9 gr% to 10.2 gr%, an increase in platelet counts and reduction of organomegaly (Barton et al 1990). Subsequently, 12 non-splenectomized type I Gaucher patients, eight children and four adults, were treated with this preparation. Ten patients received 60 U/kg body weight every 2 weeks, while two patients with more severe disease manifestations received the same dose on a weekly basis. All 12 patients showed an increase in hemoglobin levels and reduction of splenic volume; 7 patients experienced a reduction in hepatomegaly and 10 of the 12 patients showed increase in platelet counts. The treatment was well tolerated without any significant adverse effects (Barton et al 1991a). On the basis of this study the FDA approved alglucerase (Ceredase™, Genzyme, MA, USA) in April 1991.

The unprecedented and daunting high cost of the drug, over $300 000 US dollars per year of treatment for an adult Gaucher patient, stimulated an attempt to achieve therapeutic results at a lower cost. There are at least three theoretical reasons why alglucerase may be more effective when given frequently in small amounts than when given as a large bolus at infrequent intervals:

1. Large doses will quickly saturate receptors and since the infused enzyme has an intravascular half-life of only about 10 minutes, most of the infused enzyme would be wasted;

2. There may be stages in the maturation of a monocyte to a macrophage that are optimal for treatment. Infrequent infusions might miss this critical stage for some cells;

3. There may be a maximum rate at which a cell can catabolize glucocerebrosidase, and exceeding the amount of enzyme that can achieve this rate would waste the excess.

Because of these considerations, enzyme was administered at frequent intervals in our early trials (Beutler 1981, Beutler et al 1980, Dale & Beutler 1982) and one of us (E Beutler) devised an alternative protocol wherein much lower doses of alglucerase (2.3 U/kg body weight) were given but at more frequent intervals (three times weekly) (Beutler 1991, 1993b, Figueroa et al 1992, Beutler et al 1993a). The results of this regimen, known as the 'low-dose high-frequency' protocol, were comparable to those reported by the investigators who used the original 'high-dose low-frequency' protocol (Fallet et al 1992, Pastores et al 1993, Barton et al 1991a). The lack of consensus as to whether a high dose was justified and whether high frequency resulted in low patient compliance, is still evident today, despite the confirmatory results obtained in large groups of patients using the same low-dose high frequency schedule (Mistry et al 1992, Zimran et al 1992b, 1994, Beutler et al 1993a, Hollak et al 1993a; Beutler 1993a, Zevin et al 1993). It is clear that this treatment is fully effective in patients of all ages and genotypes, severe and less severe disease, and in patients with or without a spleen (Figs 1 and 2). Although skeletal responses occur slowly in patients receiving any dose schedule, the rate of improvement of skeletal disease appears to be the same in patients receiving low-dose therapy as those receiving high-dose therapy (Beutler et al 1994a). It is interesting and important that although many objections have been raised to the use of the 'low-dose high-frequency' protocol (Barton et al 1993, Moscicki & Taunton-Rigby 1993, Barranger 1993), none of those objecting have presented evidence of treatment failures using this approach. Indeed, Hollack et al (1993b) have shown that even one-half of the dose that is usually given as 'low-dose high-frequency' therapy is quite effective.

While the most obvious differences between the two regimens of therapy concern the cost of treatment and convenience, there is a third aspect which involves the theoretical underpinning of the mode of therapy. Barton has suggested that there is only one single type of macrophage receptor for glucocerebrosidase, and it is not saturated at doses below 100 U/kg (Barton et al 1991a,b). On the other hand, Sato and Beutler (1993) have clearly demonstrated the existence of at least two types of mannose-dependent receptors for glucocerebrosidase: a low number of high-affinity receptors limited to macrophages and a high number (approximately 20-fold higher) of low-affinity receptors. These latter receptors are also more widely distributed in that they exist on peripheral blood leukocytes and on endothelial cells. According to these findings, most of the enzyme that is infused at high doses will be bound to the less specific receptor, whereas the enzyme infused in low doses will preferentially bind to the mannose-specific receptors, thereby ensuring greater efficacy. Study of uptake of high concentrations (60 U/kg) of enzyme infused into patients undergoing orthopedic surgery has shown that hardly any of the enzyme can be found in marrow-rich bone samples removed immediately after enzyme infusion. Indeed, the amount of enzyme detected is less than 2% of the amount of that would be expected if the enzyme were not targeted but merely uniformly distributed to all body cells (Beutler & Kuhl 1994). Therefore, it is evident that alglucerase is not, as has been claimed, macrophage targeted, and that the means by which the therapeutic effect of this preparation is exerted is far from clear.

One of the unexplained aspects of alglucerase therapy is the development of antibodies in some of the patients; 10–15% of those treated with high-dose levels of the enzyme (Pastores et al 1993, Richards et al 1993). In general, those patients who developed antibodies did not have to discontinue treatment. Most cases were asymptomatic while others had some allergic reaction including rash and pruritus, which responded well to antihistamines. There were two episodes of apparent anaphylaxis, both in patients treated by high doses, one of them following an unintentionally rapid infusion of the enzyme (Richards et al 1993). A single patient, who developed blocking antibodies, is currently undergoing a detailed immunological evaluation (Moscicki, personal communication). Interestingly, we observed a smaller percentage (approximately 5%) of seropositive patients among those treated by the low-dose regimen (Zimran et al 1994), and have not observed any but the most minor allergic reactions in the few patients who seroconverted. At present, it is too early to state whether or not these preliminary observations have any significance with regard to safety of the treatment. Of note is a recent report on the clinical implications of the hCG (human chorionic gonadotrophin) contamination of alglucerase, within the context of the low-dose regimen (Cohen et al 1994). Treated patients had higher β-hCG levels (albeit well within the normal range) than untreated Gaucher patients who served as controls; this finding may also suggest the possibility that giving smaller doses of alglucerase may contribute an additional margin of safety.

Regardless of which protocol is chosen, there are common clinical observations in patients treated with alglucerase that are shared by all

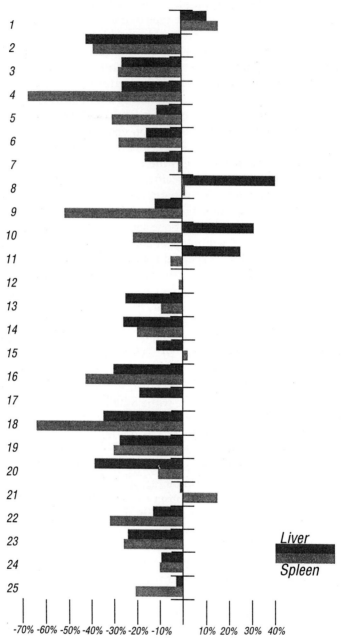

Fig. 1. Percent changes from baseline of liver and spleen volumes (measured by ultrasound) following 6 months of alglucerase therapy. Data are from Gaucher disease patients treated at Shaare-Zedek Medical Center. Volumes were evaluated by ultrasound. The first 15 patients are children of which No. 8 has type III Gaucher disease. All other patients have type I disease. The remaining patients are adults over the age of 18 years. No corrections were made for changes in body weight or height as a result of growth.

physicians with experience in enzyme replacement therapy; these are enumerated below:

1. Alglucerase is a relatively safe, effective drug for the correction of the hematological complications of Gaucher disease and for the reduction of both splenomegaly and hepatomegaly.

2. The increase in hemoglobin levels is more rapid and more pronounced than the increase in platelet counts in patients with massively enlarged spleens. A dramatic response in platelet counts is seen in the relatively rare patients who have undergone splenectomy and are thrombocytopenic.

3. The skeletal response to alglucerase lags behind the aforementioned responses and may require 3 years or more before significant radiological changes in the bones are observed.

4. Patients differ markedly in their clinical response to therapy, and factors such as age, sex, ethnic origin, genotype or general clinical severity, cannot adequately predict the individual response to treatment.

In May 1994 a new form of human derived recombinant 'macrophage-targeted' glucocerebrosidase was approved by the FDA; this preparation, known as imiglucerase (Cerezyme™, Genzyme Inc., MA), was produced in order to ensure unlimited supply of the enzyme, to further improve the safety of therapy and finally, in the future, to potentially reduce the cost of treatment. Clinical trials with this enzyme were conducted in two modes, the first at the NIH in Bethesda and in Mount Sinai Hospital in New York, comparing in a double-blind trial alglucerase to imiglucerase, both at high doses of 60 U/kg body weight every other week;15 patients in each group. The second mode was at Shaare-Zedek Medical Center in Jerusalem, comparing low-dose imiglucerase on two schedules of administration: once every 2 weeks versus 3 times a week. Imiglucerase was found to be safe and effective and no significant differences were found between the efficacy of any of the doses or dosage schedules tested.

KEY POINTS FOR CLINICAL PRACTICE

- Gaucher Disease is the most common glycolipid storage disorder, occurring in approximately 1:1000 Jewish births, and less frequently in other populations.

- Three major forms of Gaucher disease have been delineated. Type 1 is characterized by the absence of primary neurologic involvement, while types II and III are neuronopathic forms of the disease.

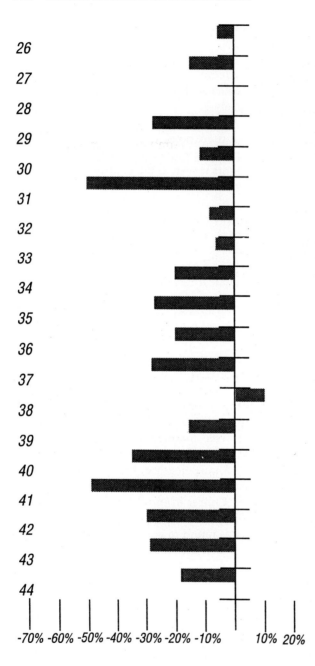

Fig. 2. Percent changes from baseline of liver volumes in splenectomized patients. Presented are data of 19 splenectomized Gaucher patients treated at Shaare-Zedek Medical Center. Volumes were evaluated by ultrasound as described previously. The first (No. 26) was 16 years old, the remainder are adults.

- The clinical manifestations of Gaucher disease are directly or indirectly related to the accumulation of the glycolipid glucocerebroside in macrophages throughout the body. The most prominent sites of involvement are liver, spleen, and bone.

- Over 50 different mutations have been documented in Gaucher disease. In the Jewish population, the most common of these is 1226G. This mutation protects against neuronopathic disease. In contrast, the common panethnic 1448C mutation can be associated with neuronopathic disease.

- Enzyme replacement therapy, now commercially available, is effective in the treatment of Gaucher disease. Small doses of enzyme (15–30 U/kg/month) give results that are indistinguishable from the large doses (60–130 U/kg/month) that are often used. Because of the high cost of enzyme replacement therapy, we recommend that therapy be started with a dose no higher than 30 U/kg/month.

- Gaucher disease will be a good candidate for gene transfer therapy in the future.

REFERENCES

Aker M, Zimran A, Abrahamov A et al 1993 Abnormal neutrophil chemotaxis in Gaucher disease. Br J Haematol 83: 187–191
Amstutz H C 1973 The hip in Gaucher disease. Clin Orthop 90: 83–89
Ashkenazi A, Zaizov R, Matoth Y 1986 Effect of splenectomy on destructive bone changes in children with chronic (Type I) Gaucher disease. Eur J Pediatr 145: 138–141
Barneveld R A, Keijzer W, Tegelaers F P W et al 1983 Assignment of the gene coding for human beta-glucocerebrosidase to the region q21–q31 of chromosome 1 using monoclonal antibodies. Hum Genet 64: 227–231
Barranger J A 1993 Editor's comments. Gaucher Clinical Perspectives 1: 16
Barton N W, Furbish F S, Murray G J et al 1990 Therapeutic response to intravenous infusions of glucocerebrosidase in a patient with Gaucher disease. Proc Natl Acad Sci USA 87: 1913–1916
Barton N W, Brady R O, Dambrosia J M et al 1991a Replacement therapy for inherited enzyme deficiency—Macrophage-targeted glucocerebrosidase for Gaucher disease. N Engl J Med 324: 1464–1470
Barton N W, Brady R O, Murray G J et al 1991b Enzyme-replacement therapy for Gaucher disease: Reply. N Engl J Med 325: 1811
Barton N W, Brady R O, Dambrosia J M 1993 Treatment of Gaucher disease. N Engl J Med 328: 1564–1565
Beighton P, Goldblatt J, Sacks S 1982 Bone involvement in Gaucher disease. In: Desnick R J, Gatt S, Grabowski G A (eds) Gaucher disease: a century of delineation and research. Alan R. Liss, Inc., New York, p 107
Belchetz P E, Crawley J C W, Braidman I P et al 1977 Treatment of Gaucher disease with liposome-entrapped glucocerebroside: Beta-glucosidase. Lancet 2: 116–117
Bernard R, Payan H, Maestraggi T et al 1961 Maladie de Gaucher du nourrison a manifestations cerebrales predominates. Etude anatomoclinique. Pediatrie 16: 285–289
Bernstein J, Sheldon W E 1959 A note on the development of Gaucher cells in a newborn infant. J Pediatr 55: 577
Beutler E 1977a Gaucher disease in an asymptomatic 72-year-old. JAMA 237: 2529
Beutler E 1977b Newer aspects of some interesting lipid storage diseases: Tay-Sachs and Gaucher diseases. West J Med 126: 46–54

Beutler E 1981 Enzyme replacement therapy. TIBS Rev. 6: 95–97
Beutler E 1988a Gaucher disease: new developments. In: Fairbanks V F (ed) Current hematology and oncology. Year Book Medical Publishers, Inc., Chicago, p 6:1
Beutler E 1988b Gaucher Disease. Blood Rev 2: 59–70
Beutler E 1991 Gaucher disease. N Engl J Med 325: 1354–1360
Beutler E 1992 Gaucher disease: New molecular approaches to diagnosis and treatment. Science 256: 794–799
Beutler E 1993a Gaucher disease as a paradigm of current issues regarding single gene mutations of humans. Proc Natl Acad Sci USA 90: 5384–5390
Beutler E 1993b Modern diagnosis and treatment of Gaucher disease. Am J Dis Child 147: 1175–1183
Beutler E 1994 Gaucher disease. In: Advances in Genetics, Friedmann T, ed. San Diego, Academic Press inc, pp17-49
Beutler E, Gelbart T 1990 Gaucher disease associated with a unique KpnI restriction site: identification of the amino acid substitution. Ann Hum Genet 54: 149–153
Beutler E, Gelbart T 1993 Gaucher disease mutations in non-Jewish patients. Br J Haematol 85: 401–405
Beutler E, Gelbart T 1994a Two new Gaucher disease mutations. Hum Genet 93: 209–210
Beutler E, Gelbart T 1994b Erroneous assignment of Gaucher disease genotype as a consequence of a complete gene deletion. Hum Mutat 4: 212–216
Beutler E, Grabowski G 1995 Gaucher disease. In: Scriver C R, Beaudet A L, Sly W S, Valle D (eds) The metabolic basis of inherited disease. McGraw-Hill Publishing Company, New York, p 2641
Beutler E, Kuhl W, Vaughan LM 1995 Failure of alglucerase infused into Gaucher disease patients to localize in marrow macrophages. Molecular Medicine 1: 320-324
Beutler E, Demina A, Gelbart T et al 1994a The clinical course of treated and untreated Gaucher disease. A study of 45 patients. Blood Cells Mol Dis 21: 86-108
Beutler E, Gelbart T, Demina A 1994b Glucocerebrosidase (GBA) mutations in Gaucher disease. Mol Med 1: 82–92
Beutler E, Dale G L, Guinto E et al 1977 Enzyme replacement therapy in Gaucher disease: Preliminary clinical trial of a new enzyme preparation. Proc Natl Acad Sci USA 74: 4620–4623
Beutler E, Dale G L, Kuhl W 1980 Replacement therapy in Gaucher disease. In: Desnick R J (ed.) Enzyme therapy in genetic diseases: 2. Alan R. Liss, Inc., New York, p 369
Beutler E, Sorge J A, Zimran A et al 1988 The molecular biology of Gaucher disease. In: Salvayre R, Douste-Blazy L, Gatt S (eds) Lipid storage disorders. Biological and medical aspects. Plenum Press, New York, p 19
Beutler E, Kay A, Saven A et al 1991a Enzyme replacement therapy for Gaucher disease. Blood 78: 1183–1189
Beutler E, Gelbart T, Kuhl W et al 1991b Identification of the second common Jewish Gaucher disease mutation makes possible population based screening for the heterozygote state. Proc Natl Acad Sci USA 88: 10544–10547
Beutler E, West C, Gelbart T 1992a Polymorphisms in the human glucocerebrosidase gene. Genomics 12: 795–800
Beutler E, Gelbart T, Kuhl W et al 1992b Mutations in Jewish patients with Gaucher disease. Blood 79: 1662–1666
Beutler E, Figueroa M, Koziol J 1993a Treatment of Gaucher disease. N Engl J Med 328: 1567
Beutler E, Gelbart T, West C 1993b Identification of six new Gaucher disease mutations. Genomics 15: 203–205
Boklan B F, Sawitsky A 1976 Factor IX deficiency in Gaucher disease. An in vitro phenomenon. Arch Intern Med 136: 489–492
Brady R O 1966 The sphingolipidoses. N Engl J Med 275: 312–318
Brady R O, Barton N W 1994 Development of effective enzyme therapy for metabolic storage disorders. Int Pediatr 9: 175–180
Brady R O, Pentchev P G, Gal A E et al 1974 Replacement therapy for inherited enzyme deficiency. Use of purified glucocerebrosidase in Gaucher disease. N Engl J Med 291: 989–993
Brady R O, Barton N W, Grabowski G A 1993 The role of neurogenetics in Gaucher disease. Arch Neurol 50: 1212–1224

Brady R O, Murray G J, Barton N W 1994 Modifying exogenous glucocerebrosidase for effective replacement therapy in Gaucher disease. J Inherited Metab Dis 17: 510–519

Brinn L, Glabman S 1962 Gaucher disease without splenomegaly. Oldest patient on record with review. NY State J Med 62: 2346–2354

Burns G F, Cawley R J, Flemans R J et al 1977 Surface marker and other characteristics of Gaucher cell. J Clin Pathol 30: 981–988

Burstein Y, Zakuth V, Rechavi G et al 1987 Abnormalities of cellular immunity and natural killer cells in Gaucher disease. J Clin Lab Immunol 23: 149–151

Carlson D E, Busuttil R W, Giudici T A et al 1990 Orthotopic liver transplantation in the treatment of complications of type I Gaucher disease. Transplantation 49: 1192–1194

Chabas A, Cormand B, Burguera J et al 1993 Enzymatic and molecular studies in an unusual case of Gaucher disease with cardiovascular calcifications. Second International Duodecim Symposium, Finland 69

Choy F Y M, Wei C, Applegarth D A et al 1994 A new missense mutation in glucocerebrosidase exon 9 of a non-Jewish Caucasian type 1 Gaucher disease patient. Hum Mol Genet 3: 821–823

Christomanou H, Kleinschmidt T, Braunitzer G 1987 N-terminal amino acid sequence of a sphingolipid activator protein missing in a new human Gaucher disease variant. Biol Chem Hoppe Seyler 368: 1193–1196

Christomanou H, Chabás A, Pámpols T et al 1989 Activator protein deficient Gaucher disease. A second patient with the newly identified lipid storage disorder. Klin Wochenschr 67: 999–1003

Cohen I J, Katz K, Freud E et al 1992 Long-term follow-up of partial splenectomy in Gaucher disease. AM J Surg 164: 345–347

Cohen Y, Elstein D, Abrahamov A et al 1994 HCG contamination of alglucerase: Clinical implications in low-dose regimen. Am J Hematol 47: 235–236

Conradi N G, Sourander P, Nilsson O et al 1984 Neuropathology of the Norbottnian type of Gaucher disease: Morphological and biochemical studies. Acta Neuropathol (Berlin) 65: 99–100

Dale G L, Beutler E 1982 Enzyme therapy in Gaucher disease: Clinical trials and model system studies. In: Crawford M A, Gibbs D A, Watts R W E (eds) Advances in the treatment of inborn errors of metabolism. John Wiley and Sons, New York, p 77

DeDuve C 1964 From cytases to lysosomes. Fed Proc 23: 1045–1049

Diamond J M 1994 Jewish lysosomes. Nature 368: 291–292

DuCerf C, Bancel B, Caillon P et al 1992 Orthotopic liver transplantation for type 1 Gaucher disease. Transplantation 53: 1141–1143

Edwards W D, Hurdey H P, Partin J R 1983 Cardiac involvement by Gaucher disease documented by right ventricular endomyocardial biopsy. Am J Cardiol 52: 654

Eyal N, Wilder S, Horowitz M 1990 Prevalent and rare mutations among Gaucher patients. Gene 96: 277–283

Eyal N, Firon N, Wilder S et al 1991 Three unique base pair changes in a family with Gaucher disease. Hum Genet 87: 328–332

Fallet S, Sibille A, Mendelson R et al 1992 Enzyme augmentation in moderate to life-threatening Gaucher disease. Pediatr Res 31: 496–502

Fellows K E, Grand R J, Colodny A H et al 1975 Combined portal and vena caval hypertension in Gaucher disease: The value of preoperative venography. J Pediatr 87: 739–743

Figueroa M L, Rosenbloom B E, Kay A C et al 1992 A less costly regimen of alglucerase to treat Gaucher disease. N Engl J Med 327: 1632–1636

Firon N, Eyal N, Horowitz M 1990 Genotype assignment in Gaucher disease by selective amplification of the active glucocerebrosidase gene. Am J Hum Genet 46: 527–532

Fleshner P R, Aufses A H Jr, Grabowski G A et al 1991 A 27-year experience with splenectomy for Gaucher disease. Am J Surg 161: 69–75

Gaucher P C E 1882 De l'epithelioma primitif de la rate, hypertrophie idiopathique del la rate san leucemie. Thesis, Paris

Ginsberg H, Grabowski G A, Gibson J C et al 1984 Reduced plasma concentrations of total, low density lipoprotein and high density lipoprotein cholesterol in patients with Gaucher type I disease. Clin Genet 26: 109–116

Glenn D, Gelbart T, Beutler E 1994 Tight linkage of pyruvate kinase (*PKLR*) and glucocerebrosidase (*GBA*) genes. Hum Genet 93: 635–638

Goldblatt J, Beighton P 1985 Obstetric aspects of Gaucher disease. Br J Obstet Gynaecol 92: 145–149

Goldblatt J, Sacks S, Dall D et al 1988 Total hip arthoplasty in Gaucher disease. Long-term prognosis. Clin Orthop 228: 94–98

Granovsky-Grisaru S, Aboulafia Y, Diamont Y Z et al 1995 Gynecologic and obstetric aspects of Gaucher disease: A survey of 53 patients. Am J Obstet Gynecol 172: 1284–1290

Graves P N, Grabowski G A, Eisner R et al 1988 Gaucher disease type 1: Cloning and characterization of a cDNA encoding acid β-glucosidase from an Ashkenazi Jewish patient. DNA 7: 521–528

Groen J, Garrer A H 1948 Adult Gaucher disease with special reference to the variation in its clinical course and value of sternal puncture as an aid to its diagnosis. Blood 3: 1221–1227

Groth C G, Dreborg S, Öckerman P A et al 1971 Splenic transplantation in a case of Gaucher disease. Lancet 1: 1260–1264

Groth C G, Collste H, Dreborg S et al 1979 Attempts at enzyme replacement in Gaucher disease by renal transplantation. Acta Paediator Scand 68: 475–479

Guzzetta P C, Ruley E J, Merrick H F W et al 1990 Elective subtotal splenectomy. Indications and results in 33 patients. Ann Surg 211: 34–42

He G-S, Grabowski G A 1992 Gaucher disease: A G^{+1}–A^{+1} IVS2 splice donor site mutation causing exon 2 skipping in the acid β-glucosidase mRNA. Am J Hum Genet 51: 810–820

He G-S, Grace M E, Grabowski G A 1992 Gaucher disease: Four rare missense mutations enclouding F2131, F289Y, T3231 and R463C in type I variants. Hum Mutat 1: 423–427

Hermann G, Shapiro R S, Abdelwahab I F et al 1993 MR imaging in adults with Gaucher disease type I: Evaluation of marrow involvement and disease activity. Skeletal Radiol 22: 247–251

Hill S C, Reinig J W, Barranger J A et al 1986 Gaucher disease: Sonographic appearance of the spleen. Radiology 160: 631–634

Hill S C, Damaska B M, Ling A et al 1992 Gaucher disease: Abdominal MR imaging findings in 46 patients. Radiology 184: 561–566

Hobbs J R, Shaw P J, Jones K H et al 1987 Beneficial effect of pre-transplant splenectomy on displacement bone marrow transplantation for Gaucher syndrome. Lancet 1: 1111–1115

Hollak C E M, Aerts J M F G, van Oers M H J 1993a Treatment of Gaucher disease. N Engl J Med 328: 1565–1566

Hollak C E M, Aerts J M F G, van Weely S et al 1993b Enzyme supplementation therapy for type I Gaucher disease. Efficacy of very low dose alglucerase in 12 patients. Blood 82 (Suppl.1): 33a

Hollak C E M, van Weely S, van Oers M H J et al 1994 Marked elevation of plasma chitotriosidase activity. A novel hallmark of Gaucher disease. J Clin Invest 93: 1288–1292

Hong C M, Ohashi T, Yu X J et al 1990 Sequence of two alleles responsible for Gaucher disease. DNA Cell Biol 9: 233–241

Horev G, Kornreich L, Hadar H et al 1991 Hemorrhage associated with 'bone crises' in Gaucher disease identified by magnetic resonance imaging. Skeletal Radiol 20: 479–482

Horowitz M, Wilder S, Horowitz Z et al 1989 The human glucocerebrosidase gene and pseudogene: Structure and evolution. Genomics 4: 87–96

Hsia D Y Y, Naylor J, Bigler J A 1962 The genetic mechanism of Gaucher disease. In: Aronson S M, Volk B W (eds) Cerebral sphingolipidoses. Academic Press, New York

James S P, Stromeyer F W, Chang C et al 1981 Liver abnormalities in patients with Gaucher disease. Gastroenterology 80: 126–133

James S P, Stromeyer F W, Stowens D W et al 1982 Gaucher disease: Hepatic abnormalities in 25 patients. In: Desnick R J, Gatt S, Grabowski G A (eds) Gaucher disease: a century of delineation and research. Alan R Liss Inc, New York, p 131

Kawame H, Eto Y 1991 A new glucocerebrosidase-gene missense mutation responsible for neuronopathic Gaucher disease in Japanese patients. Am J Hum Genet 49: 1378–1380

Kawame H, Hasegawa Y, Eto Y et al 1992 Rapid identification of mutations in the glucocerebrosidase gene of Gaucher disease patients by analysis of single-strand conformation polymorphisms. Hum Genet 90: 294–296

Kolodny E H, Ullman M D, Mankin H J et al 1982 Phenotypic manifestations of Gaucher disease: clinical features in 48 biochemically verified Type I patients and comment on Type II patients. In: Desnick R J, Gatt S, Grabowski G A (eds) Gaucher disease: a Century of delineation and research. Alan R Liss, Inc., New York, p 33

Latham T, Grabowski G A, Theophilus B D M et al 1990 Complex alleles of the acid β-glucosidase gene in Gaucher disease. Am J Hum Genet 47: 79–86

Latham T E, Theophilus B D M, Grabowski G A et al 1991 Heterogeneity of mutations in the acid β-glucosidase gene of Gaucher disease patients. DNA Cell Biol 10: 15–21

Laubscher K H, Glew R H, Lee R E et al 1993 A new exon 9 mutation in Gaucher disease detected by denaturing gradient gel electrophoresis. Am J Hum Genet 53 (Suppl): Abstract 1190
Le N A, Gibson J C, Rubinstein A et al 1988 Abnormalities in lipoprotein metabolism in Gaucher type I disease. Metabolism 37: 240–245
Lee R E 1982 The Pathology of Gaucher disease. In: Desnick R J, Gatt S, Grabowski G A (eds) Gaucher disease: a Century of delineation and research. Alan R. Liss, Inc., New York, p 177
Lee R E, Yousem S A 1988 The frequency and type of lung involvement in patients with Gaucher disease. Lab Invest 58: 54
Lenzner C, Jacobasch G, Reis A et al 1994 Trinucleotide repeat polymorphism at the PKLR locus. Hum Mol Genet 3: 523
Lieberman J, Beutler E 1976 Elevation of serum angiotensin-converting enzyme in Gaucher disease. N Engl J Med 294: 1442–1444
Liel Y, Rudich A, Nagauker-Shriker O et al 1994 Monocyte dysfunction in patients with Gaucher disease: Evidence for interference of glucocerebroside with superoxide generation. Blood 83: 2646–2653
Mankin H J, Doppelt S H, Rosenberg A E et al 1990 Metabolic bone disease in patients with Gaucher disease. In: Avioli L V, Krane S M (eds) Metabolic bone disease and clinically related disorders. W B Saunders, Philadelphia, p 730
Markin R S, Skultety F M 1984 Spinal cord compression secondary to Gaucher disease. Surg Neurol 21: 341–346
Matoth Y, Fried K 1965 Chronic Gaucher disease. Clinical observations on 34 patients. Isr J Med Sci 1: 521–530
Mazor M, Wiznitzer A, Pinku A et al 1986 Gaucher disease in pregnancy associated with portal hypertension. Am J Obstet Gynecol 154: 1119–1120
Mistry P K, Davies S, Corfield A et al 1992 Successful treatment of bone marrow failure in Gaucher disease with low-dose modified glucocerebrosidase. Quart J Med 83: 541–546
Morimoto S, Martin B M, Yamamoto Y et al 1989 Saposin A: Second cerebrosidase activator protein. Proc Natl Acad Sci USA 86: 3389–3393
Moscicki R A, Taunton-Rigby A 1993 Treatment of Gaucher disease. N Engl J Med 328: 1564
Nilsson O, Grabowski G A, Ludman M D et al 1985 Glycosphingolipid studies of visceral tissues and brain from type 1 Gaucher disease variants. Clin Genet 27: 443–450
Nishimura R N, Barranger J A 1980 Neurologic complications of Gaucher disease type 3. Arch Neurol 37: 92–93
Ohshima T, Sasaki M, Matsuzaka T et al 1993 A novel splicing abnormality in a Japanese patient with Gaucher disease. Hum Mol Genet 2: 1497–1498
Pastores G M, Sibille A R, Grabowski G A 1993 Enzyme therapy in Gaucher disease type 1: Dosage efficacy and adverse effects in thirty-three patients treated for 6 to 24 months. Blood 82: 408–416
Patterson M C, Horowitz M, Abel R B et al 1993 Isolated horizontal supranuclear gaze palsy as a marker of severe systemic involvement in Gaucher disease. Neurology 43: 1993–1997
Pelini M, Boice D, O'Neil K et al 1994 Glucocerebrosidase treatment of type I Gaucher disease with severe pulmonary involvement. Ann Intern Med 121: 196–197
Pratt P W, Estren F, Kochwa S 1968 Immunoglobulin abnormalities in Gaucher disease. Report of 16 cases. Blood 31: 633–640
Rappeport J M, Ginns E I 1984 Bone-marrow transplantation in severe Gaucher Disease. N Engl J Med 311: 84–88
Richards S M, Olson T A, McPherson J M (1993) Antibody response in patients with Gaucher disease after repeated infusion with macrophage-targeted glucocerebrosidase. Blood 82: 1402–1409
Ringdén O, Groth C-G, Erikson A et al 1988 Long-term follow-up of the first successful bone marrow transplantation in Gaucher disease. Transplantation 46: 66–70
Rose J S, Grabowski G A, Barnett S H et al 1982 Accelerated skeletal deterioration after splenectomy in Gaucher type 1 disease. Am J Roentgenol 139: 1202–1204
Ross L 1969 Gaucher cells in kidney glomeruli. Arch Path (Chicago) 87: 164–167
Sato Y, Beutler E 1993 Binding, internalization, and degradation of mannose-terminated glucocerebrosidase by macrophages. J Clin Invest 91: 1909–1917
Schnabel D, Schröder M, Sandhoff K 1991 Mutation in the sphingolipid activator protein 2 in a patient with a variant of Gaucher disease. FEBS Lett 284: 57–59
Seligsohn U, Zitman D, Many A et al 1976 Coexistence of factor XI (plasma thromboplastin antecedent) deficiency and Gaucher disease. Isr J Med Sci 12: 1448–1452

Shiran A, Brenner B, Laor A et al 1993 Increased risk of cancer in patients with Gaucher disease. Cancer 72: 219–224

Shoenfeld Y, Berliner S, Pinkhas J et al 1980 The association of Gaucher disease and dysproteinemias. Acta Haematol (Basel) 64: 241–243

Shoenfeld Y, Gallant L A, Shaklai M et al 1982 Gaucher disease. A disease with chronic stimulation of the immune system. Arch Pathol Lab Med 106: 388–391

Sibille A, Eng C M, Kim S-J et al 1993 Phenotype/genotype correlations in Gaucher disease type I: Clinical and therapeutic implications. Am J Hum Genet 52: 1094–1101

Sidransky E, Sherer D M, Ginns E I 1992a Gaucher disease in the neonate: A distinct Gaucher phenotype is analogous to a mouse model created by targeted disruption of the glucocerebrosidase gene. Pediatr Res 32: 494–498

Sidransky E, Tsuji S, Stubblefield B K et al 1992b Gaucher patients with oculomotor abnormalities do not have a unique genotype. Clin Genet 41: 1–5

Smanik E J, Tavill A S, Jacobs G H et al 1993 Orthotopic liver transplantation in two adults with Niemann-Pick and Gaucher diseases: Implications for the treatment of inherited metabolic disease. Hepatology 17: 42–49

Smith R L, Hutchins G M, Sack G H, Jr. et al 1978 Unusual cardiac, renal and pulmonary involvement in Gaucher disease. Interstitial glucocerebroside accumulation, pulmonary hypertension and fatal bone marrow embolization. Am J Med 65: 352–360

Soffer D, Yamanaka T, Wenger D A et al 1980 Central nervous system involvement in adult-onset Gaucher disease. Acta Neuropathol (Berlin) 49: 1–6

Sorge J, Gelbart T, West C et al 1985 Heterogeneity in type I Gaucher disease demonstrated by restriction mapping of the gene. Proc Natl Acad Sci USA 82: 5442–5445

Sorge J A, West C, Kuhl W et al 1987 The human glucocerebrosidase gene has two functional ATG initiator codons. Am J Hum Genet 41: 1016–1024

Sorge J, Gross E, West C et al 1990 High level transcription of the glucocerebrosidase pseudogene in normal subjects and patients with Gaucher disease. J Clin Invest 86: 1137–1141

Starzl T E, Demetris A J, Trucco M et al 1993 Chimerism after liver transplantation for type IV glycogen storage disease and type 1 Gaucher disease. N Engl J Med 328: 745–749

Stowens D W, Teitelbaum S L, Kahn A J et al 1985 Skeletal complications in Gaucher disease. Medicine (Baltimore) 64: 310–322

Svennerholm L, Dreborg S, Erikson A et al 1982 Gaucher disease of the Norrbottnian type (type III). Phenotypic manifestations. In: Desnick R J, Gatt S, Grabowski G A (eds) Gaucher disease: a century of delineation and research. Alan R Liss, Inc., New York, p 67

Tamari I, Motro M, Neufeld H N 1983 Unusual pericardial calcification in Gaucher disease. Arch Intern Med 143: 2010–2011

Teton J B, Treadwell N C 1957 Gaucher disease in pregnancy. Am J Obstet Gynecol 74: 1363–1366

Theise N D, Ursell P C 1990 Pulmonary hypertension and Gaucher disease: logical association or mere coincidence? Am J Pediatr Hematol Oncol 12: 74–76

Theophilus B D M, Latham T, Grabowski G A et al 1989 Comparison of RNase A, chemical cleavage, and GC-clamped denaturing gradient gel electrophoresis for the detection of mutations in exon 9 of the human acid β-glucosidase gene. Nucl Acids Res 17: 7707–7722

Tripp J H, Lake B D, Young E et al 1977 Juvenile Gaucher disease with horizontal gaze palsy in three siblings. J Neurol Neurosurg Psychiatry 40: 470–478

Tsuji S, Choudary P V, Martin B M et al 1987 A mutation in the human glucocerebrosidase gene in neuronopathic Gaucher disease. N Engl J Med 316: 570–575

Tsuji S, Martin B M, Barranger J A et al 1988 Genetic heterogeneity in type 1 Gaucher disease: Multiple genotypes in Ashkenazic and non-Ashkenazic individuals. Proc Natl Acad Sci USA 85: 2349–2352, 5708

Tsutsumi A 1982 A case of Gaucher disease with corneal opacities. Ganka Rhinshoiho (Japanese) 76: 1730–1733

Turpin J C, Dubois G, Brice A et al 1987 Parkisonian syndrome in a patient with type I (adult) Gaucher disease. In: Salvayre R, Douste-Blazy L, Gatt S (eds) Lipid storage disorders: biological and medical aspects. Plenum Press, New York, p 103

Tuteja R, Tuteja N, Lilliu F et al 1994 Y418C: A novel mutation in exon 9 of the glucocerebrosidase gene of a patient with Gaucher disease creates a new Bgl I site. Hum Genet 94: 314–315

Tybulewicz V L J, Tremblay M L, LaMarca M E et al 1992 Animal model of Gaucher disease from targeted disruption of the mouse glucocerebrosidase gene. Nature 357: 407–410
Uchiyama A, Tomatsu S, Kondo N et al 1994 New Gaucher disease mutations in exon 10: A novel L444R mutation produces a new *Nci*I site the same as L444P. Hum Mol Genet 3: 1183–1184
Uyama E, Takahashi K, Owada M et al 1992 Hydrocephalus, corneal opacities, deafness, valvular heart disease, deformed toes and leptomeningeal fibrous thickening in adult siblings: A new syndrome associated with beta-glucocerebrosidase deficiency and a mosaic population of storage cells. Acta Neurol Scand 86: 407–420
Walley A J, Harris A 1993 A novel point mutation (D380A) and a rare deletion (1255del55) in the glucocerebrosidase gene causing Gaucher disease. Hum Mol Genet 2: 1737–1738
Wigderson M, Firon N, Horowitz Z et al 1989 Characterization of mutations in Gaucher patients by cDNA cloning. Am J Hum Genet 44: 365–377
Wilson E R, Barton N W, Barranger J A 1985 Vascular involvement in type 3 neuronopathic Gaucher disease. Arch Pathol Lab Med 64: 82–84
Winkelman M D, Banker B Q, Victor M et al 1983 Non-infantile, non-neuronopathic Gaucher disease: A clinicopathologic study. Neurology 33: 994–1008
Yosipovitch Z, Katz K 1990 Bone crisis in Gaucher disease—An update. Isr J Med Sci 26: 593–595
Young K R 1985 Obstetric aspects of Gaucher disease. Br J Obstet Gynaecol 92: 993–996
Zevin S, Abrahamov A, Hadas-Halpern I et al 1993a Adult-type Gaucher disease in children: Genetics, clinical features and enzyme replacement therapy. Quart J Med 86: 565–573
Zimran A, Horowitz M 1994 RecTL: A complex allele of the glucocerebrosidase gene associated with a mild clinical course of Gaucher disease. Am J Med Genet 50: 74–78
Zimran A, Sorge J, Gross E et al 1989 Prediction of severity of Gaucher disease by identification of mutations at DNA level. Lancet 2: 349–352
Zimran A, Sorge J, Gross E et al 1990a A glucocerebrosidase fusion gene in Gaucher disease. Implications for the molecular anatomy, pathogenesis and diagnosis of this disorder. J Clin Invest 85: 219–222
Zimran A, Gelbart T, Beutler E 1990b Linkage of the Pvu II polymorphism with the common Jewish mutation for Gaucher disease. Am J Hum Genet 46: 902–905
Zimran A, Kay A C, Gelbart T et al 1992a Gaucher disease: Clinical, laboratory, radiologic and genetic features of 53 patients. Medicine (Baltimore) 71: 337–353
Zimran A, Abrahamov A, Goldberg M et al 1992b Home treatment with intravenous enzyme replacement therapy for patients with Gaucher disease. Blood 80 (Suppl. 1): 428a
Zimran A, Abrahamov A, Gross-Tsur V et al 1993a A unique form of Gaucher disease in Arabs characterized by oculomotor apraxia and valvular heart disease. Second International Duodecim Symposium, Finland 107
Zimran A, Abrahamov A, Aker M et al 1993b Correction of neutrophil chemotaxis defect in patients with Gaucher disease by low-dose enzyme replacement therapy. Am J Hematol 43: 69–71
Zimran A, Elstein D, Kannai R et al 1994b Low-dose enzyme replacement therapy for Gaucher disease: Effects of age, sex, genotype, and clinical features on response to treatment. Am J Med 97: 3–13
Zimran A, Elstein D, Shiffman R et al 1995 A reappraisal of partial splenectomy in type I Gaucher disease—a collaborative long-term followup study of 24 patients. J Pediatr: 126: 596–597
Zlotogora J, Sagi M, Zeigler M et al 1989 Gaucher disease type I and pregnancy. Am J Med Genet 32: 475–477

6

Treatment of acute myeloid leukaemia in elderly patients

M. Baudard   R. Zittoun

Most of the first reports on treatment results in acute myeloid leukaemia (AML) dealt with patients less than 60 years of age. Nowadays a review of the literature, with many published studies on elderly patients, gives a better picture of the epidemiological reality of AML. Better knowledge of the drugs available and of their side effects, development of new therapeutic agents and improvement of supportive care have reduced the initial reluctance of physicians to treat elderly AML patients.

The incidence of AML increases with age and more than 55% of AML patients are aged 60 years or more at time of diagnosis (Brincker 1985, Cartwright & Staines 1992). Because of the current ageing of our populations and since more elderly patients are referred to specialized departments than previously, the management of elderly AML patients constitutes a major challenge for haemato-oncologists. Prognosis is poorer in elderly than in younger patients, both when achievement of complete remission (CR) and overall survival are considered (Swirsky et al 1986, Preisler et al 1987, Zittoun et al 1989, Tucker et al 1990, Wahlin et al 1991). The introduction of induction regimens combining an anthracycline with cytosine arabinoside has led to an improvement in the results of treatment in young adult AML patients. In older patients treatment dose intensity remains a matter of controversy and therapeutic attitudes vary from high-dose chemotherapy to palliative treatment.

The main objectives of this chapter are:

1. To report the results of current conventional induction in elderly patients and the attempts to overcome marked treatment toxicity and leukaemia resistance, which are characteristic of this age-group

2. To highlight the influence of patient selection on treatment results

3. To address the question of whether poor prognosis in elderly patients is caused by peculiar leukaemic cell properties or host-related factors

4. To review therapeutic alternatives and to address the role of palliative care especially in patients with smouldering AML.

CONVENTIONAL INDUCTION IN ELDERLY PATIENTS

Correlation between age and treatment results

Despite the discrepancies from one study to another, the results of conventional chemotherapeutic induction are clearly poorer in AML patients aged 60 years or more than in younger patients, both when achievement of CR and overall survival (Fig. 1) and are considered. Current combinations of cytosine arabinoside (AraC) and an anthracycline yield CR in 65–75% of patients less than 60 years of age (Gale & Foon 1986, Vogler et al 1992, Wiernik et al 1992, Cassileth et al 1993). A few authors reported similar CR rates in older patients (Reiffers et al 1980, Foon et al 1981, Lui Yin 1988, Hutchinson et al 1992) but in most larger studies and cooperative group trials only 40–50% of elderly patients enter CR, with most of the CR (80%) being achieved after a single

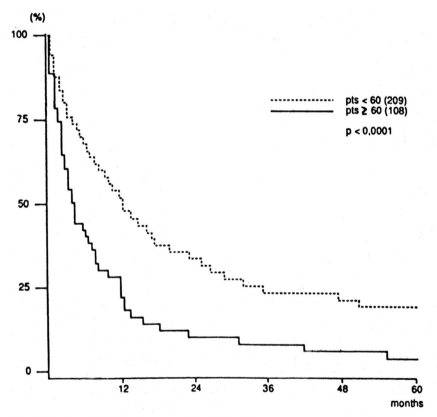

Fig. 1 Overall survival following conventional induction treatment: comparison between elderly and younger patients. In the study by Baudard et al (1994), the overall survival of 108 consecutive elderly patients who received conventional chemotherapeutic induction has been compared to that of 209 patients aged less than 60 years admitted to the same department during the same 10 year period. (Reproduced with permission from Baudard et al (1994), p 85, Fig. 2.)

Table 1. Recent large studies on conventional induction regimen in elderly AML patients

References	Age (years)	No. of patients	% CR	% ED*	Median CR duration (months)	Median survival duration (months)
Büchner et al (1985)	60–78	143	51	33	13	-
Rees et al (1986)	≥60	305	47	-	-	-
Preisler et al (1987)	>60	104	41	-	11.6	3.6
Zittoun et al (1989)	60–65	77	53	27	-	-
Arlin et al (1990)	≥60	99	41	10	7.7–9.9	1.7–3.3
Tucker et al (1990)	60–76	88	28	48	12	2
Stein et al (1990)	60–86	194	38	-	-	-
Dillman et al (1991)	60–83	100	41	27	-	2.5
Löwenberg et al (1991)	>60	407	45	14	-	7.5
Vogler et al (1992)	>60	111	57	-	-	6.9–7.8
Wiernik et al (1992)	>60	83	46	-	-	3.4
Johnson et al (1993)	60–81	104	58	11	11**	9
Rowe et al (1993)	55–70	118	54	17	-	4.5–10.8
Baudard et al (1994)	60–94	108	33	21	9.7**	3.5
Stone et al (1994)	≥60	347	51	26	-	-

*median disease free survival
CR, complete remission, ED, early death

induction course (Table 1). About 30% of the elderly patients die within the induction period (either before completion of chemotherapy administration or during treatment-related hypoplasia) and 15–25% survive without entering CR. As for CR rate there is a broad variability in reported treatment-related death rates, from 11% (Johnson et al 1993) to 48% (Tucker et al 1990).

Several studies have highlighted the significant relationship between increasing age and decreased probability of attaining CR, with a CR rate of 42–52% in the 60–69 year age group and of less than 30% in patients aged 70 or more (Swirsky et al 1986, Rees et al 1986, Baudard et al 1994). There is a particularly marked drop of CR rate (7%) and a high mortality rate (43%) in patients aged 75 or more (Baudard et al 1994). Whereas many patients more than 75 or 80 years should be excluded from intensive chemotherapy, conventional induction may be beneficial to elderly patients between 60 and 70 years of age. However, physicians are confronted by two major problems: increased patient vulnerability and greater resistance to chemotherapy in this age group compared with younger patients.

Attempts to reduce the toxicity of conventional induction

A main concern in the design of induction treatment for elderly patients is the dose intensity of anthracyclines. The dose of daunorubicin (DNR) administered to elderly patients ranges from 30 to 70 mg/m^2/day for 3 days. Since Yates et al (1982) and Kahn et al (1984) demonstrated that DNR dose reduction resulted in lower induction death rate and better overall survival in elderly patients without compromising the probability of CR, an attenuated DNR dose (30–45 mg/m^2/day for 3 days) has been adopted in most subsequent protocols for patients over 60 years of age. However, when dosage is reduced, treatment may become inadequate. The high proportion of patients, reported in recent studies, surviving induction without entering CR might partly be the result of reduced treatment efficacy secondary to a decrease in DNR dose. Therefore, reduction of DNR dose has not been adopted universally and, in some trials, elderly patients have received doses similiar to those administered to younger patients.

Substitution of DNR by other intercalating agents, which might have a better therapeutic index, has been evaluated. DNR is preferred over doxorubicin because of its reduced toxicity especially to the gastro-intestinal tract (Yates et al 1982). Amsacrine and aclarubicine did not prove to be superior to DNR (Stein et al 1990, Montastruc et al 1990). Zorubicine might be as effective as DNR and less toxic, especially to the mucous membranes and heart, and therefore be beneficial in elderly patients (Marty et al 1987). Compared with DNR, idarubicin may induce higher CR rates but mainly in patients younger than 60 years of age (Wiernik et al 1992, Berman 1993) and the role of the oral form of idarubicin has still to be defined (Harousseau et al 1989). At present, mitoxantrone, an anthracedione, seems to be the more promising drug. In several comparative studies, CR rate was higher in patients receiving mitoxantrone than in those administered DNR (Arlin et al 1990, Löwenberg et al 1991); mitoxantrone-containing regimens may also be associated with a shorter median time to CR, a lower need for supportive care, a longer remission duration and a longer survival (Arlin et al 1990). The toxicity of mitoxantrone compared to DNR is still open to question (Löwenberg et al 1991, Johnson & Liu Yin 1993).

Major improvements in supportive care have resulted in improved tolerance of induction-related myelosuppression. The possibility of accelerating the recovery of normal haemopoiesis with recombinant colony stimulating factors (CSFs) has been evaluated since the late 1980s. In most trials CSF therapy reduced the duration of neutropenia by a few days (Estey 1994). For example, in a recent large double-blind comparison between GM-CSF and placebo in 388 patients aged 60 or more (Stone et al 1995) the median duration of neutropenia was slightly shorter ($P=0.02$) in the patients who received GM-CSF (15 days) than in those who received placebo (17 days); no difference in the rate of documented infections was observed. Since, in vitro, some CSFs increase the fraction of leukaemic cells in S-phase (targets for AraC) and might also affect intracellular drug pharmacology favourably (Löwenberg & Touw 1993), the question of whether CSFs might enhance treatment efficacy has also been raised. However, no significant influence on CR rate, CR duration or survival duration has been demonstrated so far except in the study of Dombret et al (1995). In some cases GM-CSF and G-CSF enhance blast cell proliferation in vitro without promoting leukaemic cell differentiation; therefore the innocuousness of CSF administration has been questioned. In many of the cases where growth factor administration could have been responsible for accelerated leukaemic regrowth abrogation of CSF treatment reversed the effect (Löwenberg & Touw 1993). Therefore, the real benefit of CSF administration is difficult to assess. More studies are needed, especially with regard to the optimum timing of CSF administration (before, during or after induction administration).

Attempts to overcome leukaemia resistance

'High'-dose (3 g/m^2 twice daily for 4–5 days, Lazarus et al 1989), 'attenuated high-dose' (1.5 g/m^2 or 2.0 g/m^2 twice daily for 4 days, Kahn et al 1989) or 'intermediate-dose' (500 mg/m^2 twice daily for 6 days, Letendre et al 1989) AraC have been used in AML to overcome resistance, but their major toxicity limits their use in elderly patients, who are particularly at risk of neurotoxicity. In contrast to younger patients, the addition of etoposide to a DNR-AraC combination appears to be of no advantage in the elderly (Bishop et al 1990); addition of vincristine or thioguanine has also not proved to be effective (Büchner et al 1985, Rees et al 1986). However, these issues remain controversial. For example, Shepherd et al (1993) reported a high CR rate (78%) and a relatively low treatment toxicity in 23 patients aged 60 or more who received a combination of intermediate dose AraC (1.5 g/m^2 per day for 3 days) combined with mitoxantrone and etoposide.

AML resistance may be the result of overexpression of the P-glycoprotein (P-gp), a transmembrane protein encoded by the multidrug resistance MDR1 gene and capable of pumping out cytostatic drugs from the cytosol (Campos et al 1992). The prognostic value of P-gp expression in term of induction results has been established (Marie et al 1991, Wood et al 1994). The reversion of the multidrug resistance phenotype by P-gp antagonists such as verapamil or cyclosporine derivatives is currently being assessed in clinical trials. However, the side effects of these compounds, especially cardiac and renal, might preclude their use in elderly patients.

POST-REMISSION TREATMENT IN ELDERLY PATIENTS: ONE MORE DILEMMA

Once CR is achieved, the same difficult choice between intensive treatment with increased risk of life threatening side effects and less aggressive therapy with the risk of decreased efficacy arises. Studies on post-remission approaches in elderly patients are sparse and contradictory. In younger patients, high-dose chemotherapeutic regimens or bone marrow transplantation offer the best chance of long-term survival and cure. Allogeneic bone marrow transplantation or myeloablative therapy with autologous stem cell support are hardly feasible in patients over 60 years of age. Because of major toxicity in elderly patients, high-dose AraC-containing regimens do not demonstrate significant benefit compared with less aggressive regimens (Mayer et al 1992). Intensive induction-type consolidation may be of benefit for some selected elderly patients (Cassileth et al 1984, Liu Yin et al 1991, Jehn 1994); however, it is still unclear what intensity should be given and how many cycles of consolidation are required. The administration of haemopoietic growth factors may improve tolerance to intensive consolidation regimens. Continuous maintenance chemotherapy based on prolonged administration of AraC and 6-thioguanine offers little or no benefit if conventional induction and consolidation have been administered. However, in elderly patients unable to tolerate intensive consolidation, administration of remission maintenance chemotherapy may delay leukaemia relapse and prolong survival duration (Büchner et al 1985, Cassileth et al 1988, Champlin et al 1989, Montastruc et al 1990). The value of low-dose AraC for maintenance treatment is currently being assessed by the EORTC group: it might prolong the remission duration but not the overall survival (Suciu, personal communication). Differentiating and/or immunomodulating agents could be part of maintenance regimens. For example, bestatin, an immunomodulating agent, might be a helpful adjuvant to standard maintenance chemotherapy in elderly patients (Ota & Ogawa 1990). The side effects of other agents such as interleukin 2 given to promote an immune-mediated suppression of residual leukaemic cells (Prentice et al 1993), might limit its utilization in elderly patients for example.

Figure 2 illustrates results commonly reported in the literature: once CR has been achieved there is no significant difference in DFS between elderly and younger patients, despite a trend for a shorter DFS in the elderly. This trend is probably explained by a higher incidence of death among elderly patients during the remission period, whereas CR duration seems independent of age (Foon et al 1981, Cevreska & Gale 1987, Wahlin et al 1991). However, CR duration in elderly patients varies, according to studies, from 8 to 16 months, with a median of 10.5 months (Johnson 1992), and increasing age adversely affects the CR duration in some studies (Rees et al 1986, Walters et al 1987, Zittoun et al 1989). This may be partly explained by extended use of intensive post-remission treatment in patients less than 60 years of age, whereas less than 60% of elderly patients who achieve CR undergo such post-remission treatment (Bassan et al 1992). Moreover, post-remission programmes are rarely completed in elderly patients because of poor tolerance and/or compliance; they should be designed case by case according to the patient's clinical, biological and psychosocial background. The development of markers of the residual leukaemia might help to adapt treatment risks to required efficacy and expected result.

STUDIES ON TREATMENT RESULTS IN THE ELDERLY ARE NOT ALWAYS CONCLUSIVE

There is a broad variation in conventional induction results in the elderly from one study to another when CR rate as well as CR duration and overall survival are considered (Table 1). The definition of 'elderly' patients differs between studies, with an age limit ranging from 50 to 70 years. Age by itself is a major

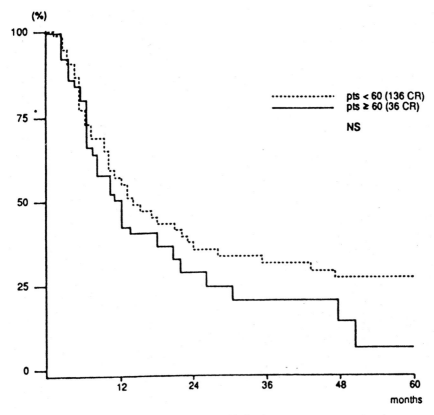

Fig. 2 Disease-free survival following conventional induction treatment: comparison between elderly and younger patients. In the study by Baudard et al (1994), 33.3% of the 108 consecutive elderly patients who received conventional induction achieved CR compared with 65.4% of the 209 younger patients admitted during the same period of time. Comparison of DFS between elderly and younger patients did not reveal any significant difference despite a trend for a shorter DFS in the elderly. (Reproduced with permission from Baudard et al (1994), p 85, Fig. 1.)

prognostic factor for response to therapy and patient outcome (Keating et al 1988, Zittoun et al 1989), and variability in the age of patients complicates comparison between different studies. Extensive series of unselected cohorts of elderly patients are rare. Advanced age reduces the probability of referral; the proportion of referred patients who receive conventional induction decreases with increasing age (from 87% in patients aged less than 60 years to 74% in patients aged 60–64 and to 19% in patients aged over 75 (Baudard et al 1994). The impact of sample size on results is also critical. For example, in 1988 Lui Yin reported an impressive CR rate of 65% in 29 patients over 60 years of age receiving a mitoxantrone-AraC combination. The subsequent inclusion of 75 more patients in the study resulted in a CR rate decrease to 58% (Johnson & Liu Yin 1993). Moreover, in most large studies, reported CR rates are lower than those observed in small series. Detailed patient eligibility criteria and pretreatment characteristics, especially the incidence of adverse prognostic factors, are not always reported. Elderly patients at higher risk are frequently excluded from remission induction evaluation either because treatment-related toxicity is judged intolerable or life expectancy is thought to be short. Several studies illustrate how selection bias may lead to optimization of published treatment results (Brincker 1985, The Toronto Leukaemia Study Group 1986, Wahlin et al 1991). In our Department, only 36% of elderly patients entered ongoing EORTC randomized trials (Baudard et al 1994). This inclusion rate was lower than expected according to the eligibility criteria. Enrolled patients presented with a significantly better physical condition and lower mean age, the incidence of MDS-AML was also statistically lower in the group of patients included in trials than in patients treated without inclusion in any kind of trial. Since there was no age limit and no restriction regarding antecedent MDS.

Difference in patient age and variations in patterns of patient selection from one study to another, small patient samples and absence of randomization in the design of some trials constitute confusing parameters which make comparisons of treatment outcome difficult.

CUMULATION OF POOR PROGNOSTIC HOST-RELATED FACTORS AND LEUKAEMIC CELL CHARACTERISTICS IN ELDERLY AML PATIENTS

Elderly patient specificities

Treatment of elderly AML patients demands recognition of many factors unique to elderly patients which cannot be exhaustively listed. We will just mention three critical factors.

Age-related changes in pharmacological parameters may contribute to increased treatment toxicity (Balducci et al 1989). Absorption and presystemic metabolism are, to a large extent, unchanged in the elderly. An age-associated decrease of serum albumin concentration may increase the bioavailability of protein-bound antineoplastic agents. The frequent increase of body fat/lean mass ratio and decrease of total body water which occur with age modify the volume of distribution and elimination half life of lipid- and water-soluble drugs. Finally, changes in hepatic metabolism and a progressive decline of renal function, the most important change associated with ageing, may reduce the clearance of major chemotherapeutic agents.

Almost 50% of elderly AML patients have a poor physical condition at the time of diagnosis, compared with one-third of younger patients (Baudard et al 1994). Poor performance status is a major adverse prognostic factor for induction results and patient outcome, limiting treatment possibilities (Rees et al 1986, Swirsky et al 1986, Sebban et al 1988, Copplestone & Prentice 1988). Such poor performance status, together with concomitant disease, increase the risk of toxicity and side effects of induction treatment and decrease the patient's ability to overcome the complications resulting from myelosuppression (Preisler et al 1987, Zittoun et al 1989). The incidence of concomitant disorders is rarely reported; in a recent series, 62% of elderly patients suffered from chronic diseases requiring specific therapeutic intervention (Bassan et al 1992).

Finally, a comparison between healthy elderly and younger subjects shows that steady-state haemopoiesis is not demonstrably impaired in elderly patients. However, the pool size of myeloid precursors appears smaller than in younger patients, and there is an impairment in the haemopoietic response to increased demand. This may contribute to the increased toxicity experienced by elderly subjects treated with cytotoxic chemotherapy (Lipschitz et al 1984). Other differences such as reduced growth factor secretion, changes in haemopoietic precursor metabolism or in the bone marrow microenvironment, may contribute to the decline of haemopoietic resources with age.

Biological characteristics of AML in the elderly

The question of whether AML in the elderly is a distinct biological entity from that seen in younger individuals has been repeatedly raised (Heinemann & Jehn 1991, Ballester et al 1992, Johnson & Liu Yin 1993). Several biological differences have been commonly reported.

The incidence of AML secondary to occupational exposure to leukaemogenic agents or to therapy or chemotherapy is higher in elderly patients, and AML with a preceding haematological disorder, in particular myelodysplasia (MDS), may include 50% of AML cases in the elderly, compared with 15% in younger patients (Hamblin 1992). Trilineage myelodysplasia is seen at the time of diagnosis in 10–20% of adults with de novo AML (Hast & Widell 1992, Kuriyama et al 1994). According to Hast & Widell, dysplastic features are more pronounced among elderly compared to younger de novo AML patients; however, Kuriyama et al did not find any correlation between age and incidence of trilineage myelodysplasia in primary AML. Treatment results are poorer in AML secondary to MDS, and in primary AML with MDS features, than in de novo AML: the CR rate is lower, remission duration and survival duration shorter, and treatment-related myelosuppression more severe and prolonged. This might be the result of unfavourable MDS-AML cell characteristics (increased expression of P-gp, involvement of a very early precursor, poor prognosis cytogenetics, proliferation dysregulation, etc.) (Sato et al 1990, San Miguel et al 1991, Masuya et al 1993).

Cytogenetic abnormalities are found in the leukaemic cells of 45–65% of AML patients regardless of age group. Abnormalities to which poor prognostic value for achievement of CR and/or CR or survival durations has been attributed (complete or partial deletion of chromosome 5 and/or 7, trisomy 8) are found more commonly in elderly patients. In contrast, the incidence of abnormal karyotypes carrying a better prognosis (t(8;21), t(15;17), inversion of chromosome 16) is higher in younger patients (Keating et al 1988, Schiffer et al 1989, Baudard et al 1994).

Malignant transformation has been considered to arise at an earlier stage of the differentiation pathway in elderly patients than in younger patients, with resulting clonal involvement of remaining mature cells and reduced numbers of normal residual haemopoietic clones capable of providing an adequate recovery from treatment-related myelosuppression (Fialkow et al 1987). Clonal remission, whose incidence is higher in the elderly (Fialkow et al 1987, 1991) could correspond to the persistence of the abnormal clone throughout remission, this 'preleukaemic clone' being capable of normal differentiation.

Compared to blasts of younger patients, elderly patient's leukaemic cells show fewer cytological and cytochemical features of differentiation: e.g. fewer Auer rods and granulocytes, and a lower maturation index (Hassan & Rees 1990). A higher incidence of differentiated leukaemia subtypes (AML3 and AML5b) has been commonly reported in younger patients (Mertelsmann et al 1980, Hassan & Rees 1990). With regard to haemoglobin level, WBC count, platelet rate, or bone marrow blast infiltration we did not find in our series (Baudard et al 1994) differences reported by others between the two age groups (Beguin et al 1985).

In vitro growth features and cytokinetics are predictive factors for patient outcome (Delmer et al 1989, Raza et al 1990). Giannoulis et al (1984) found that a poor prognosis in vitro growth pattern (such as excessive leukaemic cell cluster growth) was statistically more frequent in elderly patients but this has not been consistently confirmed (Delmer et al 1989, Löwenberg & Touw 1993). Elderly AML patients might have a higher proportion of leukaemic cells in the S+G2M phase and more rapidly cycling cells (with a shorter total cell cycle time and duration of S phase); earlier relapse in elderly patients may be caused by more rapid regrowth of leukaemic cells (Kantarjian et al 1985, Raza et al 1990). The in vitro sensitivity of CFU-L to anthracycline drugs and AraC, the antigenic phenotype of the leukaemic myeloblasts, the incidence of ras proto-oncogene mutations, and the MDR1 gene expression are all predictive parameters (Delmer et al 1989, Bradstock et al 1994, Neubauer et al 1994, Wood et al 1994). So far, however, no correlation with age has been demonstrated for these biological characteristics (Ballester et al 1992, Zhou et al 1992, Neubauer et al 1994, Baudard et al 1994).

In summary, the two most commonly reported differences of the leukaemic process in the elderly compared to younger patients, are the higher incidence of a previous haematological disorder and/or trilineage myelodysplasia and the unfavourable cytogenetics. This is of major importance since these two factors are known to be associated with a poorer outcome. Further investigations are needed to evaluate the role of leukaemia- and host-related factors.

ALTERNATIVES TO CONVENTIONAL INDUCTION

Differentiating agents represent an attractive alternative to standard myeloablative treatments

Daily administration of low dose (LD)-AraC (20 mg/m^2/day) in elderly patients induces response (CR or partial response) in 28% (Powell et al 1989) to 59% (Shtalrid et al 1987, Sebban et al 1988) of patients (Table 2). Comparing LD-AraC and conventional induction in elderly patients, Tilly et al (1990) found a similar response rate (54%) in the two groups of patients. CR rate was significantly lower in patients receiving LD-AraC (32 versus 52%), but as a consequence of the low LD-AraC-related death rate (10%) and of the long survival demonstrated by some partial responders, the overall survival in the LD-AraC group was close to that observed in patients administered conventional induction. In this series, the incidence and severity of infectious complications and transfusion requirement were lower and hospital stay shorter in the LD-AraC group. In the more recent series of Detourmignies et al (1993) LD-AraC induced a response in only 38% of the cases. Prolonged survival for partial LD-AraC responders was a rare event; 86% of patients experienced severe pancytopenia and the benefit of LD-AraC in terms of quality of life was questioned. The high incidence of myelosuppression shows that LD-AraC acts more through an ablative mechanism than through differentiation. The use of LD-AraC might compromise CR achievement and therefore shorten survival in elderly patients able to receive more myeloablative treatments. In contrast, LD-AraC is an alternative choice in patients with the greatest risk of intensive induction toxicity, namely patients with poor physical condition and advanced comorbid disease. Patients with unfavourable cytogenetic abnormalities respond poorly to conventional induction and may be better served by less aggressive approaches; however, they also demonstrate poor response to LD-AraC (Fenaux et al 1990). In a small series of patients with poor prognosis AML, 5-Aza-2'-deoxycitidine (Decitabine), a new cytosine analogue, induced a response in 40% of patients (Petti et al 1993).

The efficacy of retinoic acid as a treatment of acute promyelocytic leukaemia (AML M3) is well demonstrated. In a phase II study, this differentiating agent was administered to 18 elderly AML patients (only one of these cases being an AML3); no objective responses were observed (Kramer et al 1991). Several other agents may induce leukaemic cell differentiation in vitro: dimethyl sulfoxide, phorbol esters, gamma interferon, 1.25 dihydroxyvitamin D3, tumor necrosis factor-alpha, GM-CSF, hexamethylene bisacetamide (HMBA) etc. Some of these compounds will probably never be used clinically

Table 2. Low-dose AraC in elderly patients with newly diagnosed AML

References	Patients n	CR n(%)	PR n(%)	ED n(%)
Shtalrid et al (1987)	115	50(43)	18(16)	-
Sebban et al (1988)	22	5(23)	8(36)	2(9)
Powell et al (1989)	44	10(23)	2(5)	11(25)
Fenaux et al (1990)	40	8(20)	8(20)	9(23)
Tilly et al (1990)	41	13(32)	9(22)	4(10)
Detourmignies et al (1993)	77	13(17)	16(21)	20(26)
	339	99(29)	61(18)	46(21)

CR, complete remission; PR, partial remission; ED, early death because of their toxicity. Some have already been evaluated in phase II trial, for example HMBA, which induced some response in MDS and AML patients with morphological and cytogenetic evidence of blast differentiation (Andreef et al 1992).

Given the heterogeneity of AML, it is possible that only a subset of patients would respond to a given agent. Better knowledge of leukaemic cell biology should help to find a real differentiating agent which could be administered in place of conventional induction or be useful as adjuvant to induction and/or post-remission regimens.

Alternative myeloablative treatments

A mitoxantrone-etoposide combination could be an effective therapy. In a study by Rotche et al (1994), CR was achieved in 8 of 16 poor prognosis AML patients (15 being aged 60 or more) and Knauf et al (1994) reported a response rate of 66% in MDS-AML patients (median age: 56, range 28–67 years). Other different chemotherapeutic combinations could have a good therapeutic index: continuous infusion of DNR+carboplatin, epirubicin+VCR, fludarabine+AraC or VP16+IDAraC combinations, for example (Liso et al 1990, Archimbaud et al 1992, Gandhi 1993, Johnston et al 1994). The real therapeutic value of these regimens is still difficult to assess since most studies have been run in single centres, in poor prognosis AML (refractory, relapsed, secondary AML), on a limited number of patients and without randomized comparison with conventional induction.

The 'wait and see' strategy

In an European Organization for Research and Treatment of Cancer (EORTC) randomized trial overall survival was longer in elderly patients receiving conventional induction than in patients with treatment restricted to supportive care and palliative chemotherapy (Löwenberg et al 1989). In contrast, in the study by Bassan et al (1992) aggressive induction administration at diagnosis did not improve overall survival because of a high early death rate. Owing to increased chemotherapy toxicity, some physicians have advocated a systematic 'wait and see' strategy in elderly patients. However, mean hospital stay, transfusion requirement and quality of life of patients with treatment restricted to palliative care might not differ significantly from those of patients treated aggressively.

In practice, treatment is restricted to supportive and/or palliative care in about 25% of elderly patients because of patient- and/or family- and/or attending physician decision; median survival duration of these patients ranges from 0.8 months to 2 months depending on the study. Some elderly AML patients may show few clinical symptoms and have a prolonged survival owing to the 'smouldering' course of their disease (Rheingold et al, 1963). The actual incidence of this smouldering variant of AML is probably low, less than 5% in our experience. Smouldering AML are characterized by a good performance status at presentation, a low WBC and low circulating blast counts, a higher platelets count, a lower bone marrow blast proportion, and, more importantly, a lower incidence of abnormal karyotypes and a decreased leukaemic cell in vitro growth (Zittoun & Baudard, personal observation). In these patients, palliative chemotherapy (6-thioguanine, etoposide, etc) may be efficient enough to stop or slow down the disease evolution until the occurrence of a transformation into a more proliferative variant escaping therapeutic control.

Another important question concerns the optimum time for shifting from aggressive to palliative treatment in AML. A retrospective study from Neuss et al (1987) has identified several variables associated with adoption of palliative therapy, especially age, non-inclusion in a research protocol at presentation, female sex, absence of dependent children and secondary leukaemias. This study also highlighted that certain physicians were more likely to adopt palliative therapy than others; this questioned the weight of objective criteria and of patient preferences in the decision of abandoning aggressive treatment. The ability of elderly patients and their families to cope with the physical as well as the psychosocial impact of the disease and its treatment should remain a major factor in the medical decision.

PROGNOSTIC MODELS

A prognostic model which could help clinicians to select appropriate therapy is needed. Because most of the time, a medical decision cannot be delayed in acute leukaemia, criteria for treatment choice should be readily available at the time of presentation. However, in a second step, when biological data with assessed prognostic value (such as cytogenetic analysis, in vitro clonogenic assay, etc.) become available, the therapeutic attitude should be questioned and eventually modified. Age by itself appears to have the most consistent adverse prognostic value for response to therapy and has been incorporated into most prognostic models. Johnson et al (1993) developed a model based on four parameters (urea, performance status, peripheral blood blast count and presence of hepatomegaly) to select those elderly patients for whom intensive chemotherapy could be beneficial. According to this model aggressive treatment should not be administered if survival duration is thought to be less than 6 months. This kind of model predicting overall survival rather than remission rate may be more appropriate in elderly patients. Effective stabilization of disease, partial remission with long lasting survival may be enough to achieve worthwhile prolongation of life with an acceptable quality of life. Such a response may best be obtained without the need to expose elderly patients to the hazards of aggressive chemotherapy used in younger patients to achieve a complete remission. However, induction regimens similar to those used in patients 40–60 years old should be considered in patients aged 60–75, without adverse prognostic factors, when predicted survival duration is of 12 months or more. More studies will be needed to address the relevance of such prognostic models.

KEY POINTS FOR CLINICAL PRACTICE

- AML in the elderly is characterized by a cumulation of unfavourable host- and leukaemic cell-related features, which may explain both increased treatment toxicity and leukaemia resistance.

- Expected treatment results should be weighed against potential treatment toxicity, and treatment intensity and objectives should be tailored to patient characteristics.

- Current anthracycline-Ara-C combinations yield CR in 40–50% of patients aged 60 years or more, while 30% of the patients die within the induction period.

- Conventional chemotherapeutic induction (within a narrow range of anthracycline dose) could be the treatment of choice in patients less than 70–75 years of age with good performance status and absence of significant concomitant disease, particularly if cytogenetics are favourable and if haemopoiesis is not impaired by preceding or concomitant MDS.

- Patients with poor performance status and/or poor prognosis cytogenetic subtype may be better served by less aggressive approaches such as low-dose aracytine or 5-aza-cytidine, which could yield worthwhile haematological improvement, if not remission.

- In the few patients with true smouldering AML treatment should be limited to supportive and palliative care.

- Further improvement of supportive care, and eventually administration of haemopoietic growth factors are expected to improve treatment tolerance and to allow treatment intensification.

- Better understanding of the molecular biology of AML and of the mechanisms of drug resistance should help the development of alternative treatments.

- Patient's preferences and psychosocial background should not be neglected at the time of medical decision.

REFERENCES

Andreef M, Stone R, Michaeli J et al 1992 Hexamethylene bisacetamide in myelodysplastic syndrome and acute myelogenous leukemia: a phase II clinical trial with a differentiation-inducing agent. Blood 80: 2604–2609

Archimbaud E, Anglaret B, Thomas X et al 1992 Continuous-infusion daunorubicin and carboplatin for high-risk acute myeloid leukemia in the elderly. Leukemia 6: 776–779

Arlin Z, Case D, Moore J et al 1990 Randomized multicenter trial of cytosine arabinoside with mitoxantrone or daunorubicin in previously untreated adult patients with acute nonlymphocytic leukemia. Leukemia 4: 177–183

Balducci L, Parker M, Sexton W et al 1989 Pharmacology of antineoplastic agents in the elderly patients. Semin Oncol 16: 76–84

Ballester O, Moscinski L, Morris D et al 1992 Acute myelogenous leukemia in the elderly. JAGS 40: 277–284

Baudard M, Marie J P, Cadiou M et al 1994 Acute myelogenous leukaemia in the elderly: retrospective study of 235 consecutive patients. Br J Haematol 86: 82–91

Bassan R, Buelli M, Viero P et al 1992 The management of acute myelogenous leukemia in the elderly: ten-year experience in 118 patients. Hematol Oncol 10: 251–260

Beguin Y, Bury J, Fillet G et al 1985 Treatment of acute nonlymphocytic leukemia in young and elderly patients. Cancer 56: 2587–2592

Berman E 1993 A review of idarubicin in acute leukemia. Oncology 17: 91–98

Bishop J F, Lowenthal R M, Joshua D et al 1990 Etoposide in acute nonlymphocytic leukemia. Blood 75: 27–32 elogenous leukemia. A review. Leukemia 1: 575–579

Bradstock K, Matthews J, Benson E et al 1994 Prognostic value of immunophenotyping in acute myeloid leukemia. Blood 84: 1220–1225

Brincker H 1985 Estimate of overall treatment results in acute nonlymphocytic leukemia based on age-specific rates of incidence and of complete remission. Cancer Treat Rep 69: 5–11

Büchner T, Urbanitz D, Hiddemann W et al 1985 Intensified induction and consolidation with or without maintenance chemotherapy for acute myeloid leukemia (AML): two multicenter studies of the German AML Cooperative Group. J Clin Oncol 3: 1583–1589

Campos L, Guyotat D, Archimbaud E et al 1992 Clinical significance of multidrug resistance P-glycoprotein expression on acute nonlymphoblastic leukemia cells at diagnosis. Blood 79: 473–476

Cartwright R A, Staines A 1992 Acute leukemias. In: Fleming A T (ed) Epidemiology of haematological disease, part I. Bailliere's Clinical Haematology 5: 1–26

Cassileth P A, Begg C B, Bennett J M et al 1984 A randomized study of the efficacy of consolidation therapy in adult acute nonlymphocytic leukemia. Blood 63: 843–847

Cassileth P A, Harrington D P, Hines J D et al 1988 Maintenance chemotherapy prolongs remission duration in adult acute nonlymphocytic leukemia. J Clin Oncol 6: 583–587

Cassileth P A, Andersen J, Lazarus H M et al 1993 Autologous bone marrow transplant in acute myeloid leukemia in first remission. J Clin Oncol 11: 314–319

Cevreska L, Gale R P 1987 Prognostic factors in acute myelogenous leukemia. Hematol Blood Transf 30: 376–379

Champlin R E, Gajewski J L, Golde D W 1989 Treatment of acute myelogenous leukemia in the elderly. Semin Oncol 16: 51–56

Copplestone J A, Prentice A G 1988 Acute myeloblastic leukaemia in the elderly. Leukemia Res 12: 617–625

Delmer A, Marie J P, Thevenin D et al 1989 Multivariate analysis of prognostic factors in acute myeloid leukemia: value of clonogenic leukemic cell properties. J Clin Oncol 7: 738–746

Detourmignies L, Wattel E, Laï J L et al 1993 Is there still a role for low-dose cytosine arabinoside in de novo acute myeloid leukemia in the elderly? Ann Hematol 66: 235–240

Dillman R O, Davis R B, Green M R et al 1991 A comparative study of two different doses of cytarabine for acute myeloid leukemia: a phase III trial of Cancer and Leukemia group B. Blood 78: 2520–2526

Dombret H, Chotang C, Fenaux P et al 1995 A controlled study of recombitant human granulocyte colony-stimulating factor in elderly patients after treatment for acute myelogenous leukemia. N Engl J Med 332:1678-83

Estey E H 1994 Use of colony-stimulating factors in the treatment of acute myeloid leukemia. Blood 83: 2015–2019

Fenaux P, Lai J L, Gardin C et al 1990 Cytogenetics are a predictive factor of response to low dose ara-C in acute myelogenous leukemia (AML) in the elderly. Leukemia 4: 312

Fialkow P J, Singer J W, Raskind W H et al 1987 Clonal development, stem-cell differentiation, and clinical remissions in acute nonlymphocytic leukemia. N Engl J Med 317: 468–473

Fialkow P J, Janssen J W, Bartram C R 1991 Clonal remission in acute nonlymphocytic leukemia: evidence for a multistep pathogenesis of the malignancy. Blood 77: 1415–1417

Foon K A, Zighelboim J, Yale C et al 1981 Intensive chemotherapy is the treatment of choice for elderly patients with acute myelogenous leukemia. Blood 58: 467–470

Gale R P, Foon K A 1986 Acute myeloid leukaemia: recent advances in therapy. Clin Haematol 15: 781

Gandhi V 1993 Fludarabine for treatment of adult acute myelogenous leukemia. Leukemia and Lymphoma 11 (Suppl. 2): 7–13

Giannoulis N, Ogier C, Hast R et al 1984 Difference between young and old patients in characteristics of leukemic cells: older patients have cells growing excessively in vitro, with low antigenicity despite high HLA-DR antigens. Am J Hematol 16: 113–121

Hamblin T 1992 The treatment of acute myeloid leukaemia preceded by the myelodysplastic syndrome. Leukemia Res 16: 101–108

Harousseau J L, Rigal-Huguet F, Hurteloup P et al 1989 Treatment of acute myeloid leukemia in elderly patients with oral idarubicin as a single agent. Eur J Haematol 42: 182–185

Hassan H T, Rees J K H 1990 Relation between age and blast cell differentiation in acute myeloid leukaemia patients. Oncology 47: 439–442

Hast R, Widell S 1992 Dysplastic peripheral blood polymorphs link acute myeloblastic leukaemia in elderly to the myelodysplastic syndromes. Eur J Haematol 48: 163–167

Heinemann V, Jehn U 1991 Acute myeloid leukemia in the elderly: biological features and search for adequate treatment. Ann Hematol 63: 179–188

Hutchinson R M, Winfield D A 1992 Mitozantrone and cytosine arabinoside as first line therapy in elderly patients with acute myeloid leukaemia. Br J Haematol 80: 416–417

Jehn U 1994 Phase II-trial of double-consolidation following intensive induction treatment for improvement of survival in elderly patients with acute myeloid leukemia. Leukemia and Lymphoma 12: 435–440

Johnson P R E 1992 The biology and treatment of elderly patients with acute myeloid leukaemia. MD thesis, University of Aberdeen, Aberdeen

Johnson P R E, Liu Yin J A 1993 Acute myeloid leukaemia in the elderly: biology and treatment. Br J Haematol 83: 1–6

Johnson P R E, Hunt L P, Liu Yin J A 1993 Prognostic factors in elderly patients with acute myeloid leukaemia: development of a model to predict survival. Br J Haematol 85: 300–306

Johnston L, Damon L, Ries C et al 1994 High dose VP16 with intermediate dose Ara-C (IDAC) for high risk leukemia. Proc Annu Meet Am Soc Clin Oncol 13: A988

Kahn S B, Ebrahim K, Cassileth P et al 1989 Attenuated high-dose cytosine arabinoside in the treatment of the elderly patient with acute nonlymphocytic leukemia. Am J Clin Oncol 12: 201–204

Kahn S B, Begg C B, Mazza J et al 1984 Full dose versus attenuated dose daunorubicin, cytosine arabinoside and 6-thioguanine in the treatment of acute nonlymphocytic leukemia in the elderly. J Clin Oncol 2: 865–870

Kantarjian H M, Barlogie B, Keating M J et al 1985 Pretreatment cytokinetics in acute myelogenous leukemia: age-related prognostic implications. J Clin Invest 76: 319–324

Keating M J, Smith T L, Kantarjian H et al 1988 Cytogenetic pattern in acute myelogenous leukemia: a major reproducible determinant of outcome. Leukemia 2: 403–412

Knauf W U, Berdel W E, Ho A D et al 1994 Combination of mitoxantrone and etoposide in the treatment of myelodysplastic syndromes transformed into acute myeloid leukaemia. Leuk Lymph 12: 421–425

Kramer Z B, Boros L, Wiernik P H et al 1991 13-cis-retinoic acid in the treatment of elderly patients with acute myeloid leukemia. Cancer 67: 1484–1486

Kuriyama K, Tomonaga M, Matsuo T et al 1994 Poor response to intensive chemotherapy in de novo acute myeloid leukaemia with trilineage myelodysplasia. Br J Haematol 86: 767–773

Lazarus H M, Vogler W R, Burns C P et al 1989 High-dose cytosine arabinoside and daunorubicin as primary therapy in elderly patients with acute myelogenous leukemia. Cancer 63: 1055–1059

Letendre L, Niedringhaus R D, Therneau T M et al 1989 Treatment of acute nonlymphocytic leukemia in the elderly with intermediate high-dose cytosine arabinoside. Med Pediatr Oncol 17: 79–82

Lipschitz D A, Udupa K B, Milton K Y et al 1984 Effect of age on hematopoiesis in man. Blood 63: 502–509

Liso V, Specchia G, Pavone V et al 1990 Continuous infusion chemotherapy with epirubicin and vincristine in relapsed and refractory acute leukemia. Acta Haematol 83: 116–119

Liu Yin J A 1988 Mitozantrone in combination with ara-C for acute myeloid leukaemia in elderly patients. Proc 3rd UK Novantrone Syrup. Media Medica: 19

Liu Yin J A, Johnson P R E, Davies J M et al 1991 Mitozantrone and cytosine arabinoside as first-line therapy in elderly patients with acute myeloid leukaemia. Br J Haematol 79: 415–420

Löwenberg B, Touw I P 1993 Hematopoietic growth factors and their receptors in acute leukemia. Blood 81: 281–292

Löwenberg B, Zittoun R, Kerkhofs H et al 1989 On the value of intensive remission induction chemotherapy in elderly patients of 65 + years with acute myeloid leukemia: a randomized phase III study of the European Organisation for Research and treatment of Cancer Leukemia Group. J Clin Oncol 7: 1268–1274

Löwenberg B, Fiere D, Zittoun R et al 1991 Mitoxantron versus daunorubicin in induction of acute myelogenous leukaemia in elderly patients and low dose Ara-C versus control as maintenance. An EORTC phase III trial (AML-9). Haematologica 76 (Suppl.4): abstract 353

Marie J P, Zittoun R, Sikic B I 1991 Multidrug resistance: (mdr1) gene expression in adult acute leukemias: correlations with treatment outcome and in vitro drug sensitivity. Blood 78: 586–592

Marty M, Gisselbrecht C, Schaison G et al 1987 Place de la zorubicine dans le traitement des leucémies aiguës myéloïdes. Path Biol 35: 133

Masuya M, Kita K, Shimizu N et al 1993 Biologic characteristics of acute leukemia after myelodysplastic syndrome. Blood 81: 3388–3394

Mayer R J, Davis R B, Schiffer C A et al 1992 Comparative evaluation of intensive post-remission therapy with difference dose schedules of ara-c in adults with acute myeloid leukemia (AML): initial results of a CALGB phase III study. Proc Am Soc Clin Oncol 11: 261 (A853)

Mertelsmann R, Thaler H T, To L et al 1980 Morphological classification, response to therapy and survival in 263 adult patients with acute non-lymphoblastic leukaemia. Blood 56: 773

Montastruc M, Reiffers J, Stoppa A M et al 1990 Treatment of acute myeloid leukemia in elderly patients: the influence of maintenance therapy (BGM 84 protocol). Nouv Rev Fr Hematol 32: 147–152

Neubauer A, Dodge R K, George S L et al 1994 Prognostic importance of mutations in the *ras* proto-oncogenes in de novo acute myeloid leukemia. Blood 83: 1603–1611

Neuss M N, Feussner J R, De Long E R et al 1987 A quantitative analysis of palliative care decisions in acute nonlymphocytic leukemia. J Am Geriatr Soc 35: 125–131

Ota K, Ogawa N 1990 Randomized controlled study of chemoimmunotherapy with bestatin of acute nonlymphocytic leukemia in adults. Biomed Pharmacother 44: 93–102

Petti M C, Mandelli F, Zagonel V et al 1993 Pilot study of 5-aza-2'-deoxycytidine (Decitabine) in the treatment of poor prognosis acute myelogenous leukemia patients: preliminary results. Leukemia 7 (Suppl. 1): 36–41

Powell B, Capizzi R, Muss H B et al 1989 Low-dose Ara-C therapy for acute myelogenous leukemia in elderly patients. Leukemia 3: 23–28

Preisler H, Davis R B, Kirshner J et al 1987 Comparison of three remission induction regimens and two postinduction strategies for the treatment of acute nonlymphocytic leukemia: a Cancer and Leukemia Group B study. Blood 69: 1441–1449

Prentice H G, Macdonald I D, Hamon M D 1993 The role of immunotherapy in the treatment of acute myeloblastic leukemia: from allogeneic bone marrow transplantation to the application of interleukin 2. Cancer Treat Res: 121–134

Raza A, Preisler H D, Day R et al 1990 Direct relationship between remission duration in acute myeloid leukemia and cell cycle kinetics: a leukemia intergroup study. Blood 76: 2191–2197

Rees J K H, Gray R G, Swirski D et al 1986 Principal results of the Medical Research Council's 8th acute myeloid leukemia trial. Lancet ii: 1236–1241

Reiffers J, Raynal F, Broustet A 1980 Acute myeloblastic leukaemia in elderly patients. Cancer 45: 2816–2820

Rheingold J J, Kaufman R, Adelson E et al 1963 Smoldering acute leukaemia. N Engl J Med 268: 812–815

Rotche R, Stadtmauer E A, Luger S et al 1994 Mitoxantrone and etoposide: an effective induction regimen for poor prognosis acute myeloid leukemia (AML). Proc Annu Meet Am Soc Clin Oncol 13: A994

Rowe J M, Andersen J, Mazza J J et al 1993 Phase III randomized placebo-controlled study of granulocyte-macrophage colony stimulating factor (GM-CSF) in adult patients (55–70 years) with acute myelogenous leukemia (AML). A study of the Eastern Cooperative Oncology Group (ECOG). Blood 82 (Suppl. 1): 329a

San Miguel J F, Hernandez J M, Gonzalez-Sarmiento R et al 1991 Acute leukemia after a primary myelodysplatic syndrome: immunophenotypic, genotypic and clinical characteristics. Blood 78: 768–774

Sato H, Gottesman M M, Goldstein L J et al 1990 Expression of the multidrug resistance gene in myeloid leukemias. Leukemia Res 14: 11–22

Schiffer C A, Lee E J, Tomiyasu T et al 1989 Prognostic impact of cytogenetic abnormalities in patients with de novo acute nonlymphocytic leukemia. Blood 73: 263–270

Sebban C, Archimbaud E, Coiffier B et al 1988 Treatment of acute myeloid leukemia in elderly patients. Cancer 61: 227–231

Shepherd J D, Reece D E, Barnett M J et al 1993 Induction therapy for acute myelogenous leukemia in patients over 60 years with intermediate-dose cytosine arabinoside, mitoxantrone and etoposide. Leuk Lymphoma 9: 211–215

Shtalrid M, Lotem J, Sachs L et al 1987 Review of clinical and haematological response to low-dose cytosine arabinoside in acute myeloid leukaemia. Eur J Haematol 38: 3–11

Stein R S, Vogler W R, Winton E F et al 1990 Therapy of acute myelogenous leukemia in patients over the age of 50: a randomized southeastern cancer study group trial. Leukemia Res 14: 895–903

Stone R, Berg D, George S et al 1994 Granulocyte-macrophage colony-stimulating factor after initial chemotheraphy for elderly patients with primary acute myelogenous leukemia. N Engl J Med 332:1671-7

Swirsky D M, De Bastos M, Parish S E et al 1986 Features affecting outcome during remission induction of acute myeloid leukaemia in 619 patients. Br J Haematol 64: 435–453

The Toronto Leukemia Study Group 1986 Results of chemotherapy for unselected patients with acute myeloblastic leukaemia: effect of exclusions on interpretation of results. Lancet i: 786–788

Tilly H, Castaigne S, Bordessoule D et al 1990 Low-Dose cytarabine versus intensive chemotherapy in the treatment of acute nonlymphocytic leukemia in the elderly. J Clin Oncol 8: 272–279

Tucker J, Thomas A E, Gregory W M et al 1990 Acute myeloid leukemia in elderly adults. Hematol Oncol 8: 13–21

Vogler W R, Velez-Garcia E, Weiner R S et al 1992 A phase III trial comparing idarubicin and daunorubicin in combination with cytarabine in acute myelogenous leukemia: a Southeastern Cancer Study Group study. J Clin Oncol 10: 1103–1111

Walters R S, Kantarjian H M, Keating M J et al 1987 Intensive treatment of acute leukemia in adults 70 years of age and older. Cancer 60: 149–155

Wahlin A, Hörnsten P, Jonsson H 1991 Remission rate and survival in acute myeloid leukemia: impact of selection and chemotherapy. Eur J Haematol 46: 240–247

Wiernik P H, Banks P L C, Case D C et al 1992 Cytarabine plus idarubicin or daunorubicin as induction and consolidation therapy for previously untreated adult patients with acute myeloid leukemia. Blood 79: 313–319

Wood P, Burgess R, MacGregor A et al 1994 P-glycoprotein expression on acute myeloid leukaemia blast cells at diagnosis predicts response to chemotherapy and survival. Br J Haematol 87: 509–514

Yates J, Glidewell O, Wiernik P et al 1982 Cytosine arabinoside with daunorubicin or adriamycin for therapy of acute myelocytic leukemia: a CALGB study. Blood 60: 454–462

Zhou D C, Marie J P, Suberville A M et al 1992 Relevance of mdr1 gene expression in acute myeloid leukemia and comparison of different diagnostic methods. Leukemia 6: 879–885

Zittoun R, Jehn U, Fière D et al 1989 Alternating v repeated postremission treatment in adult acute myelogenous leukemia: a randomized phase III study (AML6) of the EORTC Leukemia Cooperative Group. Blood 73: 896–906

7

Paroxysmal nocturnal haemoglobinuria

P. Hillmen

Paroxysmal nocturnal haemoglobinuria (PNH) is an acquired haemolytic disorder which has fascinated clinical scientists for many decades. PNH was first described as a clinical entity by Paul Strübbing in 1882 (Crosby 1951). The discovery, in the late 1930s, that PNH red cells had an increased sensitivity to lysis by complement indicated that the haemolysis in PNH was the result of an intrinsic red cell defect, unlike all other acquired haemolytic anaemias. The observation that neutrophil alkaline phosphatase was decreased in PNH, suggested that haematopoietic lineages other than the erythroid series were also abnormal (Beck & Valentine 1951). This discovery led Dacie to hypothesize that PNH arose because of the expansion of an abnormal clone resulting from a somatic mutation in a multipotential haematopoietic stem cell (Dacie 1963). The first direct evidence in support of this theory was the demonstration that PNH red cells were monoclonal (Oni et al 1970).

Over the last decade, and particularly over the last 3 years, great strides have been made in the understanding of the underlying defect in PNH. These advances have in turn revealed intriguing questions regarding the pathophysiology of PNH, which remain unanswered. The aim of this chapter is to highlight these advances, to provide a framework for answering the difficult clinical questions which occur in the management of patients with PNH and to pose questions which remain to be answered, regarding the pathophysiology of PNH.

CLINICAL FEATURES

Presentation

The clinical features of classical PNH are well described (Dacie & Lewis 1972). Patients are most frequently young adults, although PNH has been described in children under the age of 10 years and in patients over 70 years of age. Both sexes appear to be affected with an equal frequency. Classical PNH presents as a haemolytic anaemia often with a gradual onset. The haemolysis is intravascular with intermittent episodes of frank haemoglobinuria which are often most evident in the mornings (nocturnal), is associated with a slightly raised bilirubin, almost invariably with decreased haptoglobins and persistent haemosiderinuria. The episodes of frank haemoglobinuria often, and in some patients only, occur in response to a trigger, such as an intercurrent infection. These episodes are often associated with abdominal pain, which may be severe and always raises the possibility of intra-abdominal thrombosis.

A minority of patients, especially those with hypoplastic PNH, never experience haemoglobinuria. These patients may present with abdominal pain and thrombocytopenia or pancytopenia. They may have little evidence to suggest haemolysis. Rarely, patients are seen with venous thrombosis as their presenting feature, particularly affecting the hepatic veins.

Course of the disease

PNH is a chronic condition. The median survival of a group of 80 patients seen at Hammersmith Hospital was approximately 10 years from the time of diagnosis. In addition, 27% of patients survive over 25 years after diagnosis (Fig. 1). The severity of the disease has a tendency to decrease with time and 12 of the 80 patients experienced a spontaneous clinical remission from their PNH between 10 and 20 years after diagnosis (Hillmen et al 1995).

Complications of PNH

Venous thrombosis is by far the most feared complication of PNH. Approximately 40% of patients with PNH will suffer from venous thrombosis at some time during their disease (see Table 1) and about one-third die as a direct result of venous thrombosis. Intra-abdominal thrombosis, in particular the Budd-Chiari syndrome (hepatic vein thrombosis), is the most frequent site.

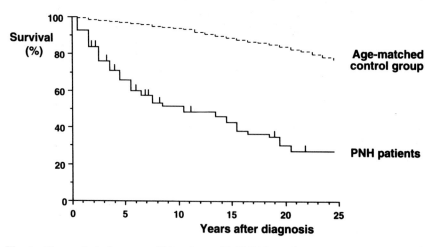

Fig. 1 The survival of a group of 80 patients with PNH from diagnosis. The median survival is 10 years. The survival of a similar group of age-matched subjects without PNH is shown for comparison.

Table 1 Sites of thrombosis in a group of 80 patients with PNH

Site of thrombosis	Number of patients
Intra-abdominal	
Hepatic vein thrombosis	8
Inferior vena caval thrombosis	3
Mesenteric vein thrombosis	4
Splenic vein thrombosis	1
Renal vein thrombosis	1
Intra-abdominal (undefined site)	1
Other venous sites	
Cerebral vein thrombosis	4
Pulmonary embolism	9
Deep vein thrombosis	7
Superficial thrombosis	3
Arterial	
Myocardial infarction	6
Cerebrovascular accident	2

Associated conditions

Aplastic anaemia

The co-existence of both PNH and aplastic anaemia (AA) in the same patient was first reported by Dacie & Gilpin (1944). The close association between these two conditions was further emphasized in reports of similar patients by Letman (1952) and Dacie & Lewis (1961). Both erythroid (BFU-E) and myeloid (CFU-GM) cultures are consistently reduced in the peripheral blood and in the bone marrow of PNH patients, even when they are not overtly aplastic (Rotoli et al 1982, Moore et al 1986). In addition, between 10 and 31% of patients with AA treated with immunosuppression eventually develop PNH as defined by a positive Ham test (Tichelli et al 1988, De Planque et al 1989, Najean & Haguenauer 1990). Recent evidence has emerged that PNH neutrophils can be detected in up to 41% of patients during follow-up for AA (Schubert et al 1994). PNH has been reported following AA resulting from various different aetiologies, such as drug-related, familial, post-hepatitic, idiopathic, etc. It is therefore improbable that the PNH was the initial diagnosis but more likely that PNH develops in a hypoplastic bone marrow. Thus, considering the rarity of both AA and PNH, the relationship between the two conditions must be significant and it appears that PNH in most, if not all, patients only develops in a background of bone marrow failure (see 'Pathophysiology of PNH' below).

Leukaemia

In view of numerous reports of leukaemia — invariably AML — developing in PNH (Rotoli & Luzzatto 1989a) it has been widely accepted that PNH is a pre-leukaemic condition. In addition, occasional patients have been reported whose leukaemic cells are deficient in GPI-linked proteins (and thus are derived from the PNH clone), (Devine et al 1987, Longo et al 1994, Stafford et al 1995). Therefore the finding that none of the 80 patients in the series followed at Hammersmith Hospital developed leukaemia might at first be surprising. A possible explanation for this apparent anomaly may lie in the relationship that both PNH and AML have with AA. Approximately 5% of patients with AA who respond to immunosuppressive therapy eventually develop AML (Tichelli et al 1988, De Planque et al 1989, Najean & Haguenauer 1990). Therefore AA predisposes to both AML and PNH, but the development of a PNH clone does not appear to increase the risk of AML above that seen in AA. In this case the incidence of leukaemia in PNH would be similar to that in AA (as appears to be the case) and would explain why a single case did not arise in a group of 80 patients.

If the presence of PNH does not predispose to leukaemia (i.e. PNH is not a preleukaemic condition) then why is the leukaemic clone frequently derived from the PNH clone? The simple explanation may be that the chance of developing a leukaemogenic mutation is the same in both the PNH and the residual aplastic stem cells, but because the PNH clone is usually numerically dominant, it is more likely to be involved in a random event (i.e. the leukaemogenic mutation) than the relatively few remaining normal stem cells. The exception (that perhaps proves the rule) is the recent report of a patient with PNH who subsequently developed myelodysplastic syndrome (MDS) and was found to have normal expression of GPI-linked proteins on his blasts. Thus the MDS in this patient was derived from the residual normal marrow and not the PNH clone (van Kamp et al 1994). Therefore the evidence suggests that the development of PNH does not increase the risk of a patient developing AML above that of an appropriate control group (patients who have recovered from aplastic anaemia without developing a PNH clone).

Considerations on management

Transfusion

There is a tendency to transfuse patients in order to maintain their haemoglobin at a certain level. This policy frequently leads to some patients receiving regular transfusions which can be largely avoided by transfusing when the anaemia is clinically significant (some patients can quite happily maintain a haemoglobin level of 7–8 g/dl).

The observation that episodes of intravascular haemolysis can follow transfusions led Dacie to transfuse patients with washed red cells in order to reduce these episodes of haemolysis (Dacie 1948). The use of washed red cells for all patients with PNH has become routine in hospitals and is probably excessive. There are relatively few reports in the literature of serious haemolytic reactions following the transfusion of PNH patients and these all appear to follow the transfusion of blood products containing plasma with an ABO isoagglutinin which is reactive against the red cells of the patients (group O plasma into group A recipients (2 cases) (Dacie & Firth 1943, Jackson et al 1992) or into a group AB recipient (1 case) (Brecher & Taswell 1989)). There are no reports in the literature of the transfusion of group-specific plasma precipitating a significant haemolytic attack. It is possible that white cells contaminating transfused blood may result in the activation of the complement pathway and, therefore, may potentially precipitate haemolysis (Sirchia et al 1970).

On balance, it would appear reasonable to transfuse patients with plasma-depleted group-specific blood products which are white-cell depleted. The routine washing of red cells is excessive and should be reserved for patients who experience problems with transfusions. This policy has been shown to be safe in a large series of patients from the Mayo clinic (Brecher & Taswell 1989).

Immunosuppressive therapy

Over the last few years the use of flow cytometry has increased the sensitivity of detection of PNH clones. Therefore the diagnosis of PNH is being established in more patients with aplastic anaemia. In addition a proportion of patients with haemolytic PNH present with or develop life-threatening cytopenias. This leads to the question: 'Are cases of pancytopenia in the presence of a PNH clone responsive to immunosuppressive therapy?'

Treatment with anti-lymphocyte globulin and/or cyclosporin A for bone marrow failure in PNH results, at least in a proportion of cases, in a haematological improvement (Kusminsky et al 1988, Nakao et al 1992, van Kamp et al 1995). There is no consistent change in the proportion of PNH cells after response. There do not appear to be any additional adverse effects in patients with PNH and there may be a better response in patients with PNH/AA rather than haemolytic PNH. Therefore the presence of a PNH clone does not alter the indications for therapy of cytopenias with immunosuppression. Unfortunately too few cases have been reported to suggest whether the chance of benefit is affected (either positively or negatively) in the presence of a PNH clone.

Bone marrow transplantation

The only curative therapy available at present for PNH is bone marrow transplantation (BMT) (Storb et al 1973, Kawahara et al 1992). BMT is only available to a small proportion of patients and carries a significant risk of morbidity and mortality. The natural history of PNH is an important factor in decisions regarding therapy in individual patients. The chance of spontaneous remission and of long-term survival in PNH must be taken into account when considering the possibility of either BMT or other novel therapies for PNH.

The indication for the vast majority of transplants reported in patients with PNH has been cytopenias; either the patients had aplastic anaemia with a small PNH clone or, more rarely, the patient developed bone marrow failure following PNH. It would appear in these patients that the indications and outcome for transplant are similar to those for severe aplastic anaemia. BMT has only been reported in a handful of patients with haemolytic PNH. It has been shown convincingly that if BMT is undertaken in a patient with PNH then myeloablative conditioning regimens are required to eradicate the PNH clone. The final decision of whether to subject a patient with a potential donor to transplantation depends on the philosophy of both the attending physician and the patient.

Thrombosis

Venous thrombosis occurs in 40% of patients and is the commonest cause of death in PNH (Hillmen et al 1995). In addition, some patients present with life-threatening thrombosis as their first thrombotic event. Therefore a reasonable case can be constructed to proceed with anticoagulation therapy in all patients with PNH, who have no contraindications, prior to their first thrombosis.

When a patient has suffered a venous thrombosis it is widely accepted that anticoagulation should be instituted and continued indefinitely. If the first thrombosis is a life-threatening Budd-Chiari syndrome (hepatic vein thrombosis) then thrombolytic therapy provides the opportunity to clear the thrombus and to improve the outcome (McMullin et al 1994).

Pregnancy

The literature regarding pregnancy in PNH largely comprises single case reports and the tendency to report eventful cases is likely to overestimate the true risk (Solal-Céligny et al 1988, Svigos & Norman 1994). Fertility in PNH appears to be normal and as PNH is caused by a somatic mutation in a haematopoietic stem cell there is no risk of transfer of the PNH abnormality to the fetus.

Maternal complications occur in approximately 50% of pregnancies, the most frequent being thrombosis, especially the Budd-Chiari syndrome. Thrombosis may occur during pregnancy or immediately after delivery following an apparently uneventful pregnancy. The other major complication which can occur is a deterioration of pancytopenia. The drop in blood counts can be quite marked and may not recover after delivery of the fetus. The maternal mortality for pregnancy in PNH is in the order of 5%. Approximately 30% of pregnancies in women with PNH result in miscarriage, which occurs with equal frequency in the second and third trimesters. The precise reason for this high rate of fetal loss is unclear. There is no increased risk of fetal abnormalities in successful pregnancies.

It is clear that the decision for a woman with PNH to become pregnant requires careful consideration and depends on the risks being fully explained to the patient. When a pregnancy occurs in a woman with PNH she should be given anticoagulant therapy in the immediate post-natal period and for several weeks post-partum (when the risk of thrombosis is greatest), assuming there is not an absolute contraindication. Anticoagulation throughout the pregnancy is also a reasonable course and should be seriously considered. It should also be remembered that such patients are particularly prone to deficiency of both folate and iron because of haemolysis and haemoglobinuria.

Contraception

There is a single case report of a patient with PNH suffering a cerebral vein thrombosis within 2 months of starting the low dose oestrogen oral contraceptive pill (Microgynon) (Stirling et al 1980). In view of this report and of the thrombotic risk associated with the use of the oral contraceptive pill it is advisable to recommend an alternative to the oral contraceptive pill in PNH.

COMPLEMENT SENSITIVITY

Ham test

The first evidence that the haemolysis in PNH was caused by the effect of a normal serum component (complement) on abnormally sensitive erythrocytes was the demonstration in 1911 that PNH erythrocytes underwent lysis in vitro when incubated with the patient's or donor serum and exposed to carbon dioxide (Hÿmans van den Bergh 1911). This eventually led to the development of the acidified serum (or Ham) test for the diagnosis of PNH (Ham & Dingle 1939). The Ham test, which relies on the demonstration that erythrocytes from patients with PNH undergo lysis when exposed to activated complement, has remained the 'gold standard' diagnostic test until the recent advent of flow cytometry.

Complement lysis sensitivity test

PNH red cells are readily lysed when opsonized with a high-titre cold antibody (anti-I) in the presence of large amounts of complement (Dacie et al 1960). Rosse & Dacie (1966) utilized this discovery to develop the complement lysis sensitivity (CLS) test which compares the amount of complement required to lyse PNH red cells with that required to lyse normal red cells. In 1973 Rosse reported the findings of the CLS test on a group of 22 patients with PNH. There are two types of PNH red cells: cells which are very sensitive to complement (10–15 times normal), known as PNH type III erythrocytes, and cells which are moderately sensitive to complement-mediated lysis (3–5 times normal), known as PNH type II erythrocytes. Perhaps a more surprising finding was that five of the patients (23%) appeared to have both PNH type III erythrocytes and PNH type II erythrocytes.

Decay accelerating factor (DAF or CD55)

DAF is a membrane-bound protein which accelerates the decay of both C3 and C5 convertase and thus regulates the activity of the complement cascade.

The first evidence that PNH cells were deficient in DAF was the finding that PNH red cells bind and convert more C3 to C3b than normal (Parker et al 1982). In 1983 it was shown that PNH red cells did not express DAF (Nicholson-Weller et al 1983, Pangburn et al 1983) and it seemed that the deficiency of DAF was responsible for the complement sensitivity of PNH erythrocytes. The description of individuals with an inherited deficiency of DAF as a result of mutations in the structural gene for DAF (the Inab phenotype) (Lin et al 1988, Tate et al 1989) disproved this inference. Individuals with the Inab phenotype were identified because they produce anti-DAF antibodies when transfused; they do not suffer any illness and, in particular, have no haemolysis. When the cells from these individuals are subjected to a Ham test they undergo little or no lysis (Merry et al 1989, Telen & Green 1989). Thus deficiency of DAF from PNH cells is not, in itself, the reason for their complement sensitivity.

Membrane inhibitor of reactive lysis (MIRL or CD59)

CD59 is a 18 kD cell-surface protein which limits the number of C9 molecules associating with the C5b–8 complex of the complement cascade and thereby inhibits the formation of the membrane attack complex (the final effector molecule of complement which mediates cell lysis). Thus CD59 is a potent inhibitor of complement-mediated cell lysis (Holguin et al 1989, Davies et al 1989, Rollins & Sims 1990). PNH cells were shown to be CD59 deficient in 1989 (Holguin et al 1989, Rollins & Sims 1990) and its deficiency was considered to be the likely cause for the complement sensitivity of PNH red cells. When normal red cells are treated with anti-CD59 they become complement sensitive in a similar fashion to PNH red cells (Davies et al 1989). In 1990 a 22-year-old man was described with repeated attacks of haemoglobinuria, persistent haemosiderinuria, twice having suffered from cerebral infarction and with a positive Ham test. His erythrocytes, granulocytes and cultured fibroblasts expressed normal levels of DAF (CD55) but were completely lacking CD59. His parents, who were first cousins, both had approximately 50% of the normal expression of CD59 (Yamashina et al 1990). The patient was shown to be homozygous for a deletion of his CD59 gene (Motoyama et al 1992). This case demonstrates that both the complement-mediated lysis in PNH and the thrombotic tendency are due largely to the deficiency of CD59, although it has to be noted that unlike classical acquired PNH his non-haemopoietic cells, including his endothelial cells, also lack CD59.

MEMBRANE DEFECT

Since the observation that neutrophil alkaline phosphatase was decreased in neutrophils from PNH patients, many more molecules have been reported to be deficient haematopoietic cells in PNH. To date at least 15 different molecules have been reported to be deficient in PNH (see Table 2). The

Table 2 Proteins deficient from PNH cells

Antigen	Year deficiency reported	Cell type
Neutrophil alkaline phosphatase (NAP)	1951	Neutrophils
Acetylcholinesterase	1956	Red cells, mature leukocytes
Decay accelerating factor (DAF or CD55)	1983	All mature haematopoietic cells
Homologous restriction factor (HRF)	1987	Red cells
Lymphocyte function-associated antigen-3 (LFA-3 or CD58)	1987	All mature haematopoietic cells
Fc receptor type III (FcγRIII or CD16)	1988	Neutrophils, NK cells, macrophages, some T-cells
Monocyte differentiation antigen, CD14	1988	Monocytes, macrophages, activated neutrophils
Membrane inhibitor of reactive lysis [(MIRL or CD59)]	1989	All mature haematopoietic cells
Blast-1 (CD48)	1990	Lymphocytes
JMH antigen	1990	Red cells, lymphocytes
CD24	1990	B-cells, neutrophils
CD67	1990	Neutrophils, eosinophils
Urokinase-type Plasminogen Activator Receptor (u-PAR)	1992	Monocytes, granulocytes
Ecto-5'-nucleotidase (CD73)	1993	Some B-cells and T-cells
CAMPATH-1 antigen (CDw52)	1993	All haemopoietic cells, highly on lymphocytes and monocytes

observation that so many molecules are deficient from PNH cells appears to be in contrast with the theory that PNH is a clonal disorder arising through a single somatic mutation occurring in a haematopoietic stem cell. The explanation for this apparent anomaly is the finding that all the proteins which are deficient PNH cells are normally attached to the cell membrane through a glycosylphosphatidyl-inositol (GPI) anchor (see Fig. 2) (Ferguson 1992). In addition, all the proteins anchored by a GPI anchor are deficient from PNH cells. Therefore if the mutation underlying PNH disrupts the GPI structure then a single mutation could account for the multiple deficiencies of PNH cells.

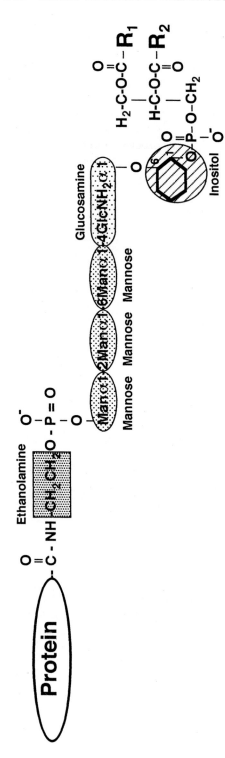

Fig. 2 Schematic representation of the conserved core of the GPI anchor. R_1 and R_2 represent different fatty acid chains which are inserted into the cell membrane. The protein is attached, via its carboxyl terminal, to the reformed GPI core in the rough endoplasmic reticulum.

DIAGNOSIS OF PNH

Flow cytometry

The Ham test has remained the 'gold standard' for the diagnosis of PNH for over 50 years. In the last few years it has been superseded by flow cytometry. A positive Ham test remains specific for a diagnosis of PNH but gives only a semi-quantitative assessment of the proportion of PNH red cells. Flow cytometric analysis of GPI-linked proteins gives an accurate estimation of the proportion of PNH cells, differentiates type II from type III erythrocytes and can be used to study the PNH defect in all haematopoietic lineages (Rosse 1990). Although a positive Ham test indicates the presence of a population of PNH erythrocytes a negative test does not exclude a small PNH clone, particularly if the neutrophils are the predominantly abnormal cells (i.e. in the clonal evolution of AA).

Flow cytometric analysis as a diagnostic test for PNH is unlike most other uses of flow cytometry because a positive test constitutes the demonstration of antigen-negative cells rather than antigen-positive cells. For this purpose any GPI-linked antigen which is normally expressed on a cell lineage of interest may be utilized (see Table 2). It is important to analyse red cells (Plesner et al 1990, Shichishima et al 1991) and neutrophils (van der Schoot et al 1990, Plesner et al 1990, Bessler & Fehr 1991) in order to demonstrate the presence of a PNH clone, and ideally two antigens for each cell type should be studied.

Antibodies

CD59 (MIRL) is expressed on all haematopoietic lineages. Anti-CD59 is readily available, can be purchased as a fluorochrome conjugate and differentiates normal from PNH cells extremely well. In addition it differentiates PNH type III red cells (complete deficiency), PNH type II red cells (partial deficiency) and normal red cells. CD55 (DAF) is also ubiquitously expressed. Unfortunately at present there is not a good commercially available antibody conjugate to CD55. CD58 (LFA-3) is expressed only in a GPI-linked form on red cells and is, therefore, a useful antibody for the analysis of red cells. However, CD58 is also expressed in a transmembrane anchored form on white cells, which renders it useless for the study of neutrophils. Anti-CD58 is available but does not clearly differentiate PNH type II red cells from normal cells. CD16 (FcγRIII) is expressed on neutrophils in a GPI-linked form and fluorochrome-conjugated anti-CD16 is readily available. In summary, at present anti-CD59 can be used to study both red cells and neutrophils with anti-CD58 for red cells and anti-CD16 for neutrophils. When a suitable anti-CD55 antibody or an equivalent antibody to an antigen expressed on both red cells and neutrophils becomes available then this will probably replace both anti-CD58 and anti-CD16.

Red cells

Three red cell patterns are seen in PNH (Fig. 3) (Rosse et al 1991, Hillmen et al 1992). The most frequent pattern (approximately 50% of cases) is a bimodal distribution with a population of cells being completely deficient in

CD59 and a residual population of normal cells (PNH III only). A small proportion of patients (about 10%) also have a bimodal distribution, with a population of cells being partially deficient in CD59 and a residual population of normal cells (PNH II only). The remaining patients have a trimodal distribution with populations of type III cells, type II cells and normal cells (PNH type II and III). Patients with only type II cells do not normally suffer from clinically apparent haemoglobinuria but remain subject to most of the complications of PNH, such as thrombosis. There appears to be a general correlation between the proportion of type III red cells and the degree of haemolysis.

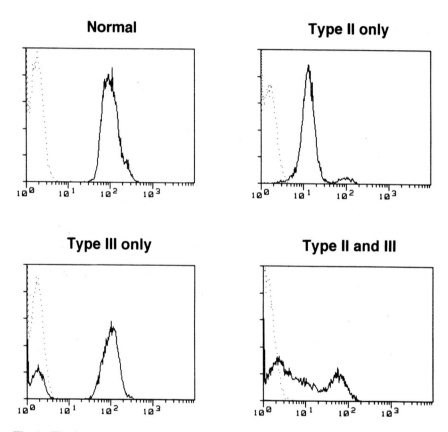

Fig. 3 The three patterns of expression of CD59 on erythrocytes which occur in patients with PNH.
PNH type III cells completely lack CD59 (fluorescence similar to the negative control antibody).
PNH type II cells are partially deficient in CD59 (fluorescence between the negative control antibody and normal CD59 expression).
PNH type III red cells only—approximately 50% of patients
PNH type II only—approximately 10% of patients
PNH type II and type III—approximately 40% of patients
Dotted line, negative control antibody; solid line, antibody to CD59; 'x' axis, fluorescence intensity; 'y' axis, number of cells.

Neutrophils

The study of GPI-linked proteins on neutrophils is a more sensitive method for the detection of small PNH clones. Even in patients who have not received transfusions, the proportion of PNH neutrophils is usually several times that of PNH red cells. This is presumably caused by the vastly reduced survival of PNH red cells compared to normal. In addition, patients who are heavily transfused may have very low proportions of PNH red cells but high proportions of PNH neutrophils (<10% PNH red cells and >90% PNH neutrophils is not unusual in such patients). Recent data has shown that a population of PNH neutrophils can be detected in up to 40% of patients after recovery from aplastic anaemia and that in many of these there are no detectable PNH red cells (Schubert et al 1994). Therefore the analysis of the GPI-linked proteins on patient's neutrophils may be the only method to detect the presence of a PNH clone in AA. CD16 is expressed on neutrophils but not on eosinophils. Therefore in normal subjects a small proportion of the granulocytes are deficient in CD16 (the eosinophils). Thus CD16 cannot be used to exclude or confirm a small population of PNH neutrophils. In addition, CD16 is only partially deficient on PNH neutrophils (although still clearly different from normal; see Fig.4). CD59 is expressed on all white cells and PNH neutrophils are completely deficient. Thus CD59 is ideal for the detection of even small populations of PNH neutrophils.

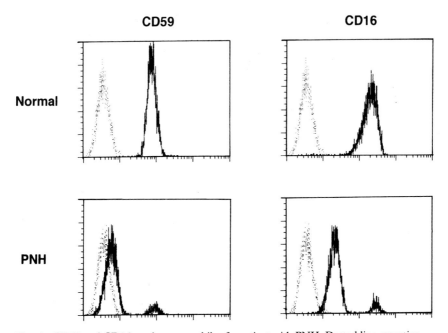

Fig. 4 CD59 and CD16 on the neutrophils of a patient with PNH. Dotted line, negative control antibody; solid line, anti-CD59 or anti-CD16; 'x' axis, fluorescence; 'y' axis, number of cells. PNH neutrophils lack CD59 (equivalent to the negative control) but express low levels of CD16.

Flow cytometric analysis of GPI-linked proteins on red cells and neutrophils is clearly superior to the Ham test in the diagnosis of PNH. A positive Ham test remains diagnostic of PNH (assuming the direct antiglobulin test is negative) and is still a useful screening test, especially for haemolytic PNH, when flow cytometry is not readily available.

GLYCOSYLPHOSPHATIDYLINOSITOL (GPI) ANCHOR

In 1960 Slein and Logan discovered that within 1 hour of rabbits being treated with a toxin from *Bacillus anthracis* there was a marked increase in their serum alkaline phosphatase. They proceeded to demonstrate that partially purified phospholipases (including phosphatidylinositol phospholipase) from both *Bacillus cereus* and *Bacillus anthracis* were capable of releasing alkaline phosphatase from both kidney and bone (Slein & Logan 1965). In the late 1970s it was found that both acetylcholinesterase and 5'nucleotidase were also released from the cell membrane in a similar fashion by phosphatidylinositol-specific phospholipase C (PI-PLC). The facts that C-type phospholipases cleave phospholipids between the phosphate and a 1, 2-diacylglycerol moiety and that PI-PLC are specific for structures containing a phosphatidylinositol suggested that these two features were largely or entirely responsible for the attachment of these proteins to the cell membrane. Low demonstrated in 1980 that PI-PLC-released alkaline phosphatase could no longer rebind to membranes and surmised that it was originally anchored through a tight linkage (Low & Zilversmit 1980), later shown to be covalent (Campbell et al 1981), to phosphatidylinositol (PI) phospholipid. Ethanolamine was found to be in amide linkage with the C-terminal α-carboxyl group of *Trypanosoma brucei* variant surface glycoprotein (VSG) and to be associated with a carbohydrate moiety. Chemical analysis of the linkage of the *Trypanosoma brucei* VSG revealed the basic residues of the anchor and, thus, led to the term 'glycosylphosphatidyl-inositol' (GPI; see Fig. 2) (Ferguson 1992). Since this discovery well over 100 proteins have been found to be anchored to the cell via a GPI structure in species from protozoa to man (Ferguson & Williams 1988).

BIOCHEMICAL DEFECT IN PNH

The biosynthesis of GPI anchors

Trypanosomes are nature's most prolific producers of GPI anchors and much of the work on the GPI biosynthetic pathway has been performed in these organisms. The pathway is similar in all species studied to date, including man. The GPI structure is synthesized in the rough endoplasmic reticulum of the cell where there is a pool of GPI precursor (Krakow et al 1986, Menon et al 1988, Mayor et al 1990). Within a few minutes of the synthesis of a protein which is destined to be GPI-linked, one of these GPI precursors is transferred *en bloc* to the protein. The protein with its GPI anchor is then transported rapidly, via the Golgi system, to the cell membrane (Bangs et al 1986,

Duszenko et al 1988). The biosynthetic pathway has been resolved by the identification of glycolipid species with physical and chemical properties consistent with being GPI precursors.

Biosynthetic block in PNH

The finding that PNH cells were unable to produce the GPI precursor provided support for the view that the PNH phenotype was caused by a block in the biosynthesis of the GPI structure (Mahoney et al 1992, Hirose et al 1992). It was possible that different steps of the complex GPI biosynthetic pathway, which involves the actions of at least 10 different gene products, might be affected in different patients, while still resulting in a similar GPI-deficient phenotype. Indeed, different mutations may have been expected to result in the PNH III and PNH II phenotypes.

The defective step in the GPI biosynthetic pathway in PNH cell lines (either T-cell lines or lymphoblastoid cell lines derived from patients with PNH) has been elucidated. In all cases the PNH defect lies at the same step in the biosynthetic pathway. This step is the transfer of N-acetyl glucosamine from UDP-N-acetyl glucosamine to phosphatidylinositol, which is the first identifiable step of the pathway (Fig. 5) (Armstrong et al 1992, Hillmen et al 1993, Takahashi et al 1993). The defect is at the same step in both PNH type III cells and type II cells (Hillmen et al 1993).

MOLECULAR DEFECT

PIG-A

In 1993 Miyata and colleagues reported the isolation of a gene named PIG-A (for Phosphatidyl Inositol Glycan complementation class A), identified by expression cloning in a GPI-deficient cell line (JY-5). JY-5 has a defect in GPI biosynthesis which is at the same step as PNH cells, and hybrids formed by the fusion of PNH cells to JY-5 have a GPI-deficient phenotype. Therefore PIG-A was a strong candidate gene for the 'PNH gene' and, as described below, PIG-A mutations have been found in over 50 patients with PNH (Takeda et al 1993, Bessler et al 1994a, Miyata et al 1994, Ware et al 1994a).

PIG-A has an open reading frame of 1452 base pairs and encodes a 484 amino acid protein. The gene consists of 6 exons and 5 introns spanning 17 kilobases and is located on the X-chromosome at Xp22.1. The PIG-A promoter region is GC-rich, a feature often associated with 'housekeeping' genes. This finding is in keeping with the discovery of GPI-anchored proteins in all tissue types. The PIG-A protein contains a 27 amino acid hydrophobic domain close to its carboxyl terminus. This is believed to be the transmembrane domain which anchors PIG-A to the rough endoplasmic reticulum where GPI anchors are synthesized (Bessler et al 1994b, Iida et al 1994).

At least three different gene products are required for the transfer of N-acetyl glucosamine to phosphatidylinositol (PIG-A, PIG-C and PIG-H). Therefore it

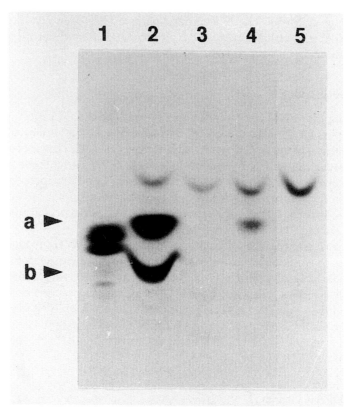

Fig. 5 Failure to transfer glucosamine onto phosphatidylinositol by PNH lymphoblastoid cell lines (LCL) indicates that the biosynthetic block in PNH is at the first detectable step of the GPI biosynthetic pathway. Incorporation of [^{3}H]N-acetyl glucosamine (GlcNAc): cell-free extracts of LCL are incubated with UDP-[^{3}H]GlcNAc and the lipid phase is then purified. The lipids are separated by thin layer chromatography (TLC). The figure is an autoradiograph following prolonged exposure (35 days) of the X-ray film to the TLC plate. Substances 'a' and 'b' are the first two intermediates of the GPI biosynthetic pathway (N-acetylglucosaminyl (α1–6) phosphatidylinositol and glucosaminyl (α1–6) phosphatidylinositol).
Lane 1 Trypanosome membranes ('a' and 'b' have slightly different positions because of differing fatty acids compared to human anchors); lane 2, normal LCL; lane 3, PNH type III LCL; lanes 4 and 5, PNH type II LCL from two different patients.
PNH type III cells incorporated no detectable N-acetylglucosamine whereas one of the two PNH type II LCL (lane 4) incorporates greatly reduced amounts.

is uncertain whether PIG-A is the glycosyl transferase, part of a transferase complex or a co-factor in the transfer. PIG-A has a 35 amino acid sequence with close homology to three other glycosyl transferases and, notably, to one other N-acetylglucosamine transferase. This evidence strongly suggests that PIG-A is the UDP-N-acetylglucosamine transferase. The PIG-A protein is orientated with this area of homology (the putative catalytic site for the glycosyl transferase activity) on the cytoplasmic side of the endoplasmic reticulum.

PIG-A has a processed pseudogene located on chromosome 12 (12q21) which has no introns, 91% homology with PIG-A and no long open reading frame (longest 236 codons). Therefore the PIG-A pseudogene is incapable of being transcribed to produce an active protein (Bessler et al 1994b).

Mutations underlying PNH

Since PIG-A is located on the X-chromosome a single mutation in the only PIG-A gene in males or in the active PIG-A in females is sufficient to cause the PNH phenotype (deficiency of GPI-linked proteins). The reason why PIG-A mutations are responsible for PNH in most, if not all, patients is that the other genes involved in the GPI biosynthetic pathway characterized to date (PIG-B, PIG-E, PIG-F and PIG-H) are located on autosomes, and two independent mutations, one at each allele of the autosomal gene, would be required to produce a GPI-deficient phenotype (Ware et al 1994b).

Mutations of PIG-A have been found in over 50 cases of PNH reported from laboratories around the world. To date, no case of PNH has been reported in which a PIG-A mutation has not been found. The mutations in different patients are extremely heterogenous, which is not unexpected as they are acquired **somatic** mutations. Approximately two-thirds of mutations found in PNH are either insertions or deletions resulting in a frameshift with early termination of transcription and, therefore, in no active gene product. The remaining mutations are single base pair substitutions. All the different mutations appear to result in little or, more often, no residual PIG-A activity.

Both PNH type III cells (complete GPI-deficiency) and PNH type II cells (partial GPI-deficiency) are caused by mutations in PIG-A (Bessler et al 1994c). However, in PNH type II the PIG-A mutations reported are single base pair substitutions rather than mutations which would result in frameshifts. This is in keeping with some residual PIG-A activity remaining in PNH type II cells. The spectrum of PIG-A mutations in AA/PNH patients and in patients with classical haemolytic PNH appears to be similar.

PATHOPHYSIOLOGY OF PNH

PNH clones, because of their increased complement sensitivity, would appear to have an intrinsic disadvantage when compared to normal. In addition the deficiency of other GPI-anchored proteins may adversely affect the growth characteristics of PNH clones. Therefore the central question to the understanding of PNH is 'Why does PNH occur at all?'

A clue to the solution of this enigma may be in the close relationship between AA and PNH. Considering the rarity of both of these conditions the discovery that as many as 40% of aplastic patients develop a PNH clone (Schubert et al 1994) and that most if not all patients with PNH have underlying bone marrow failure indicates an intimate relationship between AA and PNH.

Why should patients with AA develop PNH clones? A possible explanation was first suggested by Dacie (1980) and further developed by Rotoli

& Luzzatto (1989a,b). There is now a considerable body of evidence in support of AA being, at least in part, the result of an immunological mechanism. Furthermore, a large proportion of patients with AA experience an improvement in their condition when treated with immunosuppressive agents, such as antilymphocyte globulin or cyclosporin A. When a PNH-forming mutation occurs in a haemopoietic stem cell of a normal subject the resulting clone is at a growth disadvantage and therefore fails to thrive. However, when such a mutation occurs in a patient with AA the resulting PNH clone, presumably due to the deficiency of one or more GPI-linked proteins, is protected from the immunological attack which is responsible for the underlying bone marrow failure. Therefore in patients with aplasia the PNH clone has a growth advantage compared to the residual 'normal' haematopoiesis and is able to flourish. The PNH clone has a **selective** growth advantage. This theory implies that patients with aplasia are permissive for PNH clones. Evidence to support this theory is provided by the finding of two discrete PNH red cell populations (both types II and III), and therefore presumably more than one PNH clone, in a significant proportion of patients (37% in patients seen at Hammersmith Hospital). In addition, two discrete PNH clones with different PIG-A mutations occurring in the same patient have been reported in two patients (both only had PNH type III red cells) (Bessler et al 1994d). Thus it would appear that patients who develop PNH are permissive for the development and/or expansion of haemopoietic clones with a PNH phenotype.

The precise nature of the relative growth advantage remains unclear. The solution of this problem, as well as advancing our understanding of PNH, is likely to shed light upon the pathogenesis of aplastic anaemia and to further our understanding of normal haematopoiesis.

KEY POINTS FOR CLINICAL PRACTICE

- The median survival in PNH (prior to prophylactic anticoagulant therapy and the availability of platelet transfusions) is approximately 10 years. Twenty-seven per cent of patients survive over 25 years and approximately 15% have a spontaneous clinical remission.

- Venous thrombosis occurs in 40% of patients and is the cause of death in one-third. Therefore prophylactic anticoagulation should be seriously considered prior to an overt clinical thrombotic event.

- All blood products transfused should be of the same blood groups as the patient and should be white-cell depleted. Washed red cells are required for rare patients who experience episodes of intravascular haemolysis following transfusion.

- There is a close relationship between PNH and aplastic anaemia. PNH clones appear to have a relative growth advantage over the residual non-PNH haematopoiesis in patients with bone marrow failure. The mechanism for this growth advantage remains obscure.

- The complement sensitivity of PNH cells is a result of deficiency of CD59 from the cell membrane. CD59 deficiency is probably largely responsible for the thrombophilia in PNH.

- Flow cytometric analysis of GPI-linked proteins on red cells and neutrophils is the 'gold standard' diagnostic test for PNH. The Ham test remains a valuable diagnostic test for PNH but all positive tests should be supplemented by flow cytometry.

- PNH cells are unable to synthesize GPI anchors and are, therefore, deficient in all GPI-linked proteins. The GPI biosynthetic defect in PNH appears to be at the same step in all patients.

- The GPI-deficient phenotype of PNH is caused by a somatic mutation in the PIG-A gene of a multipotent haematopoietic stem cell. PIG-A is located on the X-chromosome and thus a single mutation is sufficient to produce the PNH phenotype. PIG-A mutations have been found to be responsible for PNH in all patients reported to date.

REFERENCES

Armstrong C, Schubert J, Ueda E et al 1992 Affected paroxysmal nocturnal hemoglobinuria T lymphocytes harbor a common defect in assembly of N-acetyl-D-glucosamine inositol phospholipid corresponding to that in class A Thy-1 murine lymphoma mutants. J Biol Chem 267: 25347–25351

Bangs J D, Andrews N W, Hart G W et al 1986 Posttranslational modification and intracellular transport of a trypanosome variant surface glycoprotein. J Cell Biol 103: 255–263

Beck W S, Valentine W N 1951 Biochemical studies on leucocytes. II. Phosphatase activity in chronic lymphatic leucemia, acute leucemia, and miscellaneous hematologic conditions. J Lab Clin Med 38: 245–253

Bessler M, Fehr J 1991 Fc III receptors (FcRIII) on granulocytes: A specific and sensitive diagnostic test for paroxysmal nocturnal hemoglobinuria (PNH). Eur J Haematol 47: 179–184

Bessler M, Mason P J, Hillmen P et al 1994a Paroxysmal nocturnal haemoglobinuria (PNH) is caused by somatic mutations in the PIG-A gene. EMBO-J 13: 110–117

Bessler M, Hillmen P, Longo L et al 1994b Genomic organization of the X-linked gene (PIG-A) that is mutated in paroxysmal nocturnal haemoglobinuria and of a related autosomal pseudogene mapped to 12q21. Hum Mol Gen 3: 751–757

Bessler M, Mason P J, Hillmen P et al 1994c Mutations in the PIG-A gene causing partial deficiency of GPI-linked surface proteins (PNH II) in patients with paroxysmal nocturnal haemoglobinuria. Br J Haem 87: 863–866

Bessler M, Mason P J, Hillmen P et al 1994d Somatic mutations and cellular selection in paroxysmal nocturnal haemoglobinuria. Lancet 343: 951–953

Brecher M E, Taswell H F 1989 Paroxysmal nocturnal hemoglobinuria and the transfusion of washed red cells: a myth revisited. Transfusion 29: 681–685

Campbell D G, Gagnon J, Reid K B M et al 1981 Rat brain Thy-1 glycoprotein. Biochem J 195: 15–30

Crosby W H 1951 Paroxysmal nocturnal haemoglobinuria: A classic description by Paul Struebing in 1882, and a bibliography of the disease. Blood 6: 270–284
Dacie J V 1948 Transfusion of saline-washed red cells in nocturnal haemoglobinuria (Marchiafava-Micheli disease). Clin Sci 7: 65–75
Dacie J V 1963 Paroxysmal nocturnal haemoglobinuria. Proc R Soc Med 56: 587–596
Dacie J V 1980 Paroxysmal nocturnal haemoglobinuria. Sangre 25: 890–895
Dacie J V, Firth D 1943 Blood transfusion in nocturnal haemoglobinuria. Br Med J 1: 626–628
Dacie J V, Gilpin A 1944 Refractory anaemia (Fanconi type). Arch Dis Childh 19: 155–162
Dacie J V, Lewis S M 1961 Paroxysmal nocturnal haemoglobinuria: variation in clinical severity and association with bone marrow hypoplasia. Br J Haem 7: 442–457
Dacie J V, Lewis S M 1972 Paroxysmal nocturnal haemoglobinuria: Clinical manifestations, haematology, and nature of the disease. Ser Haemat 5: 3–23
Dacie J V, Lewis S M, Tills D 1960 Comparative sensitivity of the erythrocytes in paroxysmal nocturnal haemoglobinuria to haemolysis by acidified normal serum and by high-titre cold antibody. Br J Haem 6: 362–371
Davies A, Simmons D L, Hale G et al 1989 CD59, an LY-6-like protein expressed in human lymphoid cells, regulates the action of the complement membrane attack complex on homologous cells. J Exp Med 170: 637–654
De Planque M M, Bacigalupo A, Wursch A et al 1989 Long-term follow-up of severe aplastic anaemia patients treated with antithymocyte globulin. Br J Haem 73: 121–126
Devine D V, Gluck W L, Rosse W F et al 1987 Acute myeloblastic leukemia in paroxysmal nocturnal hemoglobinuria. Evidence of evolution from the abnormal paroxysmal nocturnal hemoglobinuria clone. J Clin Invest 79: 314–317
Duszenko M, Ivanov I E, Ferguson M A J et al 1988 Intracellular transport of a variant surface glycoprotein in *Trypanosoma brucei*. J Cell Biol 106: 77–86
Ferguson M A J 1992 Glycosyl-phosphatidylinositol membrane anchors: The tale of a tail. Biochem Soc Trans 20: 243–256
Ferguson M A J, Williams A F 1988 Cell-surface anchoring of proteins via glycosylphosphatidylinositol structures. Annu Rev Biochem 57: 285–320
Ham T H, Dingle J H 1939 Studies on destruction of red blood cells. II. Chronic hemolytic anemia with paroxysmal nocturnal hemoglobinuria: Certain immunological aspects of the hemolytic mechanism with special reference to serum complement. J Clin Invest 18: 657–672
Hillmen P, Hows J M, Luzzatto L 1992 Two distinct patterns of glycosylphosphatidylinositol (GPI) linked protein deficiency in the red cells of patients with paroxysmal nocturnal haemoglobinuria. Br J Haem 80: 399–405
Hillmen P, Bessler M, Mason P J et al 1993 Specific defect in N-acetylglucosamine incorporation in the biosynthesis of the glycosylphosphatidylinositol anchor in cloned cell lines from patients with paroxysmal nocturnal haemoglobinuria. Proc Natl Acad Sci USA 90: 5272–5276
Hillmen P, Lewis SM, Bessler M et al 1995 Natural history of paroxysmal nocturnal hemoglobinuria. N Engl J Med 333:1253-58
Hirose S, Ravi L, Prince G M et al 1992 Synthesis of mannosylglucosaminylinositol phospholipids in normal but not paroxysmal nocturnal hemoglobinuria cells. Proc Natl Acad Sci USA 89: 6025–6029
Holguin M H, Fredrick L R, Bernshaw N J et al 1989 Isolation and characterization of a membrane protein from normal human erythrocytes that inhibits reactive lysis of the erythrocytes of paroxysmal nocturnal hemoglobinuria. J Clin Invest 84: 7–17
Hÿmans van den Bergh A A 1911 Ictère hémolytique avec crises hémoglobinuriques. Rev Méd 31: 63
Iida Y, Takeda J, Miyata T et al 1994 Characterization of genomic *PIG-A* gene: A gene for glycosylphosphatidylinositol-anchor biosynthesis and paroxysmal nocturnal hemoglobinuria. Blood 83: 3126–3131
Jackson G H, Noble R S, Maung Z T et al 1992 Severe haemolysis and renal failure in a patient with paroxysmal nocturnal haemoglobinuria. J Clin Path 45: 176–177
van Kamp H, Smit J W, van den Berg E et al 1994 Myelodysplasia following paroxysmal nocturnal haemoglobinuria: Evidence for the emergence of a separate clone. Br J Haem 87: 399–400
van Kamp H, van Imhoff G W, de Wolf J T M et al 1995 The effect of cyclosporine on haematological parameters in patients with paroxysmal nocturnal haemoglobinuria. Br J Haem 89: 79–82

Kawahara K, Witherspoon R P, Storb R 1992 Marrow transplantation for paroxysmal nocturnal hemoglobinuria. Am J Hematol 39: 283–288

Krakow J L, Hereld D, Bangs J D et al 1986 Identification of a glycolipid precursor of the *Trypanosoma brucei* variant surface glycoprotein. J Biol Chem 261: 12147–12153

Kusminsky G D, Barazzutti L, Korin J D et al 1988 Complete response to antilymphocyte globulin in a case of aplastic anemia-paroxysmal nocturnal hemoglobinuria syndrome. Am J Hematol 29: 123

Letman H 1952 Possible paroxysmal nocturnal hemoglobinuria with pronounced pancytopenia, reticulocytopenia, and without hemoglobinuria simulating aplastic anemia. Blood 7: 842–849

Lin R C, Herman J, Henry L et al 1988 A family showing inheritance of the Inab Phenotype. Transfusion 28: 427–429

Longo L, Bessler M, Beris P et al 1994 Myelodysplasia in a patient with pre-existing paroxysmal nocturnal haemoglobinuria: a clonal disease originating from within a clonal disease. Br J Haem 87: 401–403

Low MG, Zilversmit DB 1980 Role of phosphatidylinositol in attachement of alkaline phosphatase to membranes. Biochemistry 19: 3913-3918

Mahoney J F, Urakaze M, Hall S et al 1992 Defective glycosylphosphatidylinositol anchor synthesis in paroxysmal nocturnal hemoglobinuria granulocytes. Blood 79: 1400–1403

Mayor S, Menon A K, Cross G A M 1990 Glycolipid precursors for the membrane anchor of *Trypanosoma brucei* variant surface glycoproteins. J Biol Chem 265: 6164–6181

McMullin M F, Hillmen P, Jackson J et al 1994 Tissue plasminogen activator for hepatic vein thrombosis in paroxysmal nocturnal haemoglobinuria. J Int Med 235: 85–89

Menon A K, Mayor S, Ferguson M A J et al 1988 Candidate glycophospholipid precursor for the glycosylphosphatidylinositol membrane anchor of *Trypanosoma brucie* variant surface glycoproteins. J Biol Chem 263: 1970–1977

Merry A H, Rawlinson V I, Uchikawa M et al 1989 Studies on the sensitivity to complement-mediated lysis of erythrocytes (Inab phenotype) with a deficiency of DAF (decay accelerating factor). Br J Haem 73: 248–253

Miyata T, Takeda J, Iida Y et al 1993 The cloning of PIG-A, a component in the early step of GPI-anchor biosynthesis. Science 259: 1318–1320

Miyata T, Yamada N, Iida Y et al 1994 Abnormalities of *PIG-A* transcripts in granulocytes from patients with paroxysmal nocturnal hemoglobinuria. N Engl J Med 330: 249–255

Moore J G, Humphries R K, Frank M M et al 1986 Characterization of the hematopoietic defect in paroxysmal nocturnal hemoglobinuria. Exp Hematol 14: 222–229

Motoyama N, Okada N, Yamashina M et al 1992 Paroxysmal nocturnal hemoglobinuria due to hereditary nucleotide deletion in the HRF20 (CD59) gene. Eur J Immunol 22: 2669–2673

Najean Y, Haguenauer O 1990 Long-Term (5 to 20 years) evolution of nongrafted aplastic anemias. Blood 76: 2222–2228

Nakao S, Yamaguchi M, Takamatsu H et al 1992 Expansion of a paroxysmal nocturnal hemoglobinuria (PNH) clone after cyclosporine therapy for aplastic anemia/PNH syndrome. Blood 80: 2943–2944

Nicholson-Weller A, March J P, Rosenfeld S I et al 1983 Affected erythrocytes of patients with paroxysmal nocturnal hemoglobinuria are deficient in the complement regulatory protein, decay accelerating factor. Proc Natl Acad Sci USA 80: 5066–5070

Oni S B, Osunkoya B O, Luzzatto L 1970 Paroxysmal nocturnal hemoglobinuria: Evidence for monoclonal origin of abnormal red cells. Blood 36: 145–152

Pangburn M K, Schreibner R D, Muller-Eberhard H J 1983 Deficiency of an erythrocyte membrane protein with complement regulatory activity in paroxysmal nocturnal hemoglobinuria. Proc Natl Acad Sci USA 80: 5430–5434

Parker C J, Baker P J, Rosse W F 1982 Increased enzymatic activity of the alternative pathway convertase when bound to the erythrocytes of paroxysmal nocturnal hemoglobinuria. J Clin Invest 69: 337–346

Plesner T, Hansen N E, Carlsen K 1990 Estimation of PI-bound proteins on blood cells from PNH patients by quantitative flow cytometry. Br J Haem 75: 585–590

Rollins S A, Sims P J 1990 The complement-inhibitory activity of CD59 resides in its capacity to block incorporation of C9 into membrane C5b-9. J Immunol 144: 3478–3483

Rosse W F 1973 Variations in the red cells in paroxysmal nocturnal haemoglobinuria. Br J Haem 24: 327–342

Rosse W F 1990 Phosphatidylinositol-linked proteins and paroxysmal nocturnal hemoglobinuria. Blood 75: 1595–1601

Rosse W F, Dacie J V 1966 Immune lysis of normal human and paroxysmal nocturnal hemoglobinuria (PNH) red blood cells. I. The sensitivity of PNH red cells to lysis by complement and specific antibody. J Clin Invest 45: 736–748

Rosse W F, Hoffman S, Campbell M et al 1991 The erythrocytes in paroxysmal nocturnal haemoglobinuria of intermediate sensitivity to complement lysis. Br J Haem 79: 99–107

Rotoli B, Robledo R, Luzzatto L 1982 Decreased number of circulating BFU-E's in paroxysmal nocturnal hemoglobinuria. Blood 60: 157–159

Rotoli B, Luzzatto L 1989a Paroxysmal nocturnal haemoglobinuria. Bailliere's Clinical Haematology 2: 113–138

Rotoli B, Luzzatto L 1989b Paroxysmal nocturnal haemoglobinuria. Sem Haem 26: 201–207

van der Schoot C E, Huizinga T W J, van't Veer-Korthof E T et al 1990 Deficiency of glycosylphosphatidylinositol-linked membrane glycoproteins of leukocytes in paroxysmal nocturnal hemoglobinuria, description of a new diagnostic cytofluorometric assay. Blood 76: 1853–1859

Schubert J, Vogt H G, Zielinska-Skowronek M et al 1994 Development of the glycosylphosphatidylinositol-anchoring defect characteristic for paroxysmal nocturnal hemoglobinuria in patients with aplastic anemia. Blood 83: 2323–2328

Shichishima T, Terasawa T, Hashimoto C et al 1991 Heterogenous expression of decay accelerating factor and CD59/membrane attack complex inhibition factor on paroxysmal nocturnal haemoglobinuria (PNH) erythrocytes. Br J Haem 78: 545–550

Sirchia G, Ferrone S, Mercuriali F 1970 Leukocyte antigen-antibody reaction and lysis of paroxysmal nocturnal hemoglobinuria erythrocytes. Blood 36: 334–336

Slein M W, Logan G F 1960 Mechanism of action of the toxin of *Bacillus anthracis*. J Bacteriol 80: 77–85

Slein M W, Logan G F 1965 Characterization of the phospholipases of *Bacillus cereus* and their effects on erythrocytes, bone, and kidney cells. J Bacteriol 90: 69–81

Solal-Céligny P, Tertian G, Fernandez H et al 1988 Pregnancy and paroxysmal nocturnal hemoglobinuria. Arch Int Med 148: 593–595

Stafford H A, Nagarajan S, Weinberg J B et al 1995 PIG-A, DAF and protooncogene expression in paroxysmal nocturnal haemoglobinuria-associated acute myelogenous leukaemia blasts. Br J Haem 89: 72–78

Stirling M L, Tenton R J, Summerling M D 1980 Cerebral vein thrombosis and the contraceptive pill in paroxysmal nocturnal haemoglobinuria. Scott Med J 25: 243

Storb R, Evans R S, Thomas E D et al 1973 Paroxysmal nocturnal haemoglobinuria and refractory marrow failure treated by marrow transplantation. Br J Haem 24: 743–750

Svigos J M, Norman J 1994 Paroxysmal nocturnal haemoglobinuria and pregnancy. Aust N Z J Obstet Gynaecol 34: 104–106

Takahashi M, Takeda J, Hirose S et al 1993 Deficient biosynthesis of N-acetylglucosaminyl-phosphatidylinositol, the first intermediate of glycosyl phosphatidylinositol anchor biosynthesis, in cell lines established from patients with paroxysmal nocturnal hemoglobinuria. J Exp Med 177: 517–521

Takeda J, Miyata T, Kawagoe K et al 1993 Deficiency of the GPI anchor caused by a somatic mutation of the *PIG-A* gene in paroxysmal nocturnal hemoglobinuria. Cell 73: 703–711

Tate C G, Uchikawa M, Tanner M J A et al 1989 Studies on the defect which causes absence of decay accelerating factor (DAF) from the peripheral blood cells of an individual with the Inab phenotype. Biochem J 261: 489–493

Telen M J, Green A M 1989 The Inab phenotype: Characterization of the membrane protein and complement regulatory defect. Blood 74: 437–441

Tichelli A, Gratwohl A, Wursch A et al 1988 Late haematological complications in severe aplastic anaemia. Br J Haem 69: 413–418

Ware R E, Rosse W F, Howard T A 1994a Mutations within the *Piga* gene in patients with paroxysmal nocturnal hemoglobinuria. Blood 83: 2418–2422

Ware R E, Howard T A, Kamitani T et al 1994b Chromosomal assignment of genes involved in glycosylphosphatidylinositol anchor biosynthesis: Implications for the pathogenesis of paroxysmal nocturnal hemoglobinuria. Blood 83: 3753–3757

Yamashina M, Ueda E, Kinoshita T et al 1990 Inherited complete deficiency of 20-kilodalton homologous restriction factor (CD59) as a cause of paroxysmal nocturnal hemoglobinuria. N Engl J Med 323: 1184–1189

8

Automated blood cell counters

J. M. England

This chapter deals with the automated instruments used for the conventional blood cell count including the platelet count and the differential white cell count. Reticulocyte counting will also be considered because this can now be undertaken either on automated reticulocyte counters or as a special procedure on some other automated blood cell counters, i.e. the reticulocytes are stained 'off line' and then counted on the instrument.

An account will first be given of how blood counting techniques developed and became automated. The various technologies used for making the measurements will then be described. Examples will be given to show how the different technologies have been used in the automated blood counters which are available commercially. These examples will be drawn from the manufacturers who appear to have large shares of the pathology laboratory market as judged by the numbers of participants in External Quality Assessment Schemes. Manufacturers generally offer a wide range of instruments but the descriptions will be confined to the 'top of the range' models. All such instruments are fully automated, i.e. the measurements are made from whole blood without the need for the operator to dilute the blood by hand. Indeed, in order to promote safe handling, most instruments now have needle probes which pierce the cap of the blood tube so that the operator does not have to remove the cap itself. It is also common for instruments to mix the blood specimens before the samples are removed for analysis.

Automated blood counters must be properly operated. This requires them to be fully calibrated and the calibration checked both by internal quality control and external quality assessment schemes. These approaches will be described in detail. Finally, because the market is evolving so rapidly, it is necessary to understand how to evaluate new instruments or, at the very least, to critically understand evaluations undertaken by other workers.

HISTORY OF THE BLOOD CELL COUNT

Cell counting

Cell counting began in 1674 with Antonie van Leeuwenhoek using counting chambers, but the technique did not become common until there were improvements in the design both of microscopes and counting chambers in the

18th Century. However, by 1878 methods for red cell, white cell and platelet counting were well developed.

Cell sizing

Leeuwenhoek also made very early measurements of red cell size by microscopy but more accurate measurements were not made until the 19th Century when red cells, in suspension, were shown to have a diameter of 8.0 μm. Early in the 19th Century, lymphocytes, in suspension, were recognized to be smaller in diameter (5.5 μm) than neutrophils (9.5 μm); this distinction being made by Gulliver (1846) before their differential staining characteristics were described.

Differential leucocyte counting

The full white cell differential could only be undertaken once the different staining characteristics of the leucocytes had been described by Ehrlich in 1879.

Red cell indices, red cell diameter distributions and anisocytosis

The red cell indices, MCV, MCH and MCHC, were introduced by Wintrobe in 1930 and replaced rather arbitrary ratios in which the basic measurements were expressed as a percentage of normal.

Accurate red cell diameter distributions were popularized by Price Jones in 1910 and could be used as a measure of anisocytosis and to detect more than one red cell population.

Reticulocyte counting

Ehrlich was also responsible for giving the first description of the reticulocyte in 1881.

Haemoglobinometry

Primitive haemoglobin measurements were made in the 19th Century by visually matching dilutions of blood to a liquid reference. The acid haematin method was introduced by Sahli in 1895. More recently this method has been replaced by the cyanmethaemoglobin method which was introduced by Stadie (1920) and is now accepted as the reference method (ICSH, 1987).

Cyanmethaemoglobin can be quantitated either by a simple haemoglobinometer which measures absorption using a filter of suitable wavelength or by a spectrophotometer.

AUTOMATION OF THE BLOOD CELL COUNT

The development of automated blood cell counting and sizing

Though simple counting techniques had been described in the latter half of the 19th Century they were very inaccurate and even as recently as 1950 little real improvement had been made.

Early cumbersome attempts were made to automate the counting of cells in counting chambers but even if those techniques had been perfected it would still have proved difficult to automate the dilution of the blood and the filling of the counting chamber. It also proved impossible to count cells accurately by studying the electrical or optical properties of cells in suspension.

To enable cell counting to be automated, methods had to be devised for diluting the blood and delivering relatively small numbers of cells into and out of a zone, known as the 'sensing zone'. The cells could then be accurately counted as they passed through the sensing zone, provided the volume of the sensing zone was sufficiently small that it became feasible to count the cells as they passed through.

Early blood counters were semi-automated, i.e. the preparation of a suitable dilution was a manual operation and the instrument then aspirated the pre-prepared dilution. However, by the late 1960s fully automated instruments were available which aspirated samples of whole blood and performed the necessary steps to dilute and isolate the cells which were to be counted. This chapter will only deal with such fully automated instruments. Semi-automated instruments are still being produced but their use is restricted to very small laboratories because it is not cost effective to prepare dilutions by hand from large numbers of blood samples.

Early counters were described by Coulter (1956) and Crosland-Taylor (1953) but different approaches were adopted to limit the volume of the sensing zone and to perform the count itself (Table 1). In the instrument described by Coulter (1956) the cells were drawn through a narrow orifice and impedance changes were detected (Figs 1 and 2). The impedance was actually measured in a sensing zone situated between electrodes placed on either side of the orifice. Cells are insulators, relative to any saline-based diluent, so the impedance increases transiently as the cells pass through the sensing zone. These transient impedance changes form electrical impulses which can then be counted. Such systems are called aperture-impedance counters.

The instrument described by Crosland-Taylor (1953) was based on having

Table 1 Principles of blood cell counting on the early instruments

	Aperture-impedance counter	Light-scatter counter
Description of prototype	Coulter (1956)	Crosland-Taylor (1953)
Delivery of cells to sensing zone	By passage through a narrow orifice	By passage in a narrow stream created by sheath-flow
Delineation of sensing zone	By measuring impedance across the orifice	By a light beam crossing the stream of cells
Impulses used for counting as cells traverse sensing zone	Changes in impedance counted electronically	Changes in output from a photometer counted electronically

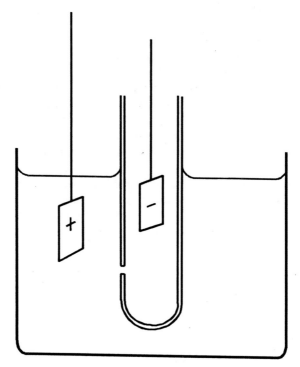

Fig. 1 Aperture-impedance counters have a tube with a small orifice. The tube is immersed in a dilution of blood cells and the cells are aspirated through the orifice. Impedance is measured between a negative electrode inside the orifice tube and a positive electrode in the dilution of blood cells.

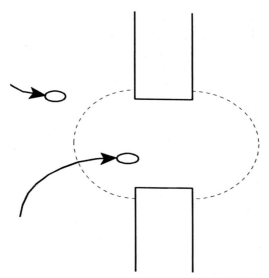

Fig. 2 The orifice on an aperture-impedance counter shown in an enlarged view. The dotted lines show the sensing zone into which the cells pass.

cells pass through a narrow beam of light. The sensing zone was restricted partly by the narrowness of the light beam and partly by delivering the cells in a very narrow stream. As the cells pass through such a sensing zone they are detected by scattering light in just the same way that airborne dust particles scatter light when a beam of light falls into a darkened room. The scattered light can then be collected by a suitable optical system and measured by a photometer (Figs 3 and 4). The transient increases in scattered light create impulses from the photometer which can then be counted electronically. Such systems are called light-scatter counters.

The impulses which were counted on the early aperture-impedance and light-scatter instruments were also used to determine cell size since, as a reasonable approximation, the size of the impulse is proportional to the size of the cell (Fig. 5). The size of the pulse can therefore also be used to discriminate

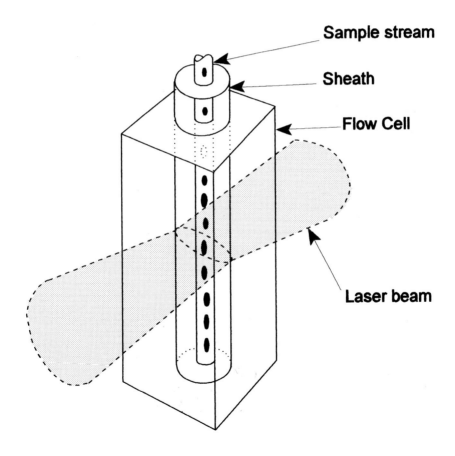

Fig. 3 The flow cell on a light-scatter counter. The cells in the sample stream are held in position by the surrounding sheath of fluid. As they pass through the flow cell they cross the laser beam.

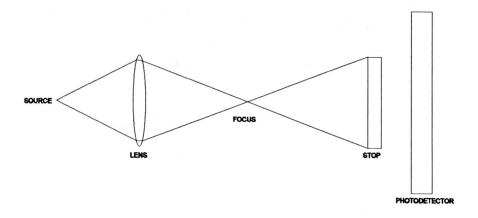

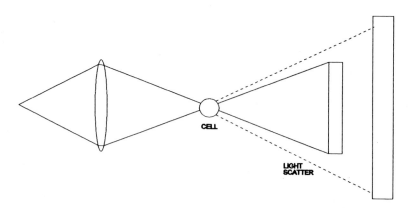

Fig. 4 The optics of light-scatter counting. In the upper diagram the light from the laser source is brought to a focus in the flow cell and then diverges. A 'stop' prevents the light falling on the photodetector. However, when a cell is at the focus (lower diagram) scattered light, shown as the dotted lines, can pass around the 'stop' and hit the photodetector.

between the cell of interest and other cells, debris or electronic noise. This process is known as thresholding (Fig. 6).

Apart from the differences in detection technologies there are important differences in how cells are delivered to the sensing zones in the two different approaches. Because the geometry has to be exactly right for light-scatter systems, the cells have to be in a very narrow stream which intersects perfectly with the light beam. Such a narrow stream is achieved by a technique known as sheath flow (Fig. 7). Cell suspensions enter the sensing zone through a narrow capillary which is surrounded by sheath fluid. The flow of the sheath fluid is adjusted to create a hydrodynamic focusing effect which forces the cell suspension to remain in a narrow stream as it passes through the centre of the sensing zone.

Although sheath flow was originally described for light-scatter systems it can also be applied to aperture-impedance systems and it has particular value in enhancing the ability of aperture-impedance systems to measure cell size as well as cell count. Enhancing the ability to measure size also means that it is easier to discriminate between different cell types, e.g. large platelets can be discriminated more easily from small red cells.

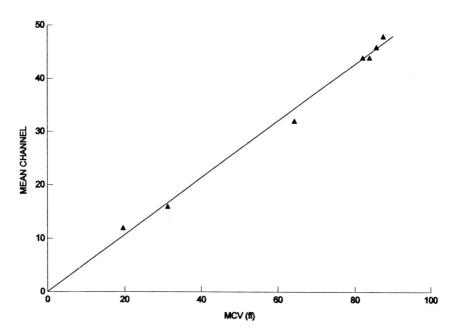

Fig. 5 The ability of an aperture-impedance counter to produce pulses proportional to red cell volume. The relationship between mean cell volume (MCV) measured independently and mean channel (an arbitrary measure of volume) on the counter is shown. The very small red cells are from a goat and a sheep.

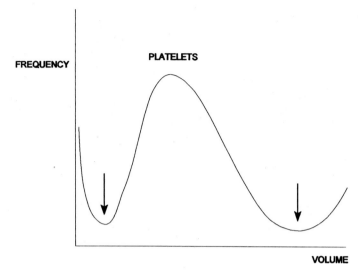

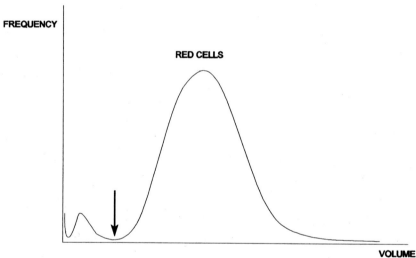

Fig. 6 The upper diagram illustrates platelet counting when thresholds (arrows) must be used to discriminate small platelets from electronic noise and large platelets from red cells. The lower diagram illustrates red cell counting when a threshold must be used to discriminate small red cells from platelets.

Cell counting in practice

Both aperture-impedance and light-scatter systems are perfectly well suited to counting red cells, platelets and total white cells and further details will be given below. But first of all it is necessary to understand the basic requirements for accurate counting of any cell type:

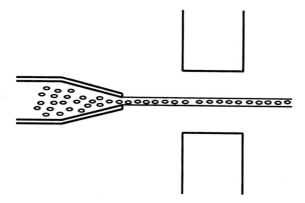

Fig. 7 Sheath flow on an aperture-impedance orifice. Compare with Fig. 2. A fine capillary is located opposite the centre of the orifice and cells are drawn from it through the centre of the orifice.

1. Whole blood is mixed, sampled and accurately diluted;

2. A known volume of that dilution must be passed through the sensing zone;

3. The cells of interest must be counted once and only once and no other cells, debris or electronic noise should contribute to the count.

The first requirement is easy to meet provided that the blood is well mixed before sampling and most instruments now do this automatically. In fully automated instruments the cap of the blood tube is pierced by a needle probe, the sample aspirated and the dilutions are then made accurately, usually by means of systems based on calibrated syringes.

The second requirement is relatively difficult to meet on an automated instrument. Most manufacturers have elected to measure counts per unit time rather than counts per unit volume of dilution. Such systems therefore have to be calibrated to convert counts per unit time to counts per unit volume. This is done by testing a blood specimen whose cell count has been determined independently and the process is explained in more detail in the section below on calibration and control.

The third requirement is of intermediate difficulty. It may sound odd to say that cells should be 'counted once' but the problem is that cells can be missed if they go through the sensing zone at virtually the same time as another cell. This problem, which is termed 'coincidence' (Fig. 8), arises from the 'dead time' in the electronics of the instrument and can usually be corrected with a suitable mathematical algorithm built into a microprocessor in the blood counter. To say that cells should be 'counted only once' sounds equally odd but the problem is that, with simple aperture-impedance counters without sheath flow, cells may recirculate in vortices just inside the orifice (Fig. 9).

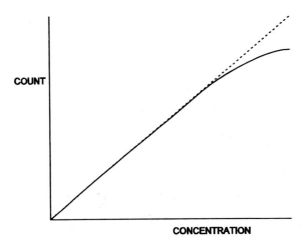

Fig. 8 The relationship between count and concentration. At high concentrations the counts begin to plateau because of coincidence.

Such recirculating cells can make a small contribution to the count even though they tend to produce smaller impulses than cells passing through the orifice. However, red cells which recirculate in this way cause signals in the platelet range and make platelet counting difficult unless 'sweep-flow' systems are in place to wash the back of the orifice and so prevent recirculation (Fig. 9). The question of discriminating the cell of interest from other cells, debris or electronic noise will be considered below for the various cell types. The methods for counting each type of cell are described below:

Red cells. These are usually counted on dilutions of whole blood with a suitable threshold set to discriminate between large platelets and small red cells (Fig. 6). Many systems do not have an upper threshold to discriminate large red cells from small white cells but the relative numbers of the two cell types means that this is usually not a problem.

Platelets. These cells can be counted on the same whole blood dilution used for red cell counting. There is usually an upper threshold to eliminate small red cells and a lower threshold to discriminate from electronic noise and debris (Fig. 6). Such simple thresholds are perfectly adequate provided the instrument has sheath flow and either aperture impedance or light scatter can be used for detection. However, if sheath flow is not used — and this is only an option with aperture-impedance counters because it is mandatory for light-scatter counters — then there is too much overlap between the signals from noise or debris and small red cells for counting to be effective with simple

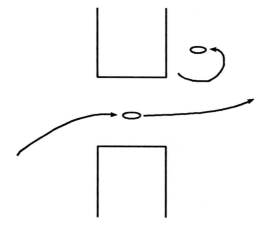
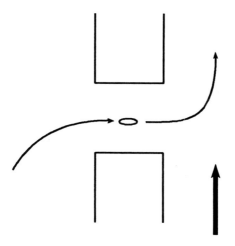

Fig. 9 On an aperture-impedance orifice some cells may recirculate just inside the orifice (upper diagram). This problem can be prevented by forcing fluid across the rear of the orifice (lower diagram). Such an arrangement is called sweep flow.

lower and upper thresholds (Fig. 10). Under these circumstances it is necessary to fit a theoretical distribution curve to the platelet volume histogram and extrapolate the platelet count from the area under the theoretical distribution.

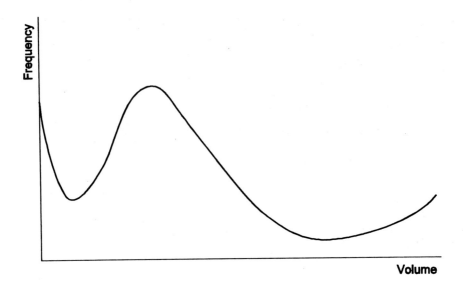

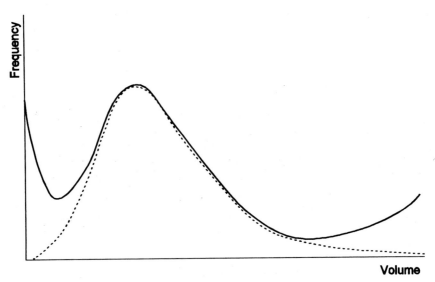

Fig. 10 Platelet counting. In the upper figure there is too much overlap to discriminate small platelets from electronic noise using a simple threshold. A lognormal curve is therefore fitted (dotted line, lower figure) and the count estimated from the area under the curve.

Total white cells. White cells cannot be counted on simple dilutions of whole blood because the red cell numbers are so relatively overwhelming. Suitable reagents therefore have to be added to lyse the red cells so that the remaining white cells can be discriminated from any remaining red cell debris. On light-scatter systems it may also be necessary to add compounds to stop the debris causing optical inference. With early systems, very strong lytic agents were used which removed most of the white cell cytoplasm so that it was actually the nuclei which were counted. More recently, however, gentler lysis is used to protect as much as possible of the cellular architecture so that it can be used as the basis for differential leukocyte counting.

Differential leucocyte counting

Early systems of differential leucocyte counting were based on differences in leucocyte volume measured by aperture impedance (England et al 1976). However, such systems are really best suited to discriminating between two classes, i.e. lymphocytes and granulocytes. Attempts to classify other cell types into a three population differential were less satisfactory and more modern approaches have now made both the two and three population differentials largely redundant.

Light scatter alone is of no value for differential leucocyte counting. Interestingly, the internal refractive index of the leucocyte, which is determined by its granules, is just as important as the true volume when determining 'apparent' leucocyte volume by light scatter. Thus, because of their granules, neutrophils appear larger than eosinophils although they actually have the same volume when measured by aperture impedance (Weil & Chused 1981).

Although light scatter alone has no useful role for differential leucocyte counting it can be used in conjunction with light absorption, when stained leucocytes are studied in suspension. The earliest work was done with peroxidase-stained leucocytes and when light scatter and absorption were simultaneously measured on a cell-by-cell basis it became possible to accurately discriminate four classes of leucocytes, i.e. neutrophils, lymphocytes, monocytes and eosinophils together with a category known as 'large unstained cells' (Fig. 11). This approach might be described as simultaneous multiparameter measurement, i.e. the two parameters of scatter and absorption undertaken on a single channel. The term 'channel' in this context, would refer to the system for diluting the blood, lysing the red cells, undertaking the peroxidase reaction and then measuring the light scatter and absorption. A single peroxidase channel made a major contribution to the differential leucocyte count but it proved to be inadequate for the differential count of basophils. The manufacturer therefore had to add on an additional channel to count these cells. Such multichannel differential white cell counting instruments have developed and are now in widespread use.

In parallel with the development of multiple channel instruments there has also been a trend to make more and more simultaneous measurements, often using a single channel. For instance, aperture-impedance systems can be enhanced to provide information on the white cell's internal constituents by using a high frequency electromagnetic probe at the same time as measuring volume. Light-scatter systems can also be enhanced by examining scatter at different angles. Finally, it is now possible to combine both aperture-impedance and light-scatter technologies, with their various refinements, into

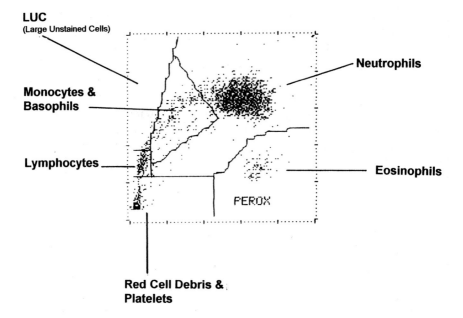

Fig. 11 Differential leucocyte counting using light scatter plotted vertically against peroxidase staining plotted horizontally. The leucocytes can be differentiated as shown. Basophils have to be estimated separately because they appear in the same 'box' as the monocytes.

a single channel. Exactly how these technologies have been used by the various instrument manufacturers will be described in the following section on modern automated blood cell counters.

Red cell indices

Although all automated blood cell counters purport to measure MCV there are other important extraneous factors which affect how the measurements are made both by aperture-impedance and light-scatter instruments. Because neither technology is perfect the various manufacturers have attempted to deal with the problems, but they have often done so in different ways.

The fundamental difficulty, which has already been mentioned, is that the impulse produced by any cell is only approximately proportional to the volume of the cell. Aberrant impulses, which do not truly represent cell size, can occur on any counter but often these impulses have an unusual characteristic which enables them to be identified by suitable electronic circuits and 'edited' out so that they do not affect the average impulse magnitude which is used as the measure of MCV. There is a particular need to edit out impulses on aperture-impedance counters without sheath flow: on such instruments cells passing near the edge of the orifice must be ignored because they produce larger impulses than cells passing through the centre of the orifice. Fortunately, such cells have a longer transit time through the orifice because flow is slower at the edge. The impulses they produce are therefore longer than they should be and so can be 'edited' out. Two cells passing through together also produce an oversize pulse but again it is longer and can be 'edited' out.

In terms of the red cell, the most serious remaining aspect, which cannot be corrected by editing, is that the MCV tends to be underestimated when the real MCHC, as measured manually (see below), is reduced. This problem affects both aperture-impedance and light-scatter systems and manufacturers have adopted different techniques to obviate the problem. These have served to reduce the magnitude of the effect although in no instance has it been eliminated. Because the red cell indices intercalculate as follows:

$$\text{MCHC} = \frac{\text{MCH}}{\text{MCV}}$$

it can be seen that an underestimated MCV will cause an overestimated MCHC. This is why, with modern blood counters, the MCHC is rarely seen to fall as much in severe iron deficiency as it used to do when measurements of haemoglobin and haematocrit were made manually and the MCHC calculated using the formula:

$$\text{MCHC} = \frac{\text{Haemoglobin}}{\text{Centrifuged haematocrit}}$$

With aperture-impedance systems there is a simple explanation for the MCV underestimation when the MCHC is low and this relates to the fact that the MCHC determines the internal viscosity of the red cell and hence its shape as it passes through the counter's orifice. The fluid shear forces in the orifice are such that the red cell adopts a 'cigar' shape (Fig. 12) but when the internal viscosity is reduced the red cell becomes shaped into a longer thinner 'cigar' and so creates a smaller impulse than it should. This is known as the effect of the 'shape factor'.

Light-scatter systems have difficulty measuring red cell volume because they are also affected by the shape of the cell and, in addition, by the cell's internal reflective index.

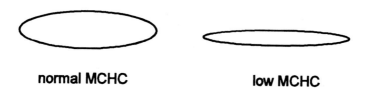

normal MCHC   **low MCHC**

Fig. 12 The cigar-shape of the red cell when deformed by fluidic forces in the aperture-impedance orifice. If the red cell has a low MCHC it forms a longer thinner 'cigar' and its volume is underestimated.

In order to minimize these complicating effects it is conventional, on light-scatter systems, to sphere and fix the red cells prior to their entry into the sensing zone. Once this has been achieved it is then possible to apply Mie theory which relates light scatter to volume and internal reflective index (Kerker 1969). The practical use of Mie theory comes by looking at low (2°–3°) and high (5°–15°) angle light scatter on a cell by cell basis. Low-angle scatter is primarily affected by volume and high-angle scatter by internal reflective index, although each are affected by both (Fig. 13). However, if both angles of scatter are plotted against each other the position of any impulse can be deconvoluted to measure the volume and haemoglobin concentration of the cell, and by averaging the measurements over many cells, the mean values, i.e. the MCV and MCHC, can be derived. When MCHC is measured on such light-scatter systems it does tend to fall more into line with the MCHC measured independently, although the agreement is still not perfect.

Red cell volume and red cell haemoglobin concentration distributions

As well as estimating MCV it is possible to produce histograms showing the distribution of red cell volume using all types of counter. Such histograms can be useful for measuring anisocytosis and for characterizing situations in which two red cell populations are present, e.g. iron deficiency responding to treatment.

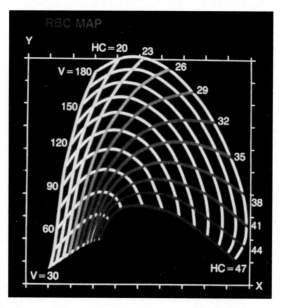

Fig. 13 Red cells. A plot of low-angle scatter vertically against high-angle scatter horizontally. The haemoglobin concentration (HC) in g/dl and the volume (V) in fl can be determined from where each cell falls on the intersecting grids.

If dual-angle light scatter is used, as explained in Figure 13 (opposite) it is possible to measure the individual haemoglobin concentration of a red cell and so construct histograms showing the distribution of cell haemoglobin concentration.

Platelet volume distributions

These can be used to determine platelet count (see above) as well as to measure the mean volume of the platelet and platelet anisocytosis (see 'new' parameters, below).

'New' parameters

Automated blood counters offer a range of so-called 'new' parameters such as red cell and platelet anisocytosis, mean platelet volume and many more reflecting other characteristics of the red cells, platelets and white cells. Unfortunately, the majority of these parameters tend to be instrument specific and parameters of the same name can compare poorly between different instruments even from the same manufacturer. It is probably for this reason that they have found little application in routine diagnostic haematology.

Many interesting studies have been published showing differences between different disorders, e.g. platelet anisocytosis in secondary thrombocytosis and thrombocythaemia. However, these differences are often not sufficient or not well enough established to become firm diagnostic criteria although they can throw some interesting light on the underlying pathophysiology.

However, all of the available new parameters have an important role inside the laboratory, even if they are not reported, because they form a useful guide as to whether the blood film should be examined.

Flagging and indications for examining a blood film

All instruments produce 'flags' which are designed to alert the operator to circumstances in which the measurements may be unreliable or in which there might be abnormal cells such as 'blasts' or nucleated red cells in the blood.

Flags must be considered, in conjunction with the 'new' parameters, any plots produced by the instrument (such as that shown in Fig. 11), the latest blood count results, any changes from the previous results and the clinical details when considering whether or not a blood film should be examined (Roberts 1991).

Reticulocyte counting

Reticulocytes stained with various dyes can either be counted on an automated instrument specifically designed for the purpose, such as the Sysmex R3000, or they can be counted on a conventional flow cytometer. More recently other automated blood cell counters have provided a reticulocyte counting option.

With these instruments the reticulocytes are stained 'off line' and then introduced into the counter for analysis.

Haemoglobinometry

Two options are in common use. The first is to convert the haemoglobin to cyanmethaemoglobin and then measure absorbance at around 540 nm. In practice, however, the cycle time on commercially available instruments is so short that full conversion is unlikely and intermediate derivatives are probably being measured.

Conversion to cyanmethaemoglobin requires the use of a Drabkin-type reagent which contains potassium cyanide and potassium ferricyanide, therefore the waste effluent from the instrument may not meet environmental standards in all the countries. Alternative 'cyanide-free' methods of measuring haemoglobin, using sodium lauryl sulphate, have been introduced on some instruments. Results appear to compare well with the cyanomethaemoglobin method (Karsan et al 1993).

MODERN AUTOMATED BLOOD CELL COUNTERS

General facilities

As explained in the introduction, this section will detail the 'top of the range' models from the manufacturers who have large shares of the pathology laboratory market, as judged by the number of participants in External Quality Assessment Schemes. Some of the models are relatively new, i.e. the market share derives from earlier instruments. As well as describing automated blood cell counters, automated reticulocyte counting will also be dealt with. The list of instruments to be considered then becomes the Abbott Cell-Dyn 3500, the Coulter STKS, the Sysmex SE9000 and R3000 and the Technicon H*3 RTX (sold in the USA as a Miles Instrument). Further information can be obtained from the manufacturers or by looking at recently published evaluations (Bentley et al 1993, Brugnara et al 1994, Drayson et al 1992, England et al 1995, Jones et al 1995, Rowan et al 1995, Warner et al 1990). Ideally, modern automated blood cell counters will do the following:

- Identify the specimen by bar code

- Mix the specimen

- Pierce the cap of the specimen tube and aspirate the sample

- Split the sample into 'channels' for the separate measurements, i.e. channels for the following:

- red cell and platelet counting and sizing
- total white cell and differential white cell counting (there may be one or more channels depending on the instrument)
- reticulocyte counting
- haemoglobinometry

- Within each channel, make the relevant dilutions, add reagents and wait until the dilution is ready for measurement

- Make measurements for each of the channels specified above

- Flag any anomalies and present suitable displays to the operator

- Check quality control using drift controls or patient means

- Transmit the data on-line to the laboratory computer system

- Be compatible with robotic systems for total laboratory automation.

All of the 'top of the range' instruments conform well to the general requirements listed above and there are relatively few distinguishing features. Most noticeable perhaps is the approach taken to reticulocyte counting. In most instances this can be performed on the automated blood cell counter as a 'semi-automated' procedure, i.e. the reticulocytes are stained off line and then aspirated by the instrument. Although one manufacturer offers the advantage of a fully automated reticulocyte counter, this means that an additional instrument has to be purchased in addition to the automated blood cell counter.

Red cell and platelet counting and sizing channel

The characteristics of this channel are shown in Table 2. No further explanation is required because the main features of this channel and the various options have already been described in the above section on automation of the blood cell count.

Total white cell and differential white cell counting channel(s)

As already explained in the section above on automation of the blood cell count, the differential white cell count may be measured on one or more channels with one or more parameters being detected in each channel. Table 3 shows the methods used on the modern automated blood cell counters with a separate line shown for each channel if an instrument has more than one.

It will be readily appreciated that conventional x–y plots can only illustrate the output of two parameters from a channel, e.g. light scatter and peroxidase

Table 2 The red cell and platelet counting and sizing channel on the modern automated blood cell counters

Instrument	Principle of measurement	Measurement of count	Flow characteristic	Number of detectors
Abbott Cell-Dyn 3500	Aperture impedance	Count/unit volume	Double orifices	One
Coulter STKS	Aperture impedance	Count/unit time	Sweep flow	Three
Sysmex SE9000	Aperture impedance	Count/unit volume	Sheath flow	One
Technicon /Miles H*3RTX	Light scatter (dual-angle 2°–3° & 5°–15°)	Count/unit time	Sheath flow	One

As explained in the text most instruments count cells per unit time and therefore have to be calibrated. If an instrument counts cells per unit volume of dilution then it is factory precalibrated and the user needs to check the calibration and call in a service engineer to effect a repair if the calibration appears to be wrong, i.e. the user cannot recalibrate the instrument.

staining on the Technicon/Miles H*3 RTX (Fig. 11). When more than two parameters are measured on a channel it can be very difficult to represent the data unless the parameters are combined, e.g. as discriminant functions, before being plotted on one or both of the axes of an x–y plot. An alternative, at least as a means of understanding the data, is to present it as a three dimensional plot. Fig. 14 shows how such a plot can be used to demonstrate white cell differentiation by aperture impedance, conductivity and light scatter on the Counter STKS.

Reticulocyte counting channel

Table 4 details the methods used for reticulocyte counting whether this is an off-line semi-automated procedure on an automated blood cell counter or a fully automated procedure on a special instrument designed for the purpose, such as the Sysmex R3000. Most instruments classify reticulocytes into several groups depending on the intensity of the RNA staining.

Haemoglobinometry channel

All of the instruments measure haemoglobin by the cyanmethaemoglobin method except the Sysmex SE9000 which uses the sodium lauryl sulphate method.

CALIBRATION, CONTROL AND EXTERNAL QUALITY ASSESSMENT

Calibration

A direct measuring instrument is one which makes measurements directly without the need for calibration. A good example of such an instrument is a

Table 3 The differential white cell counting channels on modern automated blood cell counters

Instrument	Stain	Principles of Measurement
Abbott Cell-Dyn 3500	Unstained	Light scatter at 1°–3°, 7°–11°, 70°–110° and 70°–110° depolarised (multi angle polarised scatter separation or 'MAPSS')
Coulter STKS	Unstained	Electrical impedance volume (v) Conductivity with high frequency electromagnetic probe (c) Light scatter (s) ('VCS' technology)
Sysmex SE9000	Unstained channel for lymphocytes, monocytes and granulocytes	Electrical impedance (DC) High frequency alternating current (RF) ('RF/DC' technology)
	Eosinophil channel — all other cells denucleated	DC
	Basophil channel — all other cells denucleated	DC
Technicon/Miles H*3RTX	Peroxidase stain channel — all cells except basophils	Light scatter Light absorbance
	Basophil/lobularity channel — all cells except basophils lose cytoplasm	Light scatter (dual angle as for red cells and platelets)

Table 4 The method for reticulocyte counting on modern automated blood cell counters (for abbreviations see Table 3)

Instrument	Stain	Principle of measurement
Abbott Cell-Dyn 3500	Methylene blue	'MAPSS'
Coulter STKS	New methylene blue	'VCS'
Sysmex R3000	Auramine-O	Dual angle scatter of light through green filter
Technicon/Miles H*3RTX	Oxazine-750	Dual angle scatter and absorption of light

spectrophotometer, which measures haemoglobin directly from the absorbance of cyanmethaemoglobin at 540 nm.

Automated blood cell counters are not direct measuring instruments, at least for the majority of the measurements which they make. The only exception is in terms of cell counting where two manufacturers supply instruments which measure counts per unit volume of dilution (Table 2). In this instance all a user needs to do is to check that the instrument is working correctly and call in an engineer if it is not, i.e. the user cannot recalibrate the instrument. All of the other instruments measure counts per unit time rather than counts

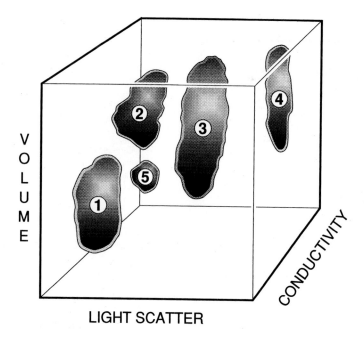

Fig. 14 Differential leucocyte counting shown as a three dimensional diagram. The cell populations are numbered as follows: 1, lymphocytes; 2, monocytes; 3, neutrophils; 4, eosinophils and 5, basophils.

per unit volume of dilution. They therefore have to be calibrated to convert counts per unit time to counts per unit volume. This is done by testing a blood specimen whose cell count per unit volume has been determined independently (see the section below on fresh blood calibrants). A calibration factor is then determined using the formula:

$$\text{Calibration factor} = \frac{\text{counts/unit volume on known blood}}{\text{counts/unit time on known blood}}$$

Once this factor has been entered into the memory of the instrument it can then calculate counts per unit volume on an unknown blood using the formula:

$$\text{Counts/unit volume on unknown blood} = \text{counts/unit time on unknown blood} \times \text{calibration factor}$$

None of the instruments are capable of directly measuring cell size, e.g. MCV and mean platelet volume. This shortcoming follows from the fact that although the impulses produced by cells are approximately proportional to cell volume the calibration factor, in this instance, is given by the formula:

$$\text{Calibration factor} = \frac{\text{volume of known cell}}{\text{size of impulse produced by known cell}}$$

and this formula cannot be predicted from first principles, i.e. from the basic physics of aperture impedance or light scatter. All instruments therefore have to be calibrated in respect of their cell volume measurements and other measurements based on MCV, i.e. PCV which is MCV times red cell count, and MCHC which is haemoglobin divided by PCV.

Similarly, the instruments have to be calibrated for haemoglobin measurements because none of them produce an absolute reading, i.e. readings based on fully converted cyanmethaemoglobin with absorbances measured spectrophotometrically. Thus the MCH also has to be calibrated, because of its link to haemoglobin, whether or not the red cell count is measured directly.

Fresh blood calibrants and reference methods

The known bloods, used to determine the calibration factors, are fresh bloods whose known values have been determined ideally by reference methods or, if the reference methods are too tedious, by suitable selected methods. Such bloods serve as calibrators. The relevant ICSH recommended methods for assigning values to fresh blood calibrators are given in Table 5.

Assigning values to preserved blood calibrants

Fresh blood calibrants have to be used as the 'gold' standard because the reference and the appropriate selected methods (Table 5) are normally only designed with fresh blood in mind. Unfortunately, however, fresh blood differs from gold in its instability! Indeed, it is only safe to assume that fresh blood is stable for 4 hours and this is often barely sufficient to determine the blood count by reference methods let alone allow time for the fresh blood to

Table 5 The methods recommended by ICSH for assigning values to fresh blood calibrants (based on ICSH 1988)

Measurement	Method
Red cell count	Semi automated aperture-impedance counter aspirating known volume through orifice using calibrated manometer and validated coincidence correction
Packed cell volume	Carefully performed microhaematocrit
Haemoglobin	Cyanmethaemoglobin determination
Red cell indices	Calculate from above measurements
White cell count	As per red cell count counting method. Count white cells after red cell lysis
Platelet count	Use a counter with sheath flow to estimate relative numbers of red cells and platelets. Measure red cell count as above and then calculate platelet count

be used to calibrate one or more automated blood cell counters. If the calibration then has to be checked, for instance on the following day, more fresh blood calibrants would have to have their values assigned and it can be seen that the process rapidly becomes extremely tedious and cost ineffective.

The solution to the problem is therefore to transfer the values from the fresh blood calibrant to a preserved blood calibrant with a much longer shelf-life, typically 30 or more days. There is only one shortcoming inherent in this process and that is that the automated blood cell counters, like the reference and selected methods, are designed with fresh blood in mind. This means that, for any given preserved and fresh blood and for any particular measurement, the ratio of preserved to fresh blood value may differ from instrument to instrument. Thus the value assigned to a preserved blood calibrant will often be instrument specific. Suitable preserved blood calibrants are available commercially, but are expensive.

Controls

From the discussion of calibration it can be seen that manufacturing fresh blood calibrants in-house will expend a lot of time, and purchasing commercial preserved blood calibrants to use day-by-day will expend a lot of money. Calibration is only cost effective, therefore, when it is strictly necessary. Indeed, as instruments have become more and more stable, much longer intervals can elapse between instrument calibration. However, the stablility of the instrument cannot be assumed and must be checked frequently. Fortunately this can be done by using a control. Controls, typically, are stable preserved bloods, but they are easy to manufacture in-house or cheaper to purchase because they do not need to have pre-assigned values. Controls should be used as follows:

1. Calibrate the instrument either with fresh blood or with a preserved blood calibrant in accordance with the manufacturers' instructions;

2. Obtain at least 20 replicate measurements on the preserved blood control and calculate the mean and SD;

3. Construct a Shewhart control chart;

4. Test the control after every 20 or so patient specimens and calculate how many SDs the result differs from the mean, using the mean and SD calculated from 2. above;

5. Plot the results on the Shewhart control chart and look for drift.

In practice, automated blood cell counters have computers with suitable software which enables them to do the relevant calculations and plot the graphs; however, the operator should still understand the basic principles of the quality control procedures which are provided.

Patient means

As an adjunct to using preserved blood controls — or some would argue as an alternative — it is possible to monitor running averages of patient means. Again automated blood cell counters are often supplied with relevant software based on the work of Korpman & Bull (1976). This work devised algorithms for calculated running means in ways which are claimed to be relatively resistant to the inclusion of abnormal bloods in the flow of patient specimens being tested.

The process of calibration either with fresh or preserved blood calibrants, and the use of controls to check for drift form the core of the internal quality control of the blood count. Such steps should be taken before the laboratory releases the results to clinicians, i.e. they are checks internal to the laboratory.

External Quality Assessment

As well as internal checks within the laboratory it is essential for the laboratory to have external checks on the reliability of its results. In the UK, laboratories requiring accreditation by CPA (UK) Ltd must participate in an External Quality Assessment Scheme (EQAS) approved by the Joint Working Group on Quality Assurance. At the time of writing the UK NEQAS(H) scheme is the only scheme with such approval.

Other countries have parallel arrangements. In the USA, for example, the Clinical Laboratory Improvement Amendments of 1988, commonly known as CLIA'88, require participation in an EQAS such as the one run by the College of American Pathologists. In the USA the equivalent term for an EQAS is a 'proficiency testing program'.

The UK National External Quality Assessment Scheme for General Haematology distributes twelve surveys a year for blood count, each containing two samples. Eight parameters are assessed: Hb, RBC, PCV, MCV, MCH, MCHC, total WBC and platelets.

The majority of samples are fresh human whole blood in CPD-A1 anticoagulant, partially fixed with a combination of formaldehyde and glutaraldehyde (Reardon et al 1991). As the blood is obtained through the National Blood Transfusion Service it has already been screened for Anti HIV 1 and 2, Anti HBsAg, Anti HCV and TPHA. The ratio of plasma to cells may be altered in the pooled material to allow for some variation in analyte levels. Donkey whole bood in ACD NIH-A anticoagulant (MCV approximately 70 fl) may also be used to simulate microcytic human blood. Antibiotics are added to ensure sterility and the blood is dispensed into sterile vials using a mixing dispensing unit (Ward et al 1975) to ensure identical aliquots of 3–4 ml volumes. The vials are closed with pierceable caps and sealed with vicose rings. These vials are acceptable for the automated sample handling systems on the majority of blood counting instruments. Each batch is checked for microbiological sterility. Samples, together with appropriate instruction and result sheets, are distributed within the UK by first class mail. The closing date for receipt of results is 5 working days from despatch and survey reports are mailed out 2 days later.

Individual results are assessed against a consensus value. The statistical techniques of Tukey (1977) are used to estimate the median and spread of the distribution of results. The population median rather than the mean is used as it is not dependent on the shape of the distribution and it is much less affected by the outlying values. The spread of the central 50% of the population between the quartiles is related to a normal Gaussian distribution to give the estimated standard deviation. This in turn is used to determine the coefficient of variation. The distance of each result from the median expressed in standard deviation units is known as the Deviation Index (DI) and is used to indicate individual performance.

$$DI = \frac{R-M}{SD \text{ (positive or negative)}}$$

R = Laboratory result
M = Median
SD = Estimated standard deviation

Different instruments and diluents used for blood cell counting may respond in different ways to the stabilized material used in the NEQAS surveys; thus there may be performance differences between the various types of counter which do not reflect behaviour with fresh EDTA blood specimens. As 'all methods' analysis will be biased by a dominant instrument, results are analysed and performance assessed within instrument group.

Typical CV percentage for the various parameters for the Coulter STKS group on a partially fixed blood sample are:

Hb	1.3%
RBC	1.5%
PCV	1.7%
MCV	1.0%
MCH	1.7%
MCHC	1.8%
WBC	2.7%
Platelets	6.1%

An example of an assessment report for a major analyser in good control is shown in Table 6.

EVALUATION

Levels of evaluation

Manufacturers of instruments will wish to evaluate prototypes and even production models prior to release to the market. Such evaluations are essentially private. Following release of the instrument to the market manufacturers will

Table 6 U.K. National External Quality Assessment Scheme for Haematology 15/03/95. A report from UK NEQAS (H) for an individual participant (reference No. 9999 to conceal identity). Restricted circulation: not for publication without permission

Results for Survey No. 9503   Participant Reference No. 9999
                               System No. 2
Sample 1: Partially Fixed Human Whole Blood   Sample Quality: Satisfactory
Sample 2: Partially Fixed Human Whole Blood   Sample Quality: Satisfactory
Haemoglobin by reference method - Sample 1: 121 g/l
                                 Sample 2: 118 g/l

Instrument	Test	Result		DI	Median	SD	CV%	N	
Coulter StkS	Hb	[g/l]							
	1	120		-0.68	121	1.48	1.2	939	All
				-0.68	121	1.48	1.2	247	Group
	2	119		-0.68	120	1.48	1.2	938	All
				-0.68	120	1.48	1.2	247	Group
Coulter StkS	RCC	$[\times 10^{12}/l]$							
	1	4.06		-0.14	4.07	0.074	1.8	895	All
				-0.36	4.08	0.056	1.4	247	Group
	2	3.90		0.00	3.90	0.067	1.7	894	All
				0.00	3.90	0.063	1.6	247	Group
Coulter StkS	PCV								
	1	0.362		-0.61	0.371	0.0148	4.0	902	All
				-0.49	0.366	0.0082	2.2	247	Group
	2	0.357		0.45	0.352	0.0111	3.2	901	All
				0.34	0.355	0.0059	1.7	247	Group
Coulter StkS	MCV	[fl]							
	1	89.1		-0.47	90.8	3.60	4.0	891	All
				-0.23	89.4	1.30	1.5	247	Group
	2	91.5		0.51	90.3	2.37	2.6	890	All
				0.98	90.7	0.82	0.9	247	Group
Coulter StkS	MCH	[pg]							
	1	29.6		-0.17	29.7	0.59	2.0	876	All
				-0.19	29.7	0.52	1.8	247	Group
	2	30.6		-0.15	30.7	0.67	2.2	875	All
				0.00	30.6	0.56	1.8	247	Group
Coulter StkS	MCHC	[%]							
	1	33.1		0.38	32.6	1.33	4.1	873	All
				0.00	33.1	0.74	2.2	245	Group
	2	33.4		-0.58	34.0	1.04	3.1	870	All
				-0.60	33.8	0.67	2.0	245	Group
Coulter StkS	WCC	$[\times 10^9/l]$							
	1	7.3		0.85	6.8	0.59	8.7	901	All
				0.68	7.0	0.44	6.3	247	Group
	2	6.6		0.27	6.5	0.37	5.7	901	All
				0.00	6.6	0.22	3.3	247	Group
Coulter StkS	PLT	$[\times 10^9/l]$							
	1	153		-0.54	163	18.5	*.*	882	All
				-0.50	160	14.1	8.8	247	Group
	2	212		0.29	209	10.4	5.0	884	All
				0.00	212	9.6	4.5	247	Group

The columns from left to right show instrument, test, sample (numbered 1 or 2), DI, median, SD, CV and number of participants. The rows show the results for each test and sample either for 'All' participants or for the particular instrument 'Group'.

wish to sponsor evaluations for publication, but it is preferable to have evaluations undertaken independently. In the UK this is done by the Medical Devices Agency (MDA), an agency of the Department of Health. The MDA contract with suitable laboratories to undertake evaluations which are then published. Recent evaluations include the Technicon H*3RTX and a robotic system manufactured by Sysmex (England et al 1995, Rowan et al 1995). Other evaluations are always being undertaken and the MDA should be contacted for further details. Full evaluations should be undertaken in accordance with an established protocol and the one described by the International Council for Standardization in Haematology (ICSH 1994) is the best one for automated blood cell counters. This protocol can be used, in an abbreviated form, if potential purchasers wish to assess particular aspects of an instrument under consideration. A very brief summary of the ICSH protocol is given below.

Scientific assessment

This part of the assessment concentrates on the measurements made by the automated blood cell counter.

Effect of dilution. It is desirable for the instrument to be linear over the usually encountered pathological range and this should be tested by using dilutions of packed cells in autologous platelet poor plasma. At the same time checks should be made to ensure that measurements, which should be independent of dilution such as the red cell indices, do not vary.

Precision and imprecision are defined by ICSH in the following way.
Precision: agreement between replicate measurements. It has no numerical value but it is recognized in terms of imprecision.
Imprecision: standard deviation or coefficient of variation of the results of a set of replicate measurements.

Checks should be performed both within and between batches of blood counts and an estimate of overall precision should be made by locating replicates randomly in a run. Such overall precision will also be affected by carry-over.

Carry-over can be assessed directly. By testing a high sample consecutively three times (i_1, i_2, i_3) followed by testing a low sample consecutively three times (j_1, j_2, j_3). Carry-over is then calculated as:

$$\frac{(j_1 - j_3)}{(i_3 - j_3)} \times 100\%$$

Comparability is defined as the ability of the instrument under evaluation to produce results which agree well with those obtained by an instrument in routine use. Comparability is not the same as accuracy (see below).

Correlation coefficients (r) should not be used to analyse such data since they give no information about comparability. For example, there would be perfect correlation (r = 1.00) if the instrument under evaluation always gave results which were 80% of those of the instrument in routine use. Instead it is better to use a paired t-test and to present the information graphically by plotting the difference between the two instruments against the result from the routine instrument. This is preferable to the approach adopted by many workers which is to plot one result against the other, a technique which results in a meaningless agglomeration of points in the centre of the graph.

Accuracy and inaccuracy are defined by ICSH in the following way:
Accuracy: a measure of agreement between the estimate of a value and the true value. Accuracy has no numerical value; it is measured as the amount of (degree of) inaccuracy.
Inaccuracy: numerical difference between the mean of a set of replicate measurements and the true value. This difference (positive or negative) may be expressed in the units in which the quantity is measured, or as a percentage of the true value.

Accuracy can only be assessed by the use of reference methods of the type used for assigning values to fresh blood calibrants (see above). As already explained such methods are very time consuming and can only be used on relatively small numbers of blood specimens. In evaluations they are best restricted to instances when very poor comparability has been observed and it is desired to see whether the instrument under evaluation or the routine instrument is correct.

Sample ageing should be assessed up to 72 hours both at 4°C (refrigeration) and at room temperature to mimic the effect of transport.

Sensitivity should be determined to abnormal samples, e.g. haemoglobins S and C, Howell-Jolly bodies, and to interferents, e.g. haemolysis, cold agglutinins.

Other analytical characteristics

Because blood counters are used for screening purposes it is important to ensure that they flag abnormal samples correctly (high sensitivity) and that they do not flag normal samples as abnormal (high specificity). Such assessments form a key part of assessing the clinical utility of the automated blood cell counter.

Safety

This is of paramount importance and checks should be made for electrical and laser hazards, moving parts and sharp edges which could injure the operator and for corrosive, toxic or carcinogenic chemicals which present a hazard in the laboratory or which cannot be safely disposed of. Finally, it is necessary to ensure that the instrument does not produce potentially infective droplets or aerosols; this is done by adding a 'safe' marker organism, such as spores of *B. subtilis*, to blood specimens and then looking for environmental contamination after they have been analysed.

Operational characteristics

This includes assessment of throughput, start up and shut down time, reliability, the quality of the user manual, the training given by the manufacturer and the costings.

ACKNOWLEDGMENTS

I am indebted to Mrs G Sanders for preparing the manuscript and to Miss J Wardle for her helpful comments. Mr P McTaggart was responsible for the illustrations.

KEY POINTS FOR CLINICAL PRACTICE

- Every large haematology laboratory should have an automated instrument to measure the blood count including platelets, reticulocytes and differential white cell count. The instrument should pre-load, identify specimens by bar code, mix, aspirate whole blood by piercing the cap of the tube, make the measurements, perform quality control checks and transmit the data on-line to the laboratory computer.

- The majority of measurements are made by delivering relatively small numbers of cells into and out of a sensing zone. Some instruments use a narrow orifice and measure impedance changes (aperture-impedance counters) whilst others have cells in sheathflow and measure scatter as they pass through a light beam (light-scatter counters).

- To undertake the differential white cell count the two basic technologies may be combined with each other and/or with additional measurements such as multi-angle scatter, absorption after peroxidase staining, high frequency electromagnetic probes, etc. Special dyes are used for reticulocyte counting.

- The basic measurements are made well on all of the instruments described although some overestimate the MCHC in hypochromic anaemias.

- Because many of the measurements are made indirectly, the instruments have to be calibrated and then controlled to ensure that there is no drift. Users should also participate in suitable external quality assessment schemes.

- The market is evolving rapidly and potential purchasers should either study an independent evaluation or undertake one themselves in accordance with a proper protocol.

REFERENCES

Bentley S A, Johnson A, Bishop C A 1993 A parallel evaluation of four automated hematology analyzers. Am J Clin Pathol 100: 626–632

Brugnara C, Hipp M J, Irving P J et al 1994 Automated reticulocyte counting and measurement of reticulocyte cellular indices. Evaluation of the Miles H*3 blood analyzer. Am J Clin Pathol 102: 623–632

Coulter W H 1956 High speed automatic blood cell counter and cell size analyzer. Proc Nat Electron Conf 12: 1034

Crosland-Taylor P J 1953 A device for counting small particles suspended in a fluid through a tube. Nature 171: 37–38

Drayson R A, Hamilton M S F, England J M 1992 A comparison of differential white cell counting on the Coulter VCS and the Technicon H1 using simple and multiple regression analysis. Clin Lab Haemat 14: 293–305

England J M, Down M C, Bashford C C et al 1976 Differential leucocyte counts on the Counter Counter Model S. Lancet 1: 1134–1135

England J M, Perry T E, McTaggart P N et al 1995 An evaluation of the Technicon H*3RTX Haematology Analyser. Medical Devices Agency, London

ICSH 1987 Recommendations for reference method for haemoglobinometry in human blood (ICSH Standard 1986) and specifications for international haemiglobincyanide reference preparation (Third edition). Clin Lab Haemat 9: 73–79

ICSH 1988 The assignment of values to fresh blood used for calibrating automated cell counts. Clin Lab Haemat 10: 203–212

ICSH 1994 Guidelines for the evaluation of blood cell analysers including those used for differential leucocyte and reticulocyte counting and cell marker applications. Clin Lab Haemat 16: 157–174

Jones R G, Faust A M, Matthews R A 1995 Quality team approach in evaluating three automated hematology analyzers with five-part differential capability. Am J Clin Pathol 103: 159–166

Karsan A, Maclaren I, Conn D et al 1993 An evaluation of hemoglobin determination using sodium lauryl sulphate. Am J Clin Pathol 100: 123–126

Kerker M 1969 The scattering of light. Academic Press, New York

Korpman R A, Bull B S 1976 The implementation of a robust estimator of the mean for quality control on a programmable calculator or laboratory computer. Am J Clin Pathol 65: 252–253

Reardon D M, Mack D, Warner B, Hutchinson D 1991 A whole blood control for blood count analysers, and source material for an external quality assessment scheme. Med Lab Sci 48: 19–26

Roberts B E 1991 Standard Haematology Practice. Blackwell Scientific Publications, Oxford

Rowan R M, Cavanagh T H, Clark P et al 1995 An evaluation of the Sysmex HS-430 Haematology System. Medical Devices Agency, London

Tukey J W 1977 Exploratory data analysis. Addison-Wesley, Reading, MA

Ward P G, Chappell D A, Fox J G C, Allen B V 1975 Mixing and bottling unit for preparing biological fluids used in quality control. Lab Prac 24: 577–583

Warner B A, Reardon D M, Marshall D P 1990 Automated haematology analysers: a four-way comparison. Med Lab Sci 47: 285–296

Weil G J, Chused T M 1981 Eosinophil autofluorescence and its use in isolation and analysis of human eosinophils using flow microfluoremetry. Blood 57: 1099–1104

9

Transplantation for patients without HLA identical siblings

J. Hows   B. Bradley

Alternative donor allogeneic bone marrow transplantation (BMT) is a major challenge for haematologists as 60% of patients in Europe, North America, Japan, Australia and New Zealand lack an HLA identical sibling. The decade from 1985 to 1995 has been the first period in the short history of BMT that using donors other than HLA identical siblings has been scientifically evaluated. Previous experience was confined to case reports and small series of patients from single centres (Hansen et al 1980, Gordon-Smith et al 1982). The dual problems of graft failure and graft versus host disease (GVHD) remain major barriers to the acceptability of BMT in the absence of an HLA identical sibling.

The purpose of this chapter is to clarify the current role of alternative donor BMT for the practising clinician against a background of rapid change. At present there are no absolute indications for alternative donor BMT except in highly specialized paediatric practice for patients with severe combined immune deficiency (SCID) (Fischer et al 1990). Whenever possible, alternative donor transplantation should be carried out in the context of clinical trials, such as those organized by the Medical Research Council, or entered into prospective clinical studies, such as the International Marrow Unrelated Search and Transplant (IMUST) Study, set up to address clinically relevant questions (Bradley et al 1989). When neither of these options are available results of alternative donor BMT may be reported to one of the international BMT registers held by the European Bone Marrow Transplantation Group (EBMTG) and the International Bone Marrow Transplant Registry (IBMTR).

With parallel advances over the past 10 years in non-allograft therapy for haematological malignancies and non-malignant haematological disorders, clinicians are faced with increasingly difficult decisions in planning the best definitive treatment for patients who lack HLA identical siblings. For example, improved supportive care including the use of haemopoietic growth factors (Bacigalupo et al 1993) combined with an immunosuppressive protocol of cyclosporin and antithymocyte globulin (Frickhoven et al 1991) has greatly improved the survival of patients with severe aplastic anaemia who lack HLA identical siblings. Furthermore, confirmation that relapse after autografting can arise from residual malignant cells in the graft (Brenner et al 1993) and the introduction of purging techniques in the clinical setting (Hurd et al 1988, Ball et al 1990, Friedman et al 1990) has led to a more scientific approach to autografting both in leukaemia and the lymphomas. An additional advance in autografting over the past 10 years is the use of autologous peripheral blood progenitor cells (PBPC). These not only give more rapid peripheral blood recovery than standard marrow autografts, thus reducing morbidity from the procedure and length of stay in hospital (Kessinger & Armitage 1991), but also make exvivo purging of malignant cells technically easier (Shpall et al 1993). Advances in autografting have yet to achieve the low incidence of disease recurrence associated with allografts, a result attributed to a graft versus leukaemia activity (Weiden et al 1979).

In the sections below we have first outlined guidelines for selecting patients and alternative donors for transplants. Secondly we have reviewed the current status of alternative donor transplantation for different haematological disorders. Finally we have highlighted future directions which we think may have an impact on alternative donor BMT.

GENERAL PRINCIPLES FOR SELECTING PATIENTS AND DONORS

The results of patients treated with alternative BMT remain inferior to those achieved for patients with the same clinical risk treated with HLA identical sibling BMT (Fig. 1A). In every case the patient's age, diagnosis, disease status (early or advanced) and the 'suitability' of the potential alternative donor should be assessed. One needs to weigh up the relative benefits of allogeneic BMT against non-allograft therapy. Some patients will choose non-allograft therapy when the risks of alternative donor BMT are properly explained. All clinicians should ask the question: 'Would allogeneic BMT be considered in this case if the patient had an HLA identical sibling?' If the answer is 'no' then treatment with alternative donor BMT should not be considered, despite frequent pressure from patients and relatives for 'something to be done'.

Patient characteristics

There are published recommendations concerning patient selection for unrelated donor BMT (Goldman 1994). Table 1 gives a simplified version of these proposals, which are disease orientated. These recommendations may also be used as guidelines for the use of partially HLA matched family donor transplants (see below). Both recipient age and disease status have been established as powerful factors predicting outcome of allogeneic BMT using alternative donors (McGlave et al 1993). The poor results of unrelated donor BMT in patients over the age of 40 years and in patients with advanced disease have been highlighted in a recent analysis from the IMUST Study (Hows et al 1993) (Figs. 1B and 1C). A major cause of morbidity and mortality after alternative donor BMT is systemic infection, often caused by viruses (Marks et al 1993). These data suggest that immune reconstitution is slow

TRANSPLANTATION WITHOUT HLA IDENTICAL SIBLINGS

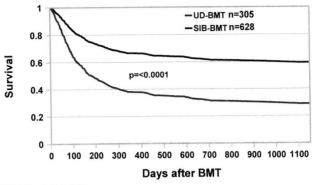

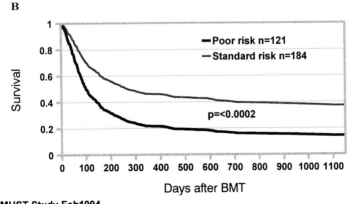

Figs 1A, B and C Estimated probability of survival after A. HLA identical sibling BMT (SIB-BMT) compared to a matched cohort of unrelated donor BMT (UD-BMT); B. UD-BMT at three different age ranges; C. UD-BMT in recipients who were poor and standard risk at the time of BMT.

and sometimes incomplete in the presence of overt or occult HLA mismatch after alternative donor BMT.

The availability of non-allograft treatment

This consideration is important and disease specific, and will be considered below in the sections addressing the role of alternative donor BMT for different haematological disorders.

HLA typing and matching

It is essential that clinical transplant units performing alternative donor BMT have strong links with an expert immunogenetics laboratory specializing in the field. Histocompatibility matching of donor and recipient has a strong influence on the outcome of allogeneic BMT. In alternative donor BMT the aim of HLA matching is to reduce the number of allo-antigens seen as 'foreign' by the recipient (host) in the graft and by the graft in the recipient. The HLA allo-antigens known to be important in BMT are the products of HLA-A,B,C (HLA Class I) genes, and HLA-DR, DQ, DP (HLA Class II) genes (Fig. 2). The impact of

Table 1. Patient criteria for unrelated donor search (assuming patient is aged less than 55 years, has given informed consent and that an accredited transplant centre has agreed to treat the patient)

Category 1: BMT by accredited unit in research programme with ethics committee approval	Category 2: BMT by accredited unit for indication generally accepted on basis of published data from other centres
ALL in CR high risk	ALL in CR high risk
AML in CR high risk	AML in CR high risk
CML in chronic phase	CML in chronic phase
MDS (RA) poor risk	MDS (RA) poor risk
Lymphoma	Lymphoma
Myeloma	Myeloma
AML relapse	
CML accelerated phase	
RAEB	
RAEB-t	
SAA (0.2×10^9/l neuts) 3–6 months post immunosuppression no response	SAA 3–6 months post immunosuppression no response
Fanconi anaemia, other congenital BM failure	Fanconi anaemia, other congenital BM failure
Inborn errors	Inborn errors
SCID, Wiskott-Aldrich syndrome	SCID, Wiskott-Aldrich syndrome
Chediack-Higashi syndrome	Chediack-Higashi syndrome
Hurler's disease	Hurler's disease
Gaucher's disease	Gaucher's disease
Osteopetrosis	Osteopetrosis
SAA (>0.2×10^9/l neuts) >6 months post immunosuppression no response	
Sickle cell disease, thalassaemia major	

Adapted from Goldman (1994)

non-HLA histocompatibility antigens on the outcome of alternative donor transplantation is currently unknown, although it is well known that mismatching can cause both graft failure and GVHD after HLA identical sibling BMT. Routinely, non-HLA allo-antigens are not matched in alternative donor selection.

Until recently, only basic HLA typing and matching methods have been required to identify HLA identical sibling donors, who are genotypically identical for both HLA haplotypes (Fig. 3A). Typing for alternative family and unrelated donors requires a much higher level of precision because of the vast polymorphism of the HLA gene region (Fig. 2). Recent studies using high resolution HLA typing and matching methods have demonstrated that 72% of unrelated donor-recipient BMT pairs thought to be matched for HLA-A, B,C, DR were in fact mismatched for one or more antigen. By implication, the number of unrelated donor-recipient BMT pairs who were as well matched as HLA identical siblings was approximately 28% (Tiercy et al 1995). The impact of HLA mismatching on survival after alternative donor BMT is considerable. Data from the IMUST Study (Bradley et al 1994) and other reports indicate that there is a highly significant reduction in survival after unrelated donor BMT compared with clinically similar cohorts of patients undergoing HLA identical sibling BMT, and an even further reduction with HLA mismatched unrelated donor BMT (Fig. 1A) (Marks et al 1993). It is unlikely that the volunteer donor pool can be enlarged significantly to increase the proportion of well matched unrelated donors, therefore a policy for intelligent mismatching is required if alternative donor BMT is to be safely extended to a higher proportion of patients. Such a policy would require both a knowledge of which HLA mismatches are associated with low allo-reactivity (Laundy & Bradley 1995), and more powerful methods for their detection (Clay et al 1991, Bradley et al 1992). It is now possible to use methods which identify

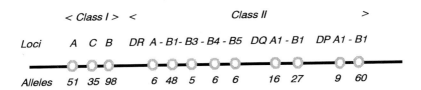

Fig. 2. Schematic diagram of an HLA haplotype showing the loci that code for histocompatibility antigens and the total number of alleles identified at each plus one for the unidentified 'null' gene (Bodmer 1994). Given that each individual inherits one allele from each parent, the theoretical number of HLA phenotypes is given by:

$(51 \times 35 \times 98 \times 6 \times 48 \times 5 \times 6 \times 6 \times 16 \times 27 \times 9 \times 60)^2 = 4.5 \times 10^{30}$

the DNA sequences of HLA alleles for typing and matching for HLA Class I and Class II. These are based on the polymerase chain reaction (PCR) followed by identification of the PCR product with oligonucleotide probes or by conformational analysis (Bidwell 1994).

Functional crossmatch tests based on the in-vitro lymphocyte alloreactivity have until recently depended on the semi-quantitative mixed lymphocyte reaction (MLR), however, this test is of limited value (Hansen et al 1994) and is being replaced by more quantitative cellular assays. These limiting dilution assays are designed to measure the frequency of cytotoxic T-lymphocyte precursor (CTL-p) cells present in the donor's blood which are specifically cytotoxic against the patient's HLA and non-HLA mismatches (Kaminski et al 1991). CTLp frequency in the peripheral blood of the donor has been shown to correlate with the probability of developing severe acute GVHD and death after unrelated donor BMT (Kaminski et al 1989, Spencer et al 1995).

Selection of partially HLA matched family donors

In clinical practice the level of acceptable HLA mismatch varies according to donor source, patient diagnosis and age. At one extreme infants with severe combined immunodeficiency (SCID) may be successfully transplanted from a one haplotype mismatch parent or sibling (refer to the section on inherited immunodeficiency below) (Fig. 3A). But this level of mismatch is unacceptable for adult leukaemia, because of a high probability of fatal graft failure (Anasetti et al 1989), and fatal GVHD (Beatty et al 1985). It is only when parents share the same or a similar HLA haplotype (Fig. 3B) that there is a reasonable probability of an acceptable family donor being found. An acceptable donor would be one who by conventional HLA-A, B, DR typing criteria is phenotypically matched with the patient, or mismatched for no more than one antigen. Beatty and colleagues have shown, in a single centre retrospective study from Seattle, that transplant survival after one antigen mismatch in young adults with acute leukaemia in remission or chronic myeloid leukaemia in chronic phase, was not significantly different from HLA identical sibling transplants for patients with the same clinical characteristics (Beatty et al 1985). In practice such donors only extend the family donor pool by 5% over that provided by HLA identical siblings.

HLA typing of the patient's extended family (blood related aunts, uncles, nieces, nephews and first cousins), with a view to finding a phenotypically matched donor, is worthwhile if the patient carries one or more common HLA haplotype (Table 2). The higher the frequency of the haplotype in the population, the higher the probability of its recurrence in the extended family (Fig. 2C). Mathematical formulae have been developed that can predict the probability of success of finding an extended family donor given prior knowledge of HLA haplotype frequencies in the associated ethnic group (Kaufman 1995). The logistic implications of commencing an extended donor search are complex and should always be discussed at the outset with an expert immunogenetics laboratory.

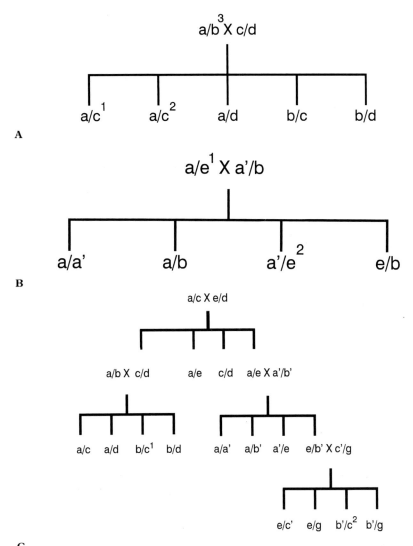

Fig. 3. Family segregation diagrams showing the different relationships between donors and recipients in different situations. The letters a, a', b, b', c, d, e and g represent single HLA haplotypes. 1 and 2 indicate donor and recipient. 3 indicates a one haplotype mismatched donor. **A.** HLA identical sibling donor BMT. Four alternative phenotypes of the children are shown with one, a/c, being duplicated to give a HLA genetically identical pair. A one haplotype mismatched BMT (see text) would involve the parent, a/b or the sibling a/d or b/c, being used as a donor for a/c. **B.** HLA phenotypically matched donor BMT using a first degree relative. Here the parental haplotypes, a and a' are identical or closely matched. The child who inherits a'/e is thus closely phenotypically matched to the parent, a/e. **C.** HLA phenotypically matched donor BMT using a distant relative discovered by extended family search. Here the phenotypically matched pair are, second uncle/aunt (b/c), and second niece/nephew (b'/c), respectively. Haplotype c is inherited in the blood line, whereas b and b' are similar but unrelated common haplotypes that recur in distant relatives of the same family. Hence the probability of success of an extended family search depends on the size of the family and whether or not the patient carries a common HLA haplotype.

Table 2. Commonest HLA Haplotypes in various ethnic groups. (Only populations where > 100 individuals were typed are included. (Imanishi 1992).

Population (Number typed)	A	Cw	B	DR	DQ	HF%*
North American Negroid (312)	36	4	53	11	1	1.1
Cornish (101)	1	7	8	3	2	8.4
Danish (122)	3	7	7	15	1	3.6
French (244)	1	7	8	3	2	2.5
German (203)	1	7	8	3	2	4.8
Greek (176)	2	4	35	11	7	2.0
Italian (483)	2	4	35	11	7	2.3
Spanish (192)	29	-**	44	7	2	3.0
USA (226)	1	7	8	3	2	4.5
Canadian (142)	1	7	8	3	2	5.2
Brazilian (286)	24	4	35	11	7	1.4
Japanese (893)	24	-	52	15	1	8.3
Korean (235)	33	-	44	13	1	4.5
Thai (235)	2	11	46	9	3	4.5
Vietnamese (140)	29	-	7	10	1	4.6
Inuit (144)	24	-	48	4	7	9.4

* haplotype frequency.   ** null or unidentified allele.

Selection of unrelated donors

The polymorphism of the HLA gene region is so extensive that when all possible theoretical phenotypes are calculated from the known alleles of the HLA-A, B, C, DR, DQ and DP loci the total exceeds 10^{30} (Fig. 2). Fortunately, because certain HLA haplotypes are conserved within populations (Table 2) the probability of donor search succeeding is greater than if HLA phenotypes were randomly distributed. Donor searches for conserved haplotypes are much more likely to succeed if directed towards geographical regions where they are known to have the highest frequency (Lonjou et al 1995), but such detailed information of the geographic distribution of HLA haplotypes is not widely available outside France.

Over the past 20 years there has been massive recruitment to unrelated donor panels worldwide, resulting in over two million HLA-typed volunteers being registered on computer files. Calculations based on the known frequency of HLA phenotypes within populations give some indication of the relationship between panel size and theoretical probability of finding an acceptably 'matched' unrelated donor (Beatty et al 1988, Bradley et al 1987). These calculations do not take into consideration the efficiency of the search procedure. The clinical situation is measurable as a probability of finding a donor within a given time. In a prospective study, 700 consecutive searches in the UK between 1989–91 were studied (Howard et al 1994). Clinical search failure was predicted by progressive disease, ethnic mismatching between the patient and the volunteer panel and an uncommon HLA phenotype. Half the searches initiated were discontinued either because the patient's condition deteriorated or logistic problems were encountered in the search procedure. Only 10% of searches resulted in BMT. In the past 5 years search procedures have improved substantially but actual donor yield is still well below the theoretical maximum with approximately 25% of searches resulting in a transplant. For ethnic and logistic reasons all searches are first performed nationally but if no donor is found the search may be extended internationally. Guidelines for international searches have recently been published by the World Marrow Donor Association (Goldman 1994). Unrelated donor searches add costs to the transplant (Ottinger et al 1994) and therefore the clinician should identify a source of funding before proceeding. Unfortunately the median time to complete an unrelated donor search is still 3–6 months which, in many cases, leads to clinical deterioration or disease progression before the patient can be transplanted.

ALTERNATIVE DONOR TRANSPLANTS FOR THE CHRONIC LEUKAEMIAS AND MYELOMA

Most experience of alternative donor transplants has to date been in chronic myeloid leukaemia (CML). Despite encouraging results for prolonging the chronic phase of the disease using alpha interferon (Allan et al 1995) and by PBPC autografting (Carella et al 1992) no cure exists for this disease apart from allogeneic BMT, but this is applicable to the minority of patients who both have a suitable donor and are under the age of 50–55 (Goldman et al 1986). Data on HLA identical sibling BMT for myeloma (Gahrton et al 1991) and chronic lymphatic leukaemia (Rabinowe et al 1993) are much more limited as the vast majority of patients are over 50 years old leaving a tiny minority eligible for allografting. Despite this, neither disease is definitely curable by non-allograft therapy, suggesting that the same principles for selecting patients for allogeneic BMT should be applied as for CML. Because of the highly experimental nature of alternative donor BMT for myeloma and chronic lymphoid leukaemia (CLL) it is suggested that these patients should be referred to transplant units with a special interest in the appropriate disorder.

Chronic myeloid leukaemia

Alternative donor BMT should whenever possible be carried out in chronic phase in the first year after diagnosis. The exception is the minority of patients whose disease can be converted to >60% Philadelphia chromosome (Ph) negativity with a 3–6 month trial of alpha interferon. This group has an excellent prognosis and should only be considered for alternative donor BMT if cytogenetic relapse occurs (Allan et al 1995). Outcome of BMT for CML in chronic phase using one antigen mismatched family donors was reported from Seattle. Leukaemia-free survival in the medium term was 40–45% and not significantly different from 'control' patients transplanted from HLA identical siblings. However, the mismatched cases were associated with a significantly higher incidence of grade II–IV and III–IV acute GVHD than the HLA identical sibling transplants (Beatty et al 1985). As previously mentioned only about 5% of patients have a suitable alternative nuclear family donor. Median time in chronic phase is in excess of 5 years giving adequate time to carry out unrelated donor searches. McGlave and colleagues (1993) reported overall disease-free survival, 2 years after unrelated donor BMT, at 27–47% for patients in chronic phase and 13–39% for patients in accelerated phase at the time of BMT. Multifactorial analysis indicated that serological HLA match (relative risk, RR, 0.60), young recipient age (RR 0.82 per decade), disease status at transplant (RR 0.69) and use of T-cell depletion for GVHD prophylaxis (RR 0.68) were favourable indicators of disease-free survival (McGlave et al 1993). Similar results have been reported by other investigators (Marks et al 1993). Of note, the incidence of graft failure is high at 10–15% (McGlave et al 1993) and the success of second salvage unrelated BMT is very low and associated with difficult ethical considerations (Goldman 1994). A practical consideration is always to cryopreserve autologous cells and to autograft the patient if graft failure occurs.

Multiple myeloma

There are few alternative donor transplants for myeloma reported in the literature. HLA identical sibling BMT provides long-term continuous remission in 40% of cases. Patients with stage I disease at diagnosis and those who only received first line chemotherapy prior to BMT have the best probability of disease-free survival (Gahrton et al 1991). Pilot studies of marrow autografts for myeloma have been disappointing because of tumour cell contamination of the graft (Samson 1992). Peripheral blood progenitor cell transplants including the use of positive selection of CD34+ cells as a purging technique are being evaluated. Unrelated donor BMT after successful first time chemotherapy with a regimen such as C-VAMP (cyclophosphamide, vincristine, adriamycin and methylprednisolone) is now an option for carefully selected patients under 40–45 years of age. This course is not recommended unless a donor matched for HLA-A, B, DR and DQ is available.

Chronic lymphatic leukaemia (CLL)

Patients under 50 years of age are rare. However, preliminary data from HLA identical sibling BMT have been reported (Rabinowe et al 1993). Most patients with CLL treated to date by sibling BMT have had poor prognosis disease, clinically or cytogenetically. Preliminary information suggests that those transplanted after debulking chemotherapy fare best. In one report, 9 of 17 patients were in continuous haematological remission with a mean follow-up of 26 months (range 4–48) after BMT (Rabinowe et al 1993). As in myeloma, results of autografting in CLL have been disappointing because of tumour cell contamination of the graft. These very preliminary data suggest that the rare patient with poor risk CLL under the age of 45–50 should be referred to a specialist transplant unit for consideration of alternative donor BMT.

ALTERNATIVE DONOR BMT FOR THE ACUTE LEUKAEMIAS AND MYELODYSPLASIA

The decision to consider alternative donor BMT depends on the patient's age, stage of disease, and whether the disease is considered good or poor risk by conventional clinical, haematological and cytogenetic criteria. For example, most haematologists would consider alternative donor BMT inappropriate in patients in first remission with AML M3, with the 15:17 translocation or AML M4 with inversion 16. In contrast, young patients with high-risk features such as ALL with Ph positivity should be considered as candidates for alternative donor BMT in first remission.

Acute myeloblastic leukaemia

Recently published data derived from prospectively randomized studies of patients of transplantable age have attempted to eliminate the effect of time censoring on comparison of the outcome of allografts from HLA identical siblings, with autografts and intensive chemotherapy alone, in patients with AML in first remission. In one study (Zittoun et al 1995) randomization between autografting and intensive chemotherapy alone in patients who lacked HLA identical sibling donors was performed immediately the patient attained complete remission. All patients with HLA identical sibling donors were allocated to consolidation with allogeneic BMT. Grafting procedures were carried out as soon as patients had recovered from consolidation chemotherapy and the outcome analysed on the basis of intention to treat, irrespective of whether individual patients actually received their assigned treatment modality. Although relapse was significantly more frequent in patients receiving intensive chemotherapy alone ($p=0.05$), survival in continuous complete remission at 5 years after attaining first remission was not different between autografting (43–53%) and allografting (51–59%). No relapses occurred in the allograft group after 2 years; longer follow-up is required to see if late relapses after autografting make this treatment inferior to allografting in the long term. As autografting appears to give similar results to allografting there is no indication for alternative donor transplantation in first remission in good or standard-risk AML. There is a need to compare the results of alternative donor BMT and autografting in high-risk AML patients in first remission defined by standard criteria and in patients with AML in second remission.

Acute lymphoblastic leukaemia

Acute lymphoblastic leukaemia (ALL) is extremely heterologous, with patient age, sex, presenting white cell count, blast cell morphology, surface immunophenotype and cytogenetics having profound effects on prognosis (Rivera & Maver 1987). A recent report from the Medical Research Council

(MRC) Working Party on Childhood Leukaemia has confirmed in the recently analysed UKALL-X study that inclusion of both early and late intensification modules provides a significant improvement in leukaemia-free survival in children under the age of 15 years with and without high risk factors (Chessells et al 1995). Overall disease-free survival at 5 years for all patients in UKALL-X was 65–76%. These data suggest that it is only children with the poorest prognostic factors including the 4:11 translocation, Ph positive disease and possibly boys with presenting white cell counts of $>100 \times 10^9/1$ who should be considered for HLA identical sibling transplants in first remission. It is not unreasonable to consider this same very high risk group for alternative donor BMT in first remission.

In young adults over 16 years of age for whom the result of intensive chemotherapy alone is less optomistic HLA identical sibling BMT in first remission is being prospectively evaluated in the MRC study UKALL-XII. The benefit of autografting seems less certain in ALL than in AML in first remission, making alternative donor BMT in first remission a reasonable option for high-risk patients. Virtually all patients under the age of 50 years with ALL in second remission are considered candidates for HLA identical sibling BMT. A recent case-controlled retrospective analysis on large numbers of individuals less than 18 years of age from the IBMTR found superior leukaemia-free survival at 5 years for patients treated by HLA identical sibling transplantation compared with those treated with recurrent intensive chemotherapy: 37–43% compared with 14–20%, respectively (Barrett et al 1994).

Preliminary data is available on unrelated donor BMT compared with HLA identical sibling BMT in young adults with poor risk ALL in first and second remission from the IMUST Study (Hows et al 1994a). At 2 years after BMT there was no significant difference in projected survival between the two groups where results had been corrected for patient age, stage of disease at BMT, transplant centre and transplant protocol, and subjected to multifactorial analysis. These preliminary data are supported by a single centre analysis of unrelated donor transplants carried out for children with high risk ALL (Cornish et al 1995). In this report a one or two antigen HLA mismatch between unrelated donor and recipient had no apparent effect on post-transplant survival. Thus adults with ALL in first and second remission and children with ALL in second remission are candidates for alternative donor BMT.

Myelodysplasia

Only a minority of patients with de novo myelodysplasia (MDS) are under 50 years old, however, an increasing number of younger patients with MDS secondary to intensive chemotherapy and/or irradiation for acute leukaemia, lymphoma and solid tumours are being identified, as are patients who develop MDS following treatment of acquired aplastic anaemia with immunosuppressive therapy. It is only over the past few years that MDS has been considered a standard indication for HLA identical sibling BMT in young patients. In the three retrospectively reported series of over 50 patients, disease-free survival at 2 years was in the range of 35–45% (Anderson et al 1993, DeWitte et al 1990, Sutton et al 1991). Refractory anaemia without excess of blasts, young patient age and short time between diagnosis and BMT were reported by the Seattle group as good prognostic factors (Anderson et al 1993). In this report 28 patients were transplanted from either phenotypically 'matched' unrelated donors or partially matched family donors. There was no detectable difference in post-transplant survival compared with those patients transplanted from HLA identical siblings. From these limited data it is reasonable to approach alternative donor BMT in MDS in the same way as in patients with CML. Both diseases are incurable apart from allogeneic BMT, so alternative donor BMT should be considered as a treatment option soon after the diagnosis is made. Patients with an excess of blasts have a poor prognosis, with a high incidence of post-transplant relapse (Anderson et al 1993). Such patients should be considered for intensive chemotherapy with the aim of reducing marrow blasts to less than 5% prior to transplantation.

ALTERNATIVE DONOR TRANSPLANTATION FOR BONE MARROW FAILURE

Severe acquired aplastic anaemia (SAA)

Results of HLA identical sibling transplantation have improved over the past decade and for patients under the age of 35–45 years BMT remains the treatment of choice, with 75–90% survival at 3–5 years post-transplant (Paquette et al 1995, Storb et al 1994). Recent analysis of the EBMTG SAA working party database of patients treated with anti-thymocyte globulin (ATG) in the early 1990s shows much improved survival compared to the 1970s and 1980s (Bacigalupo 1995, personal communication). This improvement is attributed to better immunosuppressive protocols incorporating cyclosporin and granulocyte stimulating factor, and improvement in supportive care. In this analysis, survival at 5 years was estimated at 80–85% in patients under 50 years of age. Survival after treatment with ATG is highly dependent on achieving haematological response (Paquette et al 1995). Although 15–30% of patients with SAA treated by ATG will ultimately relapse or develop clonal evolution of disease into MDS, AML, or paroxysmal nocturnal haemoglobinuria, ATG treatment-related morbidity is low and the quality of life of survivors excellent. Over the past 15 years the results of alternative donor BMT have also improved but still remain significantly inferior to HLA identical sibling BMT, with survival at 1 year post BMT of about 40% (Hows et al 1994b). These data suggest that alternative donor BMT should be reserved for patients who have failed immunosuppressive therapy and who can be included in pilot studies in specialist centres. Multicentre prospective studies are required to evaluate the results of alternative donor BMT compared with recurrent courses of immunosuppression in patients who fail to respond to one or two courses of ATG.

Fanconi anaemia

Patients with Fanconi anaemia (FA) are normally considered for HLA identical BMT before the onset of regular transfusion dependency. Transplants are usually elective as the vast majority of patients with FA can be maintained without transfusions on low-dose androgen therapy for long periods. In contrast to SAA, FA can only be treated for severe bone marrow failure by allogeneic BMT. Treatment with recombinant growth factors is disappointing in FA and not recommended as definitive therapy. Alternative donor BMT should therefore be considered as a treatment option before the patient becomes dependent on regular blood transfusions. Unfortunately data on the results of alternative donor BMT are limited because of the rarity of FA (Gluckman & Hows 1994, Hows et al 1994b).

THE GENETIC DISORDERS

Transplantable genetic disorders include congenital aplastic anaemias (see the above section on Fanconi anaemia), inherited immunodeficiency disorders, haemoglobinopathies, osteopetrosis and inborn errors of metabolism. Transplantation for this group should be carried out in specialist transplant centres where there is expertise in the diagnosis, monitoring and clinical management of the specific disorder.

Inherited immunodeficiency

The inherited immunodeficiencies were the first group of disorders to be successfully treated by allogeneic BMT (Bach et al 1968, Gatti et al 1968). Today the success rate for HLA identical sibling BMT for severe combined immunodeficiency (SCID) is 80–90%. In the majority of cases pre-graft conditioning and GVHD prophylaxis is unnecessary and full T-cell chimerism is achieved with sufficient B-cell chimerism to provide normal immune function. The success of BMT for SCID depends on carrying out the procedure as rapidly as possible after diagnosis prior to the development of life-threatening infection. For this reason the use of readily available haploidentical parental marrow has been investigated in families where the patient lacks an HLA identical sibling. Recent results of these highly mismatched transplants are good, following considerable protocol development. It is now generally accepted that pre-transplant conditioning is necessary in parental haplo-mismatched transplants. The most successful protocols also include donor T-cell depletion (Fischer et al 1990) or infusion of antibody directed against adhesion molecules such as LFA-1 (Fischer et al 1994). Using these techniques long-term survival and immune reconstitution can be achieved in 60–70% of cases (O'Reilly et al 1994). Increasing success is also attributable to improved supportive care and control of viral infections. It is unclear whether unrelated donor BMT has a significant role in the treatment of inherited immunodeficiency as the time between diagnosis and transplantation is critical and at present a delay of weeks or months in identifying a suitable donor may occur.

The haemoglobinopathies

Although results of HLA identical sibling BMT are extremely promising in beta thalassaemia major (Lucarelli et al 1993), preliminary results in experienced centres for alternative donor BMT have been less encouraging with a high incidence of transplant-related mortality and recurrent disease. Thus pilot programmes of alternative donor BMT for thalassaemia should only be carried out in specialist centres.

Sickle cell anaemia has also been successfully treated by HLA identical sibling BMT. Uncertainty regarding the selection of patients for BMT exists because of the variable phenotypic manifestations of the disease. Fifty percent of patients receiving good conventional care live beyond the age of 40 years (Chan & Schroeder 1990). Young patients were transplanted from HLA identical siblings prior to their return to a part of Africa where medical care and safety of blood transfusion therapy is suboptimal (Vermylen et al 1991). In this report 12 children were transplanted using high-dose busulphan and cyclophosphamide pre-BMT and cyclosporin as GVHD prophylaxis. All 12 patients survived, 11 with complete and one with partial chimerism; none were transfusion-dependent post-BMT. At present there are no data on alternative donor BMT in sickle cell anaemia. Pilot studies in alternative donor BMT should probably await a reduction in BMT-related morbidity and mortality.

Inborn errors of metabolism

There is a wide range of rare and very rare inborn errors of metabolism which are theoretically treatable by allogeneic bone marrow transplantation, as normal transplanted reticuloendothelial cells can produce the critical enzyme that the patient lacks. Commoner disorders include Gaucher's and Hurler's disease. Optimal timing of HLA identical sibling transplants has prevented disease progression and provided a good quality of life in well selected patients. Paediatricians specializing in this area are becoming aware that some inborn errors do not correct well after BMT and in other cases where good evidence for biochemical correction is documented there is still disease progression or significant residual clinical problems. Much more work is required in this specialized area before guidelines for alternative donor BMT can be suggested.

FUTURE DIRECTIONS

Human umbilical cord blood

Human umbilical cord blood is rich in haemopoietic stem cells and has recently been considered as an alternative source of cells for clinical transplantation (Broxmeyer et al 1989). The first successful transplant was recorded in 1989 (Gluckman et al 1989). To date 55 cord blood (CB) transplants have been carried out worldwide in children weighing up to 40 kg (Wagner et al 1994). It is not certain whether single CB donations contain sufficient stem cells to reconstitute adult recipients, although both in vivo and in vitro data are encouraging. On average, CB donations contain 15×10^8 nucleated cells (Hows et al 1992a), one-tenth of the nucleated cell dose conventionally used for marrow transplantation in adults. Using haemopoietic long-term cultures we have shown that the quality of stem cells is greater in CB compared with normal donor marrow (Hows et al 1992a). Additional studies to quantitate cord blood stem cells by limiting dilution cultures, and pre-clinical evaluation of the capacity for in vitro expansion of CB cells, are necessary before CB transplants can safely be applied to adults.

Potential advantages of CB are that cryopreserved donations are instantly available, are free from pathogenic viruses, such as cytomegalovirus, and possibly have reduced GVHD potential. In addition, CB collected after the birth of normal full-term infants is without risk to the donor (Hows et al 1992b). Efficient CB banking will depend on research, development and standardization of HLA typing, collection, processing and cryopreservation methods.

It is hoped that international links between CB banks set up at national level will shortly be established. The New York Cord Blood Bank (Rubinstein et al 1993) is already included in the Leiden publication 'Bone Marrow Donors Worldwide'. Another advantage of an international CB bank network is the potential for building up a large collection of non-Caucasian donations. Preliminary information suggests that individuals from some non-Caucasian ethnic groups may consider CB collection the most acceptable method of donation. There is wide international agreement that a pilot clinical CB transplant study is required to evaluate results in comparison with unrelated donor BMT. To perform this study a CB bank network is essential. Only if pilot transplant studies are successful should major health care resources be channelled into CB banking.

Allogeneic peripheral blood progenitor cells (PBPC)

Recent reports have appeared regarding allogeneic PBPC transplants from HLA identical sibling donors (Schmitz et al 1995). In the standard transplant setting allogeneic PBPC only provide marginal advantages in terms of speed of post-transplant peripheral blood recovery over the use of marrow from the same donor. There are no data on possible long-term donor complications after administration of recombinant haemopoietic growth factors, for example the development of leukaemia. The chance of such complications are probably small, and the early advantages to some donors, namely the avoidance of admission to hospital and a general anaesthetic, are attractive.

An exciting potential use for allogeneic PBPC in alternative donor transplantation has been reported (Aversa et al 1994). Seventeen patients with advanced leukaemia were transplanted from a combination of marrow and PBPC collected from one haplotype mismatched family members. The total dose of progenitor cells transplanted was 10-fold greater than for conventional HLA identical sibling donor BMT and the donations were treated in vitro pre-transplant to reduce the number of CD3 positive mature T-cells to less than 10^9/kg of recipient body weight. Sixteen of 17 patients engrafted as a result of the enhanced haemopoietic cell dose and only one patient developed fatal GVHD. Therefore PBPC collections can allow a large enough dose of haemopoietic cells to be given to overcome the high risk of graft failure arising from the use of T-cell depleted grafts in severely HLA mismatched transplants (O'Reilly et al 1988). It remains to be seen if these experimental transplants will be associated with a high risk of disease recurrence or post-transplant lymphoproliferative disease.

KEY POINTS FOR CLINICAL PRACTICE

Before considering alternative donor BMT the potential of non-allograft therapy should be carefully considered.

- Results of alternative donor BMT remain inferior to results of HLA identical sibling BMT with the possible exception of young patients with ALL. It follows that patients who would not have been considered for HLA identical sibling BMT should not be considered for alternative donor BMT.

- Alternative donor BMT should be carried out in accredited transplant centres with special expertise.

- Where possible, patients undergoing alternative donor BMT should be entered into clinical trials and studies or reported to an international transplant registry.

- Reduced survival after alternative donor BMT is associated with the level of HLA mismatch, increasing recipient age, stage of disease, diagnosis and choice of BMT protocol.

- Cord blood transplantation remains experimental in paediatric practice and has not yet been evaluated in adults.

REFERENCES

Allan N C, Richards S M, Shepherd P C A on behalf of the UK medical Research Council Working Parties for Therapeutic Trials in Adult Leukemia1995 UK Medical Research Council randomised Multicentre trial of interferon – αnl for chronic myeloid leukemia: improved survival irrespective of cytogenetic response. Lancet 345: 1392-1397

Anasetti C, Amos D, Beatty P G et al 1989 Effect of HLA compatibility on engraftment of

bone marrow transplants in patients with leukemia or lymphoma. N Engl J Med 320: 197–204
Anderson J E, Appelbaum F R, Fisher C D et al 1993 Allogeneic bone marrow transplantation for 93 patients with myelodysplastic syndrome. Blood 82: 677–681
Aversa F, Tabilo A, Terenzi A et al 1994 Successful engraftment of T-cell depleted haploidentical 'three loci' incompatible transplants in leukaemia patients by addition of recombinant human granulocyte colony-stimulating factor-mobilized peripheral blood progenitor cells to bone marrow inoculation. Blood 84: 3948–3955
Bach F H, Albertini R J, Anderson J L et al 1968 Bone marrow transplantation in a patient with Wiskott-Aldrich syndrome. Lancet 2: 1364–1366
Bacigalupo A, Gluckman E, Mori P G et al 1993 Antilymphocyte globulin (ALG), cyclosporin (CyA) and G-CSF in patients with acquired severe aplastic anemia (SAA): a pilot study of the EBMT SAA Working Party. Exp Hematol 21: 1081
Ball E D, Mills L E, Cornwell G G et al 1990 Autologous bone marrow transplantation for acute myeloid leukemia using monoclonal antibody-purged bone marrow. Blood 75: 1199–1206
Barrett A J, Horowitz M M, Pollock B H et al 1994 Bone marrow transplants from HLA identical siblings as compared with chemotherapy for children with acute lymphoblastic leukemia in a second remission. N Engl J Med 331: 1253–1258
Beatty P G, Clift R A, Michelson E M et al 1985 Marrow transplantation from related donors other than HLA identical siblings. N Eng J Med 313: 765–771
Beatty P G, Dahlberg S, Mickelson E M et al 1988 Probability of finding HLA matched unrelated marrow donors. Transplantation 45: 714–721
Bodmer J G, Marsh S G E, Albert E D et al 1994 Nomenclature for factors of the HLA system. Eur J Immunogen 21: 485–517
Bidwell J L 1994 Advances in DNA-based HLA-typing methods. Immunol Today 15: 303–307
Bradley B A, Gilks W R, Gore S M et al 1987 How many HLA typed volunteer donors for bone marrow transplantation (BMT) are needed to provide an effective service? Bone Marrow Transplant 2 (Suppl 11): 79
Bradley B A, Gore S M, Howard M R, Hows J M 1989 International Marrow Unrelated Search and Transplant (IMUST) Study. Bone Marrow Transplant 4 (Suppl 2): 44
Bradley B A, Clay T, Wood N A P et al 1992 DNA crossmatching for rapid selection of HLA – DR identical unrelated donors and application to DR-Dw typing. In: Tsuji K, Aizawa M, Sasazuki T (eds) HLA 1991. Oxford University Press, Oxford, pp 423–427
Bradley B A, Downie T R, Hows J M et al 1994 The impact of genetic mismatching on BMT outcome. Hum Immunol 39 (A18): 126
Brenner M K, Rill D R, Holladay M S et al 1993 Gene marking to determine whether autologous marrow infusion restores long-term haemopoiesis in cancer patients. Lancet 342: 1134–1137
Broxmeyer H E, Douglas G W, Hangoc G et al 1989 Human umbilical cord blood as a potential source of transplantable hematopoietic stem/progenitor cells. Proc Nat Acad Sci USA 86: 3828–3832
Carella A M, Pollicardo N, Raffo N R et al 1992 Intensive conventional chemotherapy can lead to a precocious overshoot of cytogenetically normal blood stem cells (BSC) in chronic myeloid leukemia and anti-lymphoblastic leukemia. Leukemia 6 (Suppl 4): 120–123
Chan D, Schroeder W A 1990 The variable expression of sickle cell disease is genetically determined. Sem Hematol 27: 360–376
Chessells J M, Bailey C, Richards S M et al 1995 Intensification of treatment and survival in ALL children with lymphoblastic leukaemia: results of UK Medical Research Council trial UKALL X. Lancet 345: 143–148
Clay T M, Bidwell J L, Howard M R, Bradley B A 1991 PCR-fingerprinting for selection of HLA matched unrelated marrow donors. Lancet 337: 1049–1052
Cornish J, Green A, Potter M N et al 1995 One hundred and thirty paediatric unrelated donor transplants. Comparable outcome using HLA mismatch. Br J Haematol 89 (Suppl 1): A3
DeWitte T, Zwaan F, Heremans J et al 1990 Bone marrow transplantation for myelodysplastic syndrome and secondary leukaemia: a survey of the Leukaemia Working Party of the European Bone Marrow Transplantation Group (EBMTG). Br J Haematol 74: 151–158
Fischer A, Landais P, Friedrich B et al 1990 European experience of bone marrow transplantation for severe combined immunodeficiency. Lancet 336: 850–854

Fischer A, Landais P, Friedrich W et al 1994 Bone marrow transplantation (BMT) in Europe for primary immunodeficiencies other than severe combined immunodeficiency: a report from the European Group for Bone Marrow Transplantation. Blood 83: 1149–1154

Frickhoven N, Kaltwasser J F, Schrezenmeier H et al 1991 Treatment of aplastic anemia with antilymphocyte globulin with or without cyclosporin. N Engl J Med 324: 1297–1304

Friedman A S, Takvorian T, Anderson K C et al 1990 Autologous bone marrow transplantation in B-cell non-Hodgkins lymphoma: very low treatment-related mortality in 100 patients in sensitive relapse. J Clin Oncol 8: 1–8

Gahrton G, Tura S, Ljungman P et al 1991 Allogeneic bone marrow transplantation in multiple myeloma. European Group for Bone Marrow Transplantation. N Engl J Med 325: 1267–1273

Gatti R A, Mewissen H J, Allen H D et al 1968 Immunological reconstitution of sex linked, lymphopenic immunological deficiency. Lancet 2: 1366–1369

Gluckman E, Hows J 1994 Bone marrow transplantation in Fanconi Anemia. In: Foreman S, Bloine K (eds) Bone Marrow Transplantation, Boston, Blackwell Scientific publications, Chapter 68 pp 902–911

Gluckman E, Broxmeyer H E, Auerbach A D et al 1989 Haematopoietic reconstitution in a patient with Fanconi Anemia by means of umbilical cord blood from an HLA identical sibling. N Engl J Med 321: 1174–1178

Goldman J M 1994 For the WMDA Executive Committee. A special report: bone Marrow transplants using volunteer donors – recommendations and requirements for a standardized practice throughout the world – 1994 update. Blood 84: 2833–2839

Goldman J M, Apperley J F, Jones L et al 1986 Bone marrow transplantation for patients with chronic myeloid leukemia. N Engl J Med 314: 202–209

Gordon-Smith E C, Fairhead S M, Chipping P M et al 1982 Bone marrow transplantation for severe aplastic anaemia using histocompatible unrelated volunteer donors. Br J Med 285: 835–837

Hansen J, Clift R A, Thomas E D 1980 Transplantation of marrow from an unrelated donor to a patient with acute leukemia. N Engl J Med 303: 565–567

Hansen J A, Anasetti C, Martin P J et al 1994 Allogeneic marrow transplantation: The Seattle experience. In: Terasaki P I, Cecka J M (eds) Clinical Transplants. UCLA Tissue Typing Laboratory, Los Angeles CA, pp 193–209

Howard M R, Gore S M, Hows J M 1994 A prospective study of factors determining the outcome of unrelated marrow donor searches. Bone Marrow Transplant 13: 389–397

Hows J M, Bradley B A, Marsh J C W 1992a Growth of human umbilical cord blood in long-term haemopoietic cultures. Lancet 340: 73–76

Hows J M, Bradley B A, Joyce D 1992b Umbilical cord blood for transplantation (letter). Lancet 340 921–922

Hows J, Bradley B, Gore S et al 1993 Prospective evaluation of unrelated donor bone marrow transplantation. Bone Marrow Transplant 12: 371–380

Hows J, Downie T, Bradley B 1994a Factors influencing outcome of unrelated donor marrow transplants. Exp Hematol 22 (Suppl): A614

Hows J M, Downie T R, Bradley B A 1994b Unrelated donor bone marrow transplantation for severe acquired aplastic anaemia. 20th Annual Meeting of the European Group for Bone Marrow Transplantation, Harrogate. (A196)

Hurd D D, Le Bien T W, Lasky L C et al 1988 Autologous bone marrow transplantation in non-Hodgkin's lymphoma: monoclonal antibodies plus complement for ex-vivo marrow treatment. Am J Med 85: 829–834

Imanashi T, Akaza T, Kimnra A et al 1992 Allele and haplotype frequencies for HLA and complement loci in various ethnic groups In: HLA 1991, proceedings of the Eleventh International Histocompatability Workshop and Conference K Tsuji, M Aizowa, T Sasusuki (eds) Oxford Science Publishers, Vol 1, Clip W15.1 pp1065-1220

Kaminski E, Hows J M, Man S et al 1989 Prediction of graft-versus-host-disease by frequency analysis of cytotoxic T cells after unrelated donor marrow transplantation. Transplantation 48: 608–613

Kaminski E, Hows J M, Goldman J M et al 1991 Optimising a limiting dilution culture system for quantitating frequencies of alloreactive cytotoxic T lymphocyte precursors. Cell Immunol 137: 88–95

Kaufman R 1995 HLA prediction model for extended family matches. Bone Marrow Transplant 15: 279–282

Kessinger A, Armitage J O 1991 The evolving role of autologous peripheral blood stem cell

transplantation following high dose chemotherapy for malignancies. Blood 77: 211–213
Laundy G J, Bradley B A 1995 The predictive value of epitope analysis in highly sensitized patients awaiting renal transplantation. Transplantation 59: 1207-1213
Lonjou C, Clayton J, Cambon-Thomsen A, Raffoux C 1995 HLA-A,B,DR haplotype frequencies in France: implications for recruitment of potential bone marrow donors. Transplantation: 60: 375-383
Lucarelli G, Galinberti M, Pokhi P et al 1993 Marrow transplantation in patients with thalassemia responsive non chelation. N Engl J Med 329: 840–844
Marks D I, Cullis J O, Ward K N et al 1993 Allogeneic bone marrow transplantation for chronic myeloid leukemia using sibling and volunteer unrelated donors: a comparison of complications in the first 2 years. Ann Intern Med 119: 207–212
McGlave P, Barsch G, Anasetti C et al 1993 Unrelated donor marrow transplantation therapy for chronic myelogous leukemia: initial experience of the National Marrow Donor Program. Blood 81: 543–550
O'Reilly R J, Kernan N A, Cunningham I et al 1988 Allogeneic transplants depleted of T cells by soybean lectin agglutination and E-rosette depletion. Bone Marrow Transplant 3: 3–10
O'Reilly R J, Friedrick W, Small T N 1994 Transplantation approaches for severe combined immunodeficiency disease, Wiskott-Aldrich Syndrome, and other lethal genetic combined immunodeficiency disorders. In: Donnall-Thomas E D (ed) Boston, Blackwell Scientific Publications, Bone Marrow Transplantation, ch 64. pp 849–874
Ottinger H, Grosse-Wilde A, Grosse-Wilde H 1994 Immunogenetic marrow donor search for 1012 patients: a retrospective analysis of strategies outcome and costs. Bone Marrow Transplant 14(4): 34–39
Paquette R L, Tebyani N, Franc M et al 1995 Long-term outcome of aplastic anemia in adults treated with antithymocyte globulin: comparison with bone marrow transplantation. Blood 85: 283–290
Rabinowe S N, Soiffer R J, Gribben J G et al 1993 Autologous and allogeneic bone marrow transplantation for poor prognosis patients with B cell chronic lymphatic leukemia. Blood 82: 1366–1376
Rivera G K, Maver A M 1987 Controversies in the management of childhood acute lymphoblastic leukaemia with reinforced early treatment and rotational combination chemotherapy. Lancet 337: 61–66
Rubinstein P, Rosenfield R E, Adamson J N, Stevens C E 1993 A review. Stored placental blood for unrelated bone marrow reconstitution. Blood 81: 1679–1691
Samson D 1992 The current position of allogeneic and autologous BMT in multiple myeloma. Leuk Lymphoma 7 (Suppl): 33–38
Schmitz N, Dreger P, Suttorp M et al 1995 Primary transplantation of allogeneic peripheral blood progenitor cells mobilized by Filgrastim (granulocyte colony-stimulating factor). Blood 85: 1666–1672
Shpall E, Jones R, Franklin W et al 1993 Transplantation of autologous CD34 positive hematopoietic progenitor cells in breast cancer patients following high dose chemotherapy. Proc Annu Soc Clin Oncol 12: 105–109
Spencer A, Brookes P A, Kaminski E et al 1995 Cytotoxic T-lymphocyte precursor frequency analyses in bone marrow transplantation with unrelated donors: value in donor selection Transplantation: 59: 1302-1308
Storb R, Etzione R, Anasetti C et al 1994 Cyclophosphamide combined with antilymphocyte globulin in preparation for allogeneic marrow transplants in patients with aplastic anemia. Blood 84: 941–950
Sutton L, LeGlond V, Le Maignan C et al 1991 Bone marrow transplantation for myelodysplastic syndrome and secondary leukemia: outcome of 86 patients. Bone Marrow Transplant 7 Suppl 2: 39
Tiercy J M, Rufer N, Breur B et al 1995 Analysis of histocompatibilities between bone marrow recipients and their unrelated 'A,B,DR matched' potential donors. Bone Marrow Transplant 15 (Suppl 2): 5104 A438
Vermylen C, Cornu G, Phillips M et al 1991 Bone marrow transplantation in sickle cell anemia. Arch Dis Child 66: 1195–1198
Wagner J E, Kernan N A, Broxmeyer H E, Gluckman E 1994 Transplantation of umbilical cord blood in 50 patients: analysis of the registry data. Blood 84 (Suppl 1): A 1564

Weiden P, Flournoy N, Thomas E D et al 1979 Anti-leukemic effect of graft-versus-host-disease in human recipients of allogeneic marrow grafts. N Engl J Med 300: 1068–1073

Zittoun R A, Mandelli R, Willemze R et al 1995 Autologous or allogeneic bone marrow transplantation compared with intensive chemotherapy in acute myelogenous leukemia. N Engl J Med 332: 217–223

10

Inhibitors and the control of thrombosis

S. R. Stone   R. W. Carrell

One of the most significant developments in haematology over the last decade has been the growth in understanding the abnormalities that contribute to premature thrombotic disease. The importance of the prothrombotic disorders reflects the high morbidity and mortality of thromboembolic disease (Goldhaber 1994). Venous thrombosis and pulmonary embolism are the cause of 10% of all hospital deaths and one-half of these are said to occur in individuals with otherwise non-fatal disorders. The statistics for mortality in the community in general are just as daunting and it is likely that at least 1 in 10 individuals has one of the multitude of genetic abnormalities that are now known to contribute to familial thrombotic disease. Yet, despite this prevalence, the problem has received comparatively little attention. One reason for the apparent lack of interest in thromboembolic disease is that we have only recently begun to understand the pathways that limit thrombosis formation. Historically, the emphasis in thrombosis and haemostasis has been on the coagulation pathway, and students have been drilled on the intrinsic and extrinsic pathways that lead to the formation of fibrin. The introduction of fibrinolytic agents for treatment of acute myocardial infarction increased our awareness of the importance of the fibrinolytic system in the control of clot formation, but it is only now that the significance of a second pathway controlling thrombosis has been realized. The importance of this anticoagulation pathway, centred on protein C, is shown by the contribution that abnormalities of its components make to the familial thrombotic disorders. Venous thrombosis before the age of 50 occurs in about 1 in 1000 of the population. However, many more than 1 in 1000 are known to be carriers of predisposing abnormalities and there is good reason to believe that premature thrombosis often results from combinations of such abnormalities (Schafer 1994).

It is useful to focus on these precisely defined prothrombotic disorders as they give a firm basis for treatment and counselling. Until 2 years ago this was, however, a frustrating exercise as the identifiable abnormalities were substantially limited to those of antithrombin, protein C and its co-factor protein S. These defects provided an explanation for only 12% of familial thrombotic diseases. This situation was transformed by the finding by Dahlbäck and colleagues (1993) of a common polymorphism, present in 5% of the population, that blocks the anticoagulant effect of activated protein C (APC). The

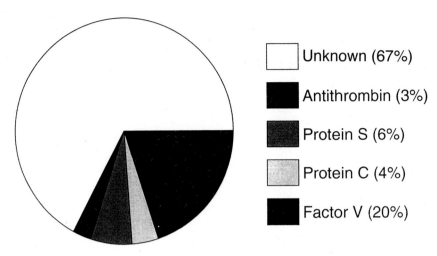

Fig. 1. Familial thrombosis. The molecular defect can now be identified in 33% of cases.

frequency of APC resistance in premature thrombotic disease is five-fold that of any other single abnormality and accounts for some 20% of the total. Therefore, we are now in a position to provide a firm diagnosis in 33% of cases (Fig. 1). This still leaves over half of such occurrences undiagnosed but there is good reason to believe that further well-defined defects will be identified, to give a good basis for a realistic diagnostic service.

At present, anticoagulation with warfarin is the only treatment of venous thrombosis in a patient with a family history of thromboembolic disease. However, once commenced, it is difficult to justify stopping this therapy, so essentially the starting of warfarin is a commitment to lifetime treatment. This long-term treatment carries with it a cumulative risk of haemorrhage, which should be justified by the best possible documentation of the underlying defect. In dealing with familial thromboembolic disease, questions will inevitably arise regarding the treatment of family members who carry the defect but who have not as yet had a thrombotic episode. In general, long-term warfarin therapy is not justifiable in the absence of a direct history of thrombosis, but coverage should be considered for at-risk periods such as pregnancy or elective surgery. This short-term coverage may be provided by heparin or better still, its low-molecular-weight forms, and the therapeutic possibilities will soon be augmented by the availability of the leech-derived anticoagulant hirudin.

In the following sections, we will discuss recent advances that have been made in identifying the genetic lesions that lead to thrombosis. The effects of such defects can only be properly understood in the context of the interplay between the coagulation, fibrinolytic and anticoagulation systems, and a brief introduction to this topic is given in the following section. We refer the reader

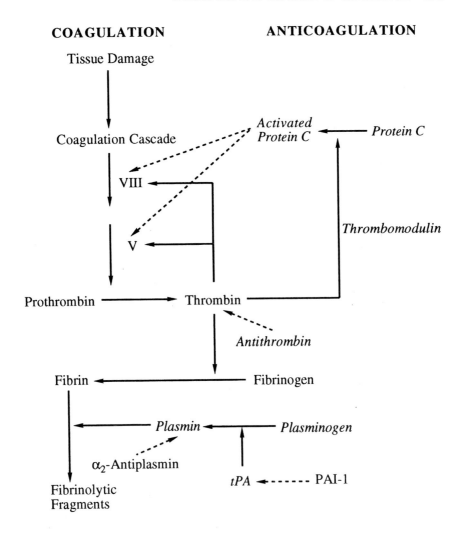

Fig. 2. Interplay of the coagulation, fibrinolysis and anticoagulation systems. Tissue damage initiates the coagulation cascade. This consists of a series of protease zymogens that are activated to active enzymes on phospholipid surfaces in the presence of protein co-factors such as factors V and VIII. Thrombin is the endproduct of the cascade and it cleaves fibrinogen to form a fibrin clot. Thrombin also activates factors V and VIII causing a further amplification of the cascade. In addition, thrombin initiates the protein C anticoagulant system which shuts down the coagulation cascade by inactivating factors Va and VIIIa. Clot formation is also limited by the fibrinolytic system. Tissue plasminogen activator (tPA) released by endothelial cells generates active plasmin which degrades the fibrin clot. The activities of proteases in the coagulation, fibrinolytic and anticoagulation systems are kept under control by serpins such as antithrombin, α_2-antiplasmin, plasminogen activator inhibitor 1 (PAI-1) and protein C inhibitor. Reactions involved in the control of the different systems are indicated by dashed lines.

to standard texts, such as that by Bloom and colleagues (1994) for a fuller description. In the final section, the recent progress in the development of new antithrombotic agents is reviewed.

BLOOD COAGULATION SYSTEM

Blood coagulation is precisely regulated to ensure the generation of a blood clot at the site of vascular injury without systemic coagulation. Injury to the endothelium triggers factors that lead to the initiation of blood clot formation. Platelets play a central role in this process. They adhere initially to subendothelial structures, which results in the expression of adhesion receptors on their surface and the recruitment of more platelets. This recruitment is promoted by the release of ADP and thromboxane A_2, which cause additional platelets to aggregate and form the platelet plug at the site of injury. Moreover, the phospholipid membranes of these activated platelets provide surfaces for the assembly of the coagulation cascade. This cascade consists of a series of serine protease zymogens, which require vitamin K for normal synthesis. The protease zymogens are sequentially converted to their active forms by limited proteolysis. This activation only proceeds efficiently in a complex containing protein co-factors, such as factors V and VIII, assembled on a phospholipid surface (Fig. 2). Exposed collagen and other negatively charged components of the subendothelial extracellular matrix catalyse the activation of factor XI which in turn initiates the intrinsic pathway of the coagulation cascade, while tissue factor, which is found on the surface of perivascular tissue cells, starts the extrinsic pathway by converting the protease factor VII into its active form. The extrinsic and intrinsic pathways converge in the prothrombinase complex, which consists of a complex of activated factors X (a protease) and V (a co-factor) assembled in the presence of calcium on a phospholipid surface (supplied by activated platelets). This complex converts prothrombin to thrombin which in turn cleaves fibrinogen to yield fibrin (Fig. 2). The proteolytic activity of thrombin is also central to the amplification of the cascade; it activates the co-factors V and VIII in a positive feedback mechanism (Davie et al 1991). Because the product of one reaction in the cascade serves as an enzyme in the next reaction of the cascade, the degree of amplification is dramatic, as shown by the results of Lawson and colleagues (1994); about 10^{-11}M factor VII in complex with tissue factor can generate 10^{-6} M thrombin in a few minutes.

FIBRINOLYTIC AND ANTICOAGULATION SYSTEMS

The endothelium plays an essential role in restricting clot formation to the site of vascular injury. Stimulation of the endothelium by factors generated upon clot formation initiates anticoagulant mechanisms. Besides its essential role in the coagulation cascade, thrombin is also important in the initiation of these anticoagulant responses. Upon stimulation by thrombin, endothelial cells secrete prostacyclin and nitric oxide which inhibit platelet aggregation. Moreover, thrombin and other factors induce endothelial cells to release tissue plasminogen activator (tPA), which initiates the fibrinolytic system by activating plasminogen to plasmin (Fig. 2). This activation reaction occurs most efficiently when both tPA and plasminogen are bound to fibrin in the clot. The plasmin generated within the clot degrades the fibrin and consequently dissolves the clot. Plasmin will also degrade fibrinogen and other coagulation factors (V and VIII) and this activity is controlled by the serpin α_2-antiplasmin (Fig. 2). Another serpin, antithrombin, controls the activity of coagulation proteases (thrombin, factors VIIa, IXa and Xa) as they are released from the site of injury. Molecules produced by the endothelium are also important in stimulating these reactions. The presence of heparin-like molecules on the endothelium greatly accelerates the inactivation of thrombin and other coagulation proteases by antithrombin.

A change in thrombin's specificity also occurs when it is bound to the co-factor thrombomodulin on the endothelial cell surface. In complex with thrombomodulin, thrombin is no longer able to cleave fibrinogen nor activate platelets, but it becomes a potent activator of protein C. Protein C is a zymogen of a serine protease that also requires vitamin K for normal biosynthesis. Activated protein C functions as an anticoagulant by cleaving, and thus inactivating, factors Va and VIIIa (Fig. 2). Another vitamin K-dependent protein, protein S, serves as a co-factor in this reaction (Esmon 1994).

GENETIC ABNORMALITIES CONTRIBUTING TO THROMBOSIS

Three major groups of genetic defects contributing to thrombosis have now been identified; these correspond to mutations in components of the protein C anticoagulant pathway, in antithrombin and in factor V. The common factor V mutation leads to a defect in its inactivation and this dysfunction of anticoagulation is referred to as activated protein C (APC) resistance. In the following sections, the salient features of these genetic defects are discussed. The reader is referred to recent reviews for more detailed treatments of these defects (Lane et al 1993, Perry 1994, Reitsma et al 1995, Dahlbäck 1995).

Protein C deficiency

The importance of the protein C anticoagulant pathway is clearly demonstrated by the association of homozygous protein C or protein S deficiency with severe, often fatal, neonatal thrombotic complications (Dahlbäck & Stenflo 1994). As observed with other deficiencies, however, the severity of the symptoms observed with homozygous protein C deficiency appears to depend on the presence of other risk factors. Milder symptoms have been reported for adults with very low or undetectable levels of protein C (Reitsma et al 1995).

Heterozygous protein C deficiency is associated with an increased risk of venous thrombosis (Dahlbäck & Stenflo 1994). Two distinct phenotypes are observed. Type I deficiency is the most common and is characterized by a parallel reduction in protein C activity and antigen levels. In type II deficiency, the antigen levels are normal but the activity of the protein C is reduced owing to synthesis of molecules with impaired function (Reitsma et al 1995). The frequency of heterozygous protein C deficiency may be as high as 1 in 200 (Miletich et al 1987). However, only a small fraction of these heterozygotes exhibit clinically overt protein C deficiency, which has a prevalence of between 1 in 16 000 to 1 in 36 000 (Broekmans & Conrad 1988; Gladson et al 1988). Thus, while heterozygous protein C deficiency is a risk factor for thrombotic disease, it is only in combination with other risk factors that the clinical symptoms become manifest. One important factor appears to be the co-inheritance of the common mutation of factor V associated with APC resistance (see below). This mutation is present with a significantly higher frequency in patients with symptomatic protein C deficiency indicating the clinically additive effects of the two defects (Koeleman et al 1994).

Activated protein C resistance

The identification of a common genetic defect that prevents the inactivation of factor V by protein C has had a major impact on coagulation laboratory practice. The abnormality is present in 5% of the population and contributes to 15-25% of premature venous thromboses. Furthermore, it is readily detectable by a straightforward screening test and can be unequivocally confirmed by one of the simpler applications of DNA technology.

The underlying defect is a mutation in factor V causing the replacement of the arginine at position 506, the site of cleavage for the degradation of activated factor V by activated protein C (APC). In the abnormal factor V, arginine 506 is substituted by a glutamine. This has been shown in a variety of European populations to be consistently due to the replacement in the gene of G to A at nucleotide 1691. A single mutation that has become established in this way in a population is termed a polymorphism and the presence in a population of a mutation that has demonstrable disadvantages, as with haemoglobin S or thalassaemia, is termed a balanced polymorphism. Therefore APC resistance is a balanced polymorphism, implying that there must have been an advantage, over millennia, which has provided a survival benefit to carriers of the abnormal factor V that is equivalent to its obvious disadvantage. With the common haemoglobinopathies, the balancing advantage was in survival against malaria; we can only surmise as to the historical advantage of the factor V mutation.

Whatever the reason for its existence, we are now left with the legacy of a defect that results in a life long risk of venous thrombosis. However, it is important to note that most of the 5% of the population who are heterozygotes for APC resistance will never have a thrombotic event in prime life (Zöller et al 1994). Although the likelihood of venous thrombosis is considerably increased in the homozygote, many of them too will be unaffected throughout their lifetime. There is now good reason to believe that most of the thromboses associated with APC resistance occur when a combination of risks exists. Individuals who also carry defects of protein C or protein S as well as APC resistance have a much higher risk of thrombosis than just with the single defect (Koeleman et al 1994, Zöller et al 1995). There is also a clear interaction of APC resistance with other acquired risk factors such as the use of oral contraceptives. Women on oral contraception have a four-fold increase in the risk of venous thrombosis but this is increased by a multiple of eight if they are also carriers of APC resistance. The combined effect is that a young woman with APC resistance who also takes oral contraceptives has a 30-fold increase in risk of thrombosis (Vandenbroucke et al 1994).

Therefore, testing for APC resistance can be carried out for two different purposes. The customary reason for thrombophilia testing is to define the cause of established thrombotic disease but the common presence of APC resistance also raises the question of preventive screening. Should we be screening groups who are placed at special risk, such as patients undergoing major orthopaedic surgery? The balance of opinion at this time would be against such screening. Perhaps the clearest case is that of women considering oral contraception; should they be tested for APC resistance? Vandenbroucke and colleagues at Leiden (1994) put the problem in perspective by calculating that the increased incidence of thrombosis in normal women on oral contraception is two events per 10 000 years of exposure and the combined risk with APC resistance is 30 events per 10 000 years. The conclusion from the Leiden group is that routine screening prior to commencing oral contraception is not justifiable, but that it should be carried out if there is a history of thrombosis, to provide information for counselling on contraceptive options.

The original finding of APC resistance followed from the observation that in some samples from patients with a history of thrombosis, the addition of APC did not prolong the standard activated partial thromboplastin time (aPTT). This is the basis for the present simple functional test for APC resistance (Dahlbäck 1995). Although the test is simple to perform, a number of precautions need to be taken to obtain results that give reproducible discrimination between normal and APC-resistant individuals. The APC-resistance test is only reliable in the absence of other gross coagulation abnormalities and it should not be carried out on samples from patients on warfarin or heparin therapy. The test can be performed on either fresh or frozen plasma samples but in either case care needs to be taken to avoid platelet contamination when preparing the plasma. With these precautions almost all the abnormal results will be caused by the common mutation in factor V but there are occasional cases, as a result of other abnormalities, that will be detected by the APC-resistance test but not by DNA-screening tests.

DNA technology provides a more precise (albeit more laborious) method of detection. The most commonly used technique depends on the change in a restriction enzyme cleavage site as a consequence of the presence of the mutation from G to A at nucleotide 1691 (Bertina et al 1994, Zöller et al

1994). Genomic DNA is extracted from buffy coat cells and then exon 10 of factor V, containing nucleotide 1691, is amplified by the polymerase chain reaction (PCR). The amplified exon 10 is normally cleaved into three fragments by the restriction nuclease *Mnl* I; but the presence of the mutation at 1691 results in loss of a cleavage site to give just the two fragments. The change in cleavage pattern, either in heterozygous or homozygous form, is readily detectable by gel electrophoresis and gives an unequivocal definition of the genotype. The results are not affected by the presence of other abnormalities of coagulation or by the use of warfarin or other anticoagulant therapies.

Dahlbäck, in his review of the tests for factor V abnormality (1995), concludes that the APC-resistance test, because of its simplicity, is the method of choice for screening, except in the case of individuals with other disorders of coagulation or those on established anticoagulation therapy. DNA-based testing should be used for these latter individuals, and also as a further procedure to define the factor V genotype with samples giving borderline or low APC ratios. If these criteria are used, some 30–50% of thrombosis patients will require both assays, but even so this still saves time when compared with a complete conversion to DNA testing. The double approach also has the advantage of detecting those few, but interesting, individuals who will have increased APC resistance owing to a cause other than the mutation of Arginine 506 in factor V.

Antithrombin deficiency

Abnormalities affecting the production or function of antithrombin are likely to be present in 1 per 2000 of the population and they are a prime or contributing cause of 3–4% of all instances of familial thrombotic disease. Over 50 such variants of antithrombin are known and they can be divided by phenotype into two main groups. As for protein C deficiency, type I variants result in the absence of the product of one allele in plasma, giving a 50% reduction in the concentration of antithrombin. This complete loss of antithrombin production from one allele is accompanied by the likelihood of a history of venous thrombosis usually commencing after the age of 16 (Olds et al 1994).

The other main class of pathological variants of antithrombin are those classified as type II; these have normal or near-normal antigenic levels in the plasma but a substantially reduced inhibitory activity. The type II variants are dysfunctional; the mutation does not primarily affect production of antithrombin, but results in a loss of its inhibitory activity. The study of these variants has also made a major contribution to our understanding of the molecular function, of the wider family of inhibitors to which antithrombin belongs — the serpins.

The serpin family includes most of the inhibitors in human plasma such as α_1-antitrypsin, antiplasmin, PAI-1 and C1-inhibitor. The whole family shares a common framework structure, illustrated in Figure 3 by the crystallographic

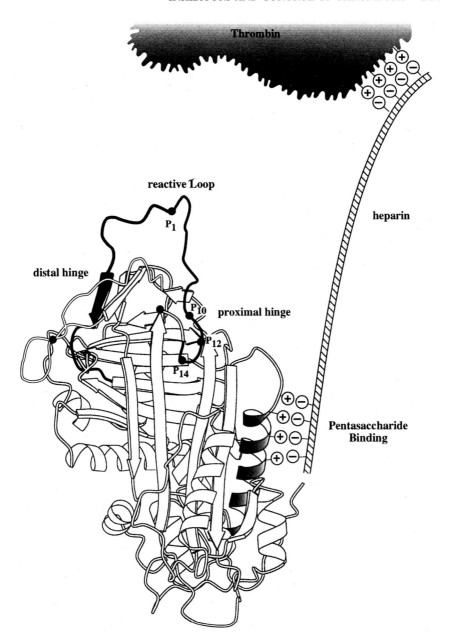

Fig. 3. Structure of antithrombin. A skeletal depiction showing the domains in which clusters of mutations causing dysfunction occur. Mutations of the loop containing the reactive centre (P_1) and its proximal hinge (P_{10}–P_{14}) hinder the mobility of the reactive centre and result primarily in a loss of inhibitory function. Mutations of the distal hinge similarly affect mobility and cause multiple 'pleotropic' dysfunctions. The heparin binding site is centred on the D helix and a diagrammatic representation shows how it binds a specific pentasaccharide sequence on heparin to provide a bridge, with the higher molecular weight heparins, that increases the efficiency of inhibition of thrombin (upper, shaded).

structure of antithrombin (Schreuder et al 1994, Carrell et al 1994). The characteristic feature is a reactive centre peptide bond, Arg–Ser393–394 in antithrombin, that acts as a pseudo substrate for the target enzyme, thrombin and factor Xa in the case of antithrombin. Although this crystallographic structure provides clues as to the mode of function of the molecule, our current knowledge is substantially based on studies of pathological variants of the plasma serpins, notably those of antithrombin (Stein & Carrell 1995). When all the mutations involved are plotted on the framework structure, they are seen to define the domains that control the unique mobility of this family of inhibitors (Fig. 3).

The reactive site of antithrombin is situated on a peptide loop that undergoes a major rearrangement when the molecule docks with thrombin or factor Xa. This conformational change is responsible for the formation of the tight complex between the protease and antithrombin and this conformational change results in the complex being taken up within minutes and catabolised in the liver. In order to form this tight complex, movement of the reactive loop has to take place at two hinges and other mobile domains. Mutations in these domains can prevent this rearrangement of the reactive loop with loss of inhibitory activity, or can allow the movement to occur prematurely, which results in a tangling of antithrombin molecules. Both the loss of inhibitory activity and the tangling of molecules to give inactive polymers of antithrombin may be accelerated by even the small changes in temperature that accompany infections (Bruce et al 1994). These points illustrate the complexity of the diseases associated with the dysfunctional antithrombins and why their presentation may be episodic and occur inconsistently, with only some affected individuals going on to develop thrombosis.

The other functional domain shown in Figure 3 is the binding site for heparin, formed by a row of positively charged amino acids that bond with the negatively charged sulphates of heparin. Specifically, the site binds a pentasaccharide sequence in the heparin which induces a conformational change that activates the inhibition of factor Xa. This occurs particularly with lower-molecular-weight heparins but the larger unfractionated heparins have an additional effect in forming a bridge with thrombin with a 1000-fold increase in the effectiveness of its inhibition (Olson & Björk 1992).

Replacements of the amino acids in the binding site for heparin on antithrombin are a frequent cause of dysfunction and are a significant contributor to familial thrombotic disease, usually in conjunction with other genetic or stress factors. Heparin, as used therapeutically, is a mixture of complex glycosaminoglycans prepared from animal extracts and it is not normally present in this form in the blood. Its nearest equivalent in the circulation is the heparan sidechains of the endothelial glycoproteins that line the capillaries and sinusoids of the circulation. These heparans contain the pentasaccharide sequence that specifically binds to antithrombin and it is an attractive but unproven proposal that they localize the inhibitor to the part of the circulation that is most vulnerable to thrombosis, the microvasculature (Marcum et al 1984).

RECENT ADVANCES IN THE DEVELOPMENT OF THROMBIN INHIBITORS AS ANTITHROMBOTIC AGENTS

Considering the central importance of thrombin in the formation of a blood clot (Fig. 2), it is not surprising that considerable effort has been expended in the search for thrombin inhibitors that would be suitable antithrombotic agents. Current antithrombin therapy is limited to two classes of compound: coumarins (e.g. warfarin) and heparins. Coumarins inhibit the generation of thrombin, while heparin catalyses the inactivation of factor Xa and thrombin by antithrombin, thus both reducing thrombin's generation and inhibiting thrombin once it is formed. Coumarins are used for long-term anticoagulation. These compounds act by inhibiting the vitamin K-dependent synthesis of γ-carboxylglutamic acid in a number of coagulation proteins, including prothrombin, protein C and factors VII, IX and X. The γ-carboxylglutamate residues of these proteins are essential for their binding to phospholipid surfaces during their activation and, thus, coumarins inhibit the production of thrombin by dampening the amplification reactions of the coagulation cascade (Fig. 2). Variability of patient response, which is complicated by the effect of other drugs and diet, necessitates careful laboratory monitoring to ensure that adequate anticoagulation is achieved without undue risk of bleeding. In addition, since the anticoagulant effect requires synthesis and turnover of plasma proteins, several days are required before stable anticoagulation is achieved. Therefore, the coumarins are not suitable antithrombotics when immediate or short-term anticoagulation is required.

Heparin is the current mainstay antithrombotic for short-term anticoagulation. However, although heparin is very effective in the prevention and treatment of thromboembolic disorders, it has several drawbacks (Weitz & Hirsh, 1993; Harker, 1994). As with the coumarins, patients have an extremely variable response to heparin, and careful laboratory monitoring of the anticoagulant response is required. This variable response is at least partly caused by the binding of heparin to plasma proteins other than antithrombin, which leads to a reduction in the amount of heparin available to accelerate the reaction of antithrombin with factor Xa and thrombin. In addition, heparin can be inactivated by platelet factor 4 and heparinase, which are released from activated platelets (Weitz & Hirsh, 1993). Some of the limitations of standard heparin have been overcome with the introduction of low-molecular-weight heparins, which are produced by controlled chemical or enzymatic degradation of standard heparin. These less heterogeneous forms of heparin exhibit less non-specific binding to plasma proteins and this probably contributes to their greater bioavailability and more predictable anticoagulant response (Hirsh & Levine, 1992).

One of the most serious limitations of heparin is its inability to catalyse the inactivation of clot-bound thrombin. After converting fibrinogen to fibrin, thrombin remains bound to fibrin via a site distinct from its active site and is still able to cleave fibrinogen as well as activate platelets and factors V and

VIII. However, this clot-bound thrombin is resistant to inactivation by the heparin–antithrombin complex. Therefore, clot-bound thrombin can amplify the coagulation cascade at sites of thrombus formation even in the presence of heparin. In contrast to heparin, the thrombin inhibitors discussed below can inactivate thrombin bound to fibrin (Weitz et al 1990).

Two factors have contributed greatly to the development of thrombin inhibitors for antithrombotic purposes. The determination of the crystal structure of thrombin has allowed the rational design of synthetic thrombin inhibitors (Stubbs & Bode, 1995) and recombinant DNA technology has allowed the production of large quantities of natural inhibitors (Johnson, 1994). For development as an antithrombotic agent, an inhibitor should bind rapidly, tightly and specifically to thrombin; it should not inhibit proteases involved in fibrinolysis (plasmin and plasminogen activators) and anticoagulation (APC). A number of different approaches have been used to identify a suitable inhibitor. The active site of thrombin is more enclosed than that of other serine proteases and this has allowed the design of small, specific inhibitors of thrombin (Tapparelli et al 1993). Because of their small size, such inhibitors have possible oral availability and, thus, could potentially be substitutes for the coumarins as long-term anticoagulants. At the moment, however, hirudin and an analogue of hirudin show the greatest promise as antithrombotic agents. Hirudin is a polypeptide of 65 amino acids which was originally isolated from the medicinal leech, but is now produced recombinantly. It binds to thrombin over an extended area in a unique manner. Hirudin occupies the active site of thrombin in an orientation that is opposite to that expected for substrates. It also binds to a positively charged surface groove (the anion-binding exosite) which is distant from the active site. Fibrinogen and the thrombin receptor also make essential interactions with this region of thrombin (Stubbs & Bode, 1995). Because of its unique interactions, hirudin binds to thrombin rapidly, tightly and specifically; it does not inhibit any other protease (Johnson, 1994). Hirudin, however, displays no appreciable oral availability and must be administered parenterally (intravenous or subcutaneous). Hirulog™ is a synthetic analogue of hirudin. It consists of a moiety based on hirudin which occupies the anion-binding exosite linked to a tetrapeptide (D-Phe-Pro-Arg-Pro) that binds to the active site of thrombin (Stubbs & Bode, 1995).

Clinical trials have investigated the use of direct thrombin inhibitors as antithrombotics in situations where the efficacy of heparin is limited. To date, the inhibitors hirudin and Hirulog™ have been studied most and the major indications that have been examined are unstable angina, coronary thrombolysis and coronary angioplasty. In all these indications, thrombin may be bound to fibrin or the extracellular matrix, and the resistance of these bound forms of thrombin to the heparin–antithrombin complex is thought to limit the efficacy of heparin. In contrast, thrombin inhibitors which are able to inhibit clot-bound thrombin, are expected to be superior to heparin in such settings. In coronary thrombolysis and unstable angina, thrombin bound to fibrin or fibrin fragments is probably one of the major causes of rethrombosis and thus thrombin inhibitors, such as hirudin and Hirulog™, should be more effective than heparin in preventing rethrombosis. Similarly, coronary angioplasty may lead to the generation of bound thrombin that is resistant to antithrombin and heparin; thrombin bound to the subendothelial extracellular matrix, exposed as a result of angioplasty, may be active but resistant to inhibition by antithrombin (Weitz & Hirsh 1993). Although most of the trials with hirudin and Hirulog™ have been relatively small, such that no definitive conclusions with respect to the efficacy and safety of these agents can be made, the results have been sufficiently promising to stimulate further development.

Although coronary artery thrombosis is the principal cause of unstable angina, treatment with heparin and thrombolytic agents has failed to provide a substantial benefit. Therefore, the results of clinical trials showing a greater efficacy for thrombin inhibitors in the treatment of unstable angina have been encouraging. For example, in a pilot trial of 166 patients, hirudin was shown to be superior to an equivalent anticoagulant dose of heparin in reducing the size of coronary thrombi as determined by angiography (Topol et al 1994).

Thrombolytic therapy has become a standard treatment for myocardial infarction. However, failure to achieve initial reperfusion and reocclusion of the infarcted artery remain the major limitations of thrombolytic therapy despite various regimens of heparin and aspirin. Anticoagulants are given during and after the administration of thrombolytic agents (tissue-plasminogen activator (tPA) or streptokinase) to accelerate the rate of recanalization and to decrease the incidence of reocclusion. Initial trials suggested that direct thrombin inhibitors were more effective as adjunctive agents in thrombolytic therapy than heparin. In a small trial (45 patients) in which Hirulog™ was compared with heparin, Hirulog™ produced a significant increase in coronary patency at 90 minutes following streptokinase treatment; vessel patency was achieved in 62% of the patients receiving Hirulog™ compared with 49% for heparin treatment (Lidon et al 1994). In combination with tPA in the TIMI 5 pilot trial, hirudin was more effective than heparin in increasing coronary patency, which was measured 18 and 36 hours after initiation of thrombolytic treatment (Cannon et al 1994). In addition, hirudin also reduced the occurrence of combined unfavourable outcomes (death, reinfarction, new congestive heart failure and shock). The results of the TIMI 6 trial suggested that hirudin was also effective in combination with streptokinase in reducing the incidence of such unfavourable occurrences (Lee, 1995). Three larger trials were initiated based on the results of these pilot trials involving hirudin in thrombolytic therapy. These trials were interrupted because of increased rates of haemorrhage with the doses of hirudin used (Antman 1994; GUSTO IIa Investigators 1994; Neuhaus et al 1994). Patients who developed a major haemorrhage had higher aPTT values, especially in the first 12 hours after thrombolysis (Antman 1994), and this parameter will be monitored in future trials. It is apparent from the results of these trials that the therapeutic range for hirudin may be smaller than previously thought. All three trials will continue with a lower (safer) dose of hirudin and we must wait to see whether the theoretical advantages of this direct thrombin inhibitor will translate into an improved clinical outcome for patients receiving thrombolytic therapy.

Although heparin is routinely used in coronary angioplasty, acute reocclusion occurs in up to 10% of cases. Platelet thrombus deposition occurs at the site of angioplasty injury and this is thought to be primarily mediated by thrombin (Harker, 1994). Therefore, it was expected that hirudin and Hirulog™ would be more effective than heparin in reducing the incidence of reocclusion. In a trial of 113 patients that compared hirudin and heparin, the hirudin group exhibited a lower incidence of myocardial infarction and/or need for emergency bypass surgery, as well as a significant reduction in the number of ischaemic events (van den Bos et al 1993). In a larger trial of 4000 patients with either unstable angina or postinfarction angina (Bittl et al 1995), Hirulog™ failed to reduce postangioplasty ischaemic complications when compared with an equivalent anticoagulant dose of heparin, but Hirulog™ treatment was associated with a significant reduction in bleeding. For the subgroup of patients with postinfarction angina, however, Hirulog™ reduced both the ischaemic and bleeding complications. Therefore, Hirulog™ appears to be a better alternative to heparin with high-risk patients. Procedures of balloon angioplasty have also been developed to allow a local application of the antithrombotic at the site of injury and such procedures appear to be a promising route of administration for thrombin inhibitors. Local delivery of hirudin in pigs significantly reduced platelet deposition and mural thrombus formation at the site of injury compared to systemic treatment with hirudin or heparin, thus reducing the reocclusion without full systemic anticoagulation (Meyer et al 1994).

One of the major advantages of hirudin and Hirulog™ over heparin is the reproducibility of their anticoagulant response. In contrast to the variable dose response observed with heparin, these inhibitors have a predictable anticoagulant response (Weitz & Hirsh, 1993; Harker, 1994). It was hoped that this predictable dose response would obviate the need for laboratory monitoring. It appears, however, that some laboratory monitoring may be necessary; after the recent problems with haemorrhage at high doses of hirudin, it has been suggested that a careful monitoring of aPTT during therapy is required (Antman, 1994; GUSTO IIa Investigators, 1994; Neuhaus et al 1994).

KEY POINTS FOR CLINICAL PRACTICE

- As many as 1 in 10 of the population have a genetic abnormality predisposing to thrombois. Premature thrombosis is likely to occur when there is a combination of these defects.

- APC resistance as a result of a mutation in the factor V gene is a major cause of thrombosis. It is carried by 1 in 20 people and contributes to 15–20% of premature thromboses.

- Familial thrombosis justifies detailed investigation. In many cases, it will be a result of the factor V Leiden mutation causing APC resistance. However, the identification of variants of antithrombin, protein C and other factors have contributed greatly to our understanding of the function of these proteins and their role in haemostasis.

- The results of recent clinical trials of the thrombin inhibitors hirudin and Hirulog™ suggest that these componds will be useful in the treatment of thrombotic conditions that are resistant to heparin therapy.

ACKNOWLEDGMENTS

The authors thank the Wellcome Trust, MRC and British Heart Foundation for research support and Drs P Coughlin and T Baglin for their comments on the manuscript.

REFERENCES

Allaart C F, Briët E 1994 Familial venous thrombophilia. In Haemostasis and thrombosis (3rd ed). Bloom A L, Forbes C D, Thomas D P, Tuddenham E G D (eds) Churchill Livingstone, Edinburgh, pp 1349–1360

Antman E M 1994 Hirudin in acute myocardial infarction. Safety report from the Thrombolysis and Thrombin Inhibition in Myocardial Infarction (TIMI) 9A Trial. Circulation 90: 1624–1630

Bertina R M, Koeleman B P C, Koster T et al 1994 Mutation in blood coagulation factor V associated with resistance to activated protein C. Nature 369: 64–67

Bittl J A, Strony J, Brinker J A et al 1995 Treatment with Bivalirudin (Hirulog) as compared with heparin during coronary angioplasty for unstable or post-infarction angina. N Engl J Med: 333: 764-769

Bloom A L, Forbes C D, Thomas D P et al 1994 Haemostasis and thrombosis (3rd edn). Churchill Livingstone, Edinburgh

van den Bos A A, Deckers J W, Heyndrickx G R et al 1993 Safety and efficacy of recombinant hirudin (CGP 39 393) versus heparin in patients with stable angina undergoing coronary angioplasty. Circulation 88: 2058–2066

Broekmans A W, Conrad J 1988 Hereditary protein C deficiency. In: Bertina R M (ed) Protein C and related proteins. Churchill Livingstone, Edinburgh, pp 160–181

Bruce D, Perry D J, Borg J-Y et al 1994 Thromboembolic disease due to thermolabile conformational changes of antithrombin Rouen-VI (187 Asn Asp). J Clin Invest 94: 2265–2274

Cannon C P, McCabe C H, Henry T D et al 1994 A pilot trial of recombinant desulfatohirudin compared with heparin in conjunction with tissue-type plasminogen activator and aspirin for acute myocardial infarction: results of the Thrombolysis in Myocardial Infarction (TIMI) 5 trial. J Am Coll Cardiol 23: 993–1003

Carrell R W, Stein P E, Fermi G et al 1994 Biological implications of a 3Å structure of dimeric antithrombin. Structure 2: 257–270

Dahlbäck B 1995 Resistance to activated protein C, the Arg506 to Gln mutation in the factor V gene, and venous thrombosis. Thromb Haemost 73: 739–742

Dahlbäck B, Carlsson M, Svensson P J 1993 Familial thrombophilia due to a previously unrecognised mechanism characterised by poor anticoagulant response to activated protein C. Proc Natl Acad Sci USA 90: 1004–1008

Dahlbäck B, Stenflo J 1994 A natural anticoagulant pathway: proteins C, S, C4b-binding protein and thrombomodulin. In: Bloom A L, Forbes C D, Thomas D P et al (eds) Haemostasis and thrombosis. Edinburgh, Churchill Livingstone, pp 671–698

Davie E W, Fujikawa K, Kisiel W 1991 The coagulation cascade: interaction, maintenance and regulation. Biochemistry 30: 10363–10370

Esmon C T 1994 Molecular events that control the protein C anticoagulanat pathway. Thromb Haemost 70: 29–35

Gladson C L, Scharrer I, Hach V et al 1988 The frequency of type I heterozygous protein S and protein C deficiency in 141 unrelated young patients with venous thrombosis. Thromb Haemost 59: 18–22

Goldhaber S Z 1994 Epidemiology of pulmonary embolism and deep vein thrombosis. In: Bloom A L, Forbes C D, Thomas D P et al (eds) Haemostasis and thrombosis (3rd edn). (eds) Churchill Livingstone, Edinburgh, pp 1327–1333

GUSTO IIa Investigators 1994 Randomized trial of intravenous heparin versus recombinant hirudin for acute coronary syndromes. Circulation 90: 1631–1637

Harker L A 1994 New antithrombotic strategies for resistant thrombotic processes. J Clin Pharmacol 34: 3–16

Hirsh J, Levine M N 1992 Low molecular weight heparins. Blood 79: 1–17

Johnson P H 1994 Hirudin: clinical potential of a thrombin inhibitor. Annu Rev Med 45: 165–177

Koeleman B P C, Reitsma P H, Allaart C F et al 1994 Activated protein C resistance as an additional risk factor for thrombosis in protein C-deficient families. Blood 84: 1031–1035

Lane D A et al 1993 Antithrombin III mutation database: first update. Thromb Haemost 70: 361–369

Lawson J H, Kalafatis M, Stram S et al 1994 A model for the tissue factor pathway to thrombin. I. An empirical study. J Biol Chem 269: 23357–23366

Lee L V 1995 Initial experience with hirudin and streptokinase in acute myocardial infarction: results of the Thrombolysis in Myocardial Infarction (TIMI) 6 trial. Am J Cardiol 75: 7–13

Lidon R M, Theroux P, Lesperance J et al 1994 A pilot, early angiographic patency study using a direct thrombin inhibitor as adjunctive therapy to streptokinase in acute myocardial infarction. Circulation 89: 1567–1572

Marcum JA, McKenney JB, Rosenberg RD 1984 Acceleration of thrombin-antithrombin complex formation in rat hindquarters by herapin-like molecules bound to the endothelium. J Clin Invest 74: 341–350

Meyer B J, Fernandez-Ortiz A, Mailhac A et al 1994 Local delivery of r-hirudin by a double-balloon perfusion catheter prevents mural thrombosis and minimizes platelet deposition after angioplasty. Circulation 90: 2474–2480

Miletich J, Sherman L, Broze G 1987 Absence of thrombosis in subjects with heterozygous protein C deficiency. N Engl J Med 317: 991–996

Neuhaus K L, von Essen R, Tebbe U et al 1994 Safety observations from the pilot phase of the randomized r-Hirudin for Improvement of Thrombolysis (HIT-III) study. A study of the Arbeitsgemeinschaft Leitender Kardiologischer Krankenhausarzte (ALKK). Circulation 90: 1638–1642

Olds R J, Lane D A, Thein S L 1994 The molecular genetics of antithrombin deficiency. Br J Haematol 87: 221–226

Olson S T, Björk I 1992 Regulation of thrombin by antithrombin and heparin cofactor II. In: Berliner L J (ed) Thrombin, structure and function. Plenum Press, New York, pp 159–217

Perry D J 1994 Antithrombin and its inherited deficiencies. Blood Reviews 8: 37–55

Reitsma P H, Bernardi F, Doig R G et al 1995 Protein C deficiency: a database of mutations, 1995 update. Thromb Haemost 73: 876–889

Schafer I A 1994 Hypercoagulable states: molecular genetics to clinical practice. Lancet 344: 1739–1742

Schreuder H A, de Boer B, Dijkema R et al 1994 The intact and cleaved human antithrombin III complex as a model for serpin-proteinase interactions. Nature Struct Biol 1: 48–54

Stein P E, Carrell R W 1995 What do dysfunctional serpins tell us about molecular mobility and disease? Nature Struct Biol 2: 96–104

Stubbs M T, Bode W 1995 The clot thickens: clues provided by thrombin structure. TIBS 20: 23–28

Tait R C, Walker I D, Perry D J et al 1994 Prevalence of antithrombin deficiency in the healthy population. Br J Haematol 87: 106–112

Tapparelli C, Metternich R, Ehrhardt C et al 1993 Synthetic low-molecular weight thrombin inhibitors: molecular design and pharmacological profile. Trends Pharmacol Sci 14: 366–376

Topol E J, Fuster V, Harrington R A et al 1994 Recombinant hirudin for unstable angina pectoris. A multicenter, randomized angiographic trial. Circulation 89: 1557–1566

Vandenbroucke J P, Koster T, Briët E et al 1994 Increased risk of venous thrombosis in oral-contraceptive users who are carriers of factor V Leiden mutation. Lancet 344: 1453–1457

Weitz J, Hirsh J 1993 New anticoagulant strategies. J Lab Clin Med 122: 364–373

Weitz J I, Hudoba M, Massel D et al 1990 Clot-bound thrombin is protected from inhibition by heparin-antithrombin III but is susceptible to inactivation by antithrombin III-independent inhibitors. J Clin Invest 86: 385–391

Zöller B, Svensson P J, He X et al 1994 Identification of the same factor V gene mutation in 47 out of 50 thrombosis-prone families with inherited resistance to activated protein C. J Clin Invest 94: 2521–2524

11

Stimulation of fetal hemoglobin synthesis using pharmacological agents

G. P. Rodgers

Sickle cell disease is a severe hemoglobin disorder originating from a single nucleotide substitution in codon 6 of the β-globin gene. This change results in the production of an abnormal hemoglobin (HbS, $\alpha_2 \beta^S_2$) that forms polymers when red blood cells are deoxygenated (Bunn & Forget 1986). Accumulation of polymer within red cells has many consequences and ultimately causes the pathognomonic irreversibly altered morphology of the cell. Polymer accumulation is irreversible, and red cells that contain substantial amounts of HbS polymer can therefore lodge in the end-arterioles, occluding vessels and causing mircoinfarction of tissues. This process presumably leads to vaso-occlusive events and irreversible tissue damage. Sickle cell disease affects nearly 1% of American Black newborns, and causes tremendous morbidity and mortality. Until recently, there was no therapy capable of preventing sickle cell vaso-occlusive events, or altering the course of this disease (Steingert 1992, Serjeant & Serjeant 1993). However, stimulation of γ-globin synthesis in patients with sickle cell disease, associated with a decrease in production of β^S chains, reduces red cell HbS concentration. This change reduces polymer formation and has now been shown unambiguously to decrease the propensity of such cells to lead to vaso-occlusive or hemolytic manifestations (see below).

Severe β-thalassemia, requiring regular blood transfusions, occurs in individuals who are homozygous for mutations and or deletions that cause a marked decrease in the rate of β-globin synthesis. Such patients usually die before the age of 25 as a direct result of cardiac iron deposition (Fosburg & Nathan 1990, Thein 1993). While chelation therapy has been shown to reduce liver iron concentration and lead to an improvement in liver function, recent evidence suggests that chelation, when begun after the age of 10 years may not always prevent the development of overt cardiac disease (Brittenham et al 1994, Olivieri 1994). Older patients, particularly those who already have evidence of cardiac disease, may not benefit from chelation; therefore, alternative forms of treatment are desperately needed.

Abundant clinical and epidemiological data now exists to support the view that elevated levels of fetal hemoglobin (HbF) abrogates the clinical manifestations of patients with sickle cell disease and β-thalassemia (Stamatoyannopoulas & Nienhuis 1992, Ley 1991, Lavelle et al 1993). Recent insights into the structure function, and developmental control of the human globin genes, coupled with several distinct yet disparate observations of the effects of certain classes of agents to 'reverse' erythroid cellular phenotype, have led to pharmacological trials to attain meaningful increases in HbF production in patients affected with these two severe β-globin disorders (Rodgers 1994). The contemporary understanding of the quantitative relationship between the abnormal molecules in the red cell — aggregates of sickle hemoglobin in the sickle cell syndromes and aggregated α-globin polypeptides in the β-thalassemia syndromes — and the extent of red cell and/or organ involvement has now enabled investigators to predict how much inhibition of these intracellular pathogenic processes might be necessary to achieve partial or total abrogation of the disease manifestations. A listing of the target goals and desired characteristics of therapeutic agents being applied to the treatment of the severe β-globin disorders with the attempt to stimulate HbF synthesis is shown in Table 1. A time line for the discovery and application of these agents is illustrated in Figure 1.

EARLY STUDIES OF FETAL HEMOGLOBIN STIMULATION

The earliest attempts to clinically effect hemoglobin switching stemmed from observations of elevated HbF levels in maternal blood during the second trimester of pregnancy, which resulted in the logical selection of human chronic gonadotropin (HCG) (Beutler 1961) as a putative HbF inducer. While the administration of either HCG (Beutler 1961) or progesterone (Beutler 1969, De Ceulaer et al 1982) to sickle cell patients leads to a transient, albeit small, rise in HbF levels, the ultimate clinical impact of these agents cannot be properly judged given the short nature of these trials.

Recent efforts to manipulate the HbF level were based on observations made in cell culture systems that eukaryotic gene expression was related (at least in part) to the extent of methylation of cytosine residues within and around the gene of inquiry. Thus, 5-azacytidine (5-Aza C), a potent inhibitor of DNA methylation, was administered to anemic primates (DeSimone et al 1982), and subsequently to patients with β-thalassemia (Ley et al 1982) and sickle cell disease (Charache et al 1983, Ley et al 1983), and was shown to markedly increase the synthesis of HbF associated with hypomethylation of the γ-globin gene promoter. DeSimone and colleagues (1982) showed that baboons, maintained chronically anemic through regular phlebotomy, after receiving subcutaneous courses of 5-Aza C consistently increased the synthesis of HbF to values as high as 70–80% (with > 90% F-cells), while reciprocally decreasing β-globin synthesis. Such dramatic changes in HbF and HbA levels implied that an apparent reversal in the normal fetal-to-adult hemoglobin switch was achievable and therefore provided the rationale for experimental application of this approach to patients with β-thalassemia and sickle cell anemia. It should be noted that in adult human and non-human primates, HbF production is limited to a subpopulation of erythrocytes (<10% in humans) termed 'F-cells' which can be detected by their ability to resist

FETAL HEMOGLOBIN SYNTHESIS 233

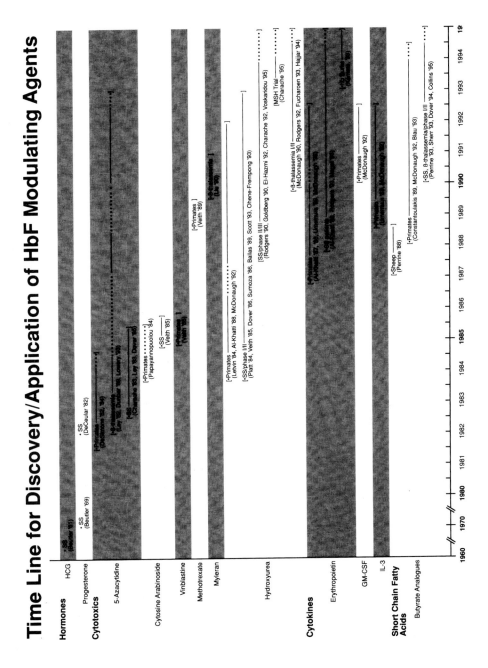

Fig. 1 Time line for the discovery and application of therapeutic agents which increase hemoglobin F in man, non-human primates, or other large animals. The major category of these agents include hormones, cytotoxics, cellular growth factors (or cytokines), and short chain fatty acids. The brackets indicate the period of time over which these studies were performed or are on-going, while the captions in parenthesis indicate the specific publications of these findings.

Table 1 Therapeutic goals and desirable characteristics of agents to modulate fetal hemoglobin synthesis

Disease	Therapeutic goals	Characteristics (both sickle cell disease and β-thalassemia agents)
Sickle cell disease	20–25% HbF >75% F-cells	Acceptable acute and long-term toxicity profile No (or minimal) effects on growth and development
β-thalassemia	>0.5 non-α-globin/α-globin biosynthetic ratio	Convenient administration schedule

alkaline denaturation (Kleihauer-Betke Method) or by immunofluorescent techniques. These 'F-cells' are derived from 'F-reticulocytes' whose numbers are normally 1–2% of the total reticulocytes.

Subsequent to these limited trials in non-human primates, several patients with β-thalassemia and sickle cell anemia were studied. Following short courses of parenteral 5-Aza C, patients have invariably shown an increase in percentage HbF and in F-cell numbers, generally within the first 2–3 days and reaching maximal levels four-to seven-fold above baseline (Charache et al 1983, Ley et al 1982, 1983). This increase in HbF production and F-cell numbers has been associated, when measured in sickle cell patients, with a decrease in the numbers of dense red cells and in the rate of hemolysis (Charache et al 1983, Dover et al 1985). In small pilot studies, other S-phase-specific drugs, such as cytosine arabinoside (Ara C) (Papayannoupoulou et al 1984 Veith et al 1985a), vinblastine (Veith et al 1985b) and myleran (Liu et al 1990), have also been found to be effective in stimulating HbF production, and because these agents do not affect methylation directly, the current view is that other factors in addition to demethylation account for induction of fetal hemoglobin in association with these therapies. However, because of their perceived carcinogenic potential, especially given the requisite chronicity of administration to maintain elevated HbF levels in these patients, the use of these types of S-phase-specific agents has recently been restricted to individuals with end-stage β-thalassemia (Dunbar et al 1989, Lowrey & Nienhuis 1993).

PHASE I/II HYDROXYUREA TRIALS

Following the demonstration that the postnatal induction of HbF in humans was both feasible and safe, attention quickly shifted to evaluating other chemotherapeutic agents with a more desirable therapeutic index. Of the several studied, hydroxyurea has emerged as the agent of choice. These studies were broadly developed to determine the relationship between toxicity and dose-scheduled treatment (Phase I), and the biological (hematological) response to hydroxyurea (Phase II).

In early Phase I/II Trials (Veith et al 1985a, Platt et al 1984, Charache et al 1987, Sumoza & Bissotti 1986) a dose of 50mg/kg hydroxyurea was selected

Table 2 Early Phase I/II hydroxyurea trials

Study	No. patients (responders)	Dose	No. days	Onset of F-retic response
Platt et al	2(2)	50mg/kg	5	48–72 h
Veith et al	2(2)	50mg/kg	5	48–72 h
Charache et al	8(4)	50mg/kg	3 or 5	48–72 h
Sumoza and Bisotti	19(16)	50mg/kg	14 to 98	ND
	7(7)	25mg/kg	>28	ND

ND = not done

based upon the results of studies in a non-human primate model. Several patients were entered into such investigations. In these trials, hydroxyurea was administered orally given on 3 to 5 consecutive days per week, while one study used hydroxyurea on a daily basis. Following such a treatment schedule, most patients showed an increase in the F-reticulocyte response, which was evident within 48–72 hours following the initiation of therapy. This rise in the percentage of F-reticulocytes invariably was associated with a increase in the F-cell numbers, and a small rise in fetal hemoglobin levels. Although there was a decrease in the absolute neutrophil count, when measured there was no change in the peripheral BFU-e HbF program obtained from the patients. Thus, these data collectively indicated that hydroxyurea therapy could influence fetal hemoglobin production in erythroid cells, presumably through mechanisms involving changes in the kinetics of the growth patterns of erythroid progenitor and precursor cells. The results of the early Phase I/II Trials with hydroxyurea are summarized in Table 2.

While the short-term toxicity in the Phase I/II trials was limited to the hematopoietic system, it was anticipated that the continuous administration of dosages in the range of 50mg/kg/day would ultimately be prohibitive. Furthermore, the potential beneficial clinical effects of HbF induction could not be judged owing to the nature of this dose-limiting toxicity.

Because of these early encouraging results, a pilot study was begun at the National Institutes of Health (NIH), in collaboration with Johns Hopkins University. The objectives of this study were to define optimal dosage schedules, and to monitor the spectrum and patterns of responses and potential predictive factors among a cohort of severe sickle cell patients hospitalized for periods of 3 to 4 months, while receiving hydroxyurea (HU). Prolonged hospitalization allowed a systematic analysis of early toxic effects, as well as the ability to exclude drug compliance as a contributory factor to (non) response. These data have been published previously (Rodgers et al 1990), and subsequently substantiated in other trials (Goldberg et al 1990, Charache et al 1992, el-Hazmi et al 1992). Figure 2 presents an update of the HbF response among 21 consecutive NIH patients entered on the HU trial, consisting of an initial in-hospital phase, and more prolonged outpatient observation periods.

Analysis of these updated data, coupled with the other Phase II/III trials (Goldberg et al 1990, Charache et al 1992, el-Hazmi et al 1992) allows one

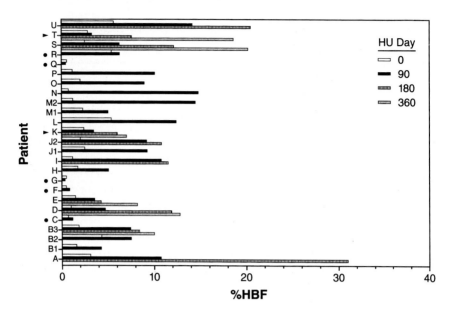

Fig. 2 The spectrum of fetal hemoglobin responses among patients treated at the National Institutes of Health, in a combination of inpatient/outpatient settings. Patients B, J, and M, were treated more than once following a period of wash-out from hydroxyurea therapy. Patients C, F, G, Q and R are considered non-responders and are indicated by a dot. Patients K and T required blood transfusions immediately before or during their first 90 days of therapy of hydroxyurea, and therefore therapy was extended for a longer period time in order to determine responsiveness.

to draw some important conclusions. First, even when drug compliance can be excluded as a variable, the positive hematological response, defined by a two-fold minimum increase from baseline in the HbF and F-reticulocyte level (Rodgers et al 1990), appears to be in the order of 75–80%, as indicated in Figure 1 (patients C, F, G, Q, R, are non-responders). Patients who are transfused before or during the course of HU therapy may take a longer period of time to evidence their response, as seen in Figure 1 (patients K and T required transfusions with the first 6 weeks of therapy and thus were followed for longer to determine their response). Second, at a fixed weekly dose (range 10–20 mg/kg) of HU, administering the dose equally divided over 4 or 7 consecutive days appears to result in a similar rate of accumulation of HbF. The HbF levels in most of the responders, though not all, were stabilized after the first 180 days (6 months) of therapy. Others with intercurrent illnesses or those requiring transfusion support may require longer periods before a plateau in HbF levels is achieved. Interestingly, in contrast to the HbF response to 5-Aza C which may be seen within days of administration, increases in HbF production with HU occurs more gradually, typically with a lag period of several weeks before measurable changes are evident. Finally, there has been no absolute correlation found between initial hematological indices, α-globin genotype or β-globin haplotype and a favorable response to hydroxyurea.

Subsequently, these observations have been confirmed and extended in single (Goldberg et al 1990, el-Hazmi et al 1992) and multi-institutional (Charache et al 1992) open-labeled trials. Goldberg and colleagues (1990) established unambiguously the improved characteristics of red cells of sickle cell patients (SS) responding to hydroxyurea, including prolonged red-cell survival, increased oxygen affinity and improved red-cell cation content. Charache and colleagues (1992) reported that among 32 SS patients treated with HU for periods up to 2 years, HbF levels increased to a mean of 14.9%, that the magnitude of the response correlated with plasma hydroxyurea levels and that hematological response appeared to presage a clinical response.

Following these observations in adult SS patients, pilot studies involving pediatric patients have also been conducted (Ohene Frempong 1993, Scott et al 1993). While the response rates in children are similar, the absolute HbF achievable may be greater. More recently, Voskaridou and co-workers (1995) have administered HU to patients with HbS/β-thalassemia, a population in whom the HbF stimulatory effects of therapy may also be greater than that observed in the adult SS population.

In contrast to the beneficial hematological and clinical effects given by hydroxyurea to approximately 80% of sickle cell patients, such treatment of transfusion-dependent β-thalassemia patients has been more disappointing (McDonagh 1990, Ley & Nienhuis 1985). However, some patients with β-thalassemia intermedia, who are not transfusion dependent, may respond to HU treatment, albeit transiently (Hajjar & Pearson 1994), by increasing their packed cell volumes (Bachir & Galactleros 1994, Zeng et al 1995). More recently, it has been observed that HU augments HbF levels and improves ineffective erythropoiesis in β-thalassemia/HbE patients (Fucharoen et al 1993).

MULTICENTER STUDY OF HYDROXYUREA

Encouraged by the results of these open-labeled studies with HU in SS patients and the general impression that a clinical response to HU often followed hematological improvement, a formal clinical trial was proposed. The objective of the investigation was to determine whether HU treatment of SS patients is associated with a significant reduction in the frequency of painful crisis, and secondarily other clinical end-points. The design was a multicenter, randomized double-blind control trial, with an expected minimum follow-up of 2 years following randomization. Twenty-one university teaching hospitals or clinics with a high volume of SS patients in the USA and Canada participated. There were 299 patients who eventually entered the trial (Charache et al 1995).

There was a lower annual rate of crisis in patients randomly assigned to the hydroxyurea treatment arm than with patients receiving placebo (median, 2.5 versus 4.5 crisis per year, P<0.001). There was also a reduction in the median time to the first and the second crisis in patients who were treated with hydroxyurea. Figure 3 shows an analysis of the cumulative crisis rate from the initiation of treatment to the first and second painful crisis, respectively.

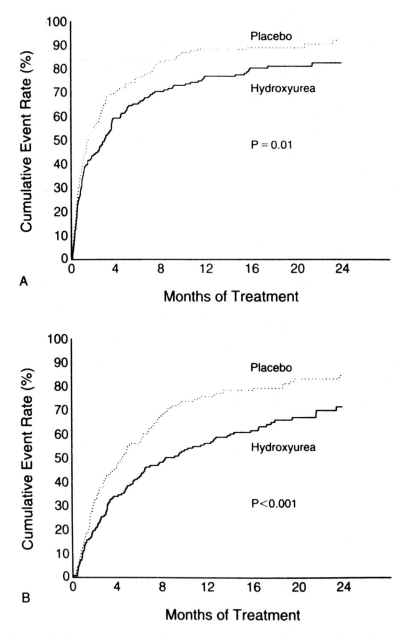

Fig. 3 Median time from the initiation of treatment to the first painful (Panel A) and second crisis (Panel B), stratified by treatment group. (Abstracted from Charache et al 1995, with permission)

Hydroxyurea-treated patients also had a significant reduction in episodes of acute chest syndrome, and required fewer blood transfusions. The treatment did not appear to be associated with any important adverse effects and it was therefore concluded that 'hydroxyrea therapy can ameliorate the clinical course of sickle cell anemia in some adults with severe symptoms defined as three or more painful crisis per year' (Charache et al 1995).

As a result of sequential analysis by a Data and Safety Monitoring Board, this study was ended by the investigators several months earlier than anticipated, and a Clinical Alert was issued by the National Heart Lung and Blood Institute on the basis of these aforementioned observations. At the present time, an accelerated review process is under way with the US Food and Drug Administration (FDA) to allow hydroxyurea to be approved for the treatment of patients severely affected with sickle cell disease. Despite these very exciting results and a desire to expedite the inclusion of severe sickle cell disease as an indication for hydroxyurea therapy, there remains several relevant questions (Schechter & Rodgers 1995) not specifically addressed in the paper by Charache and colleagues (1995).

For example, the optimal dose schedule was not defined by this study, although this trial did confirm a previous observation Rodgers et al 1990 that maximal tolerated doses of hydroxyurea may not be necessary for a therapeutic effect. Second, the Multicenter Study of Hydroxyurea (MSH) trial did not report the proportion of hydroxyurea-treated patients who failed to show a significant rise in HbF levels, nor the spectrum of HbF increments among the responders. Such data would be critical not only for determining the relationship between achievable HbF levels and clinical response, but given the myelotoxic effects of hydroxyurea and uncertain long-term toxicities, it would seem prudent not to administer this agent clinically to (hematological) non-responders. Lastly, this trial was restricted to adult sickle cell patients, and therefore any extrapolations into the pediatric population that would lead to its widespread use thereon would not be justifiable on the basis of current data. Ongoing and planned multicenter pediatric hydroxyurea trials should clarify over the next several years its role in this clinical context (Ohene-Frempong et al 1993, Scott et al 1993, de Montalembert et al 1994). Meanwhile, the findings of the MSH trial offers enough positive results to warrant the initiation (or continuation) of hydroxyurea treatment in severely affected adult patients under careful monitoring. A search for alternative agents to be used alone or in combination with hydroxyurea in eligible 'poor' responders or 'non-responders' should also be continued.

CYTOKINES (CELLULAR GROWTH FACTORS)

Because of the variability of the hemoglobin F response noted in the early trials, together with the myelotoxicity observed with chemotherapeutic agents including hydroxyurea, other agents including cytokines and non-cytotoxic therapy have been studied for their potential effects on HbF production.

Recombinant human erythropoietin (Epo) alone or in combination with hydroxyurea, has been previously shown to increase both F-cell numbers and hemoglobin F-level in non-human primates (Al-Khatti et al 1988, McDonagh et al 1992), raising the possibility that Epo may exert an additive or synergistic effect on fetal hemoglobin stimulation. A small pilot trial in sickle cell patients showed that Epo alone or in combination with hydroxyurea had no effect on hemoglobin F response (Goldberg et al 1990). More recent studies, however, have shown that concomitant administration of oral iron with Epo, the timing of the combination of Epo with hydroxyurea, and/or the absolute dose of Epo (up to 3000 IU/kg) are important variables that may determine the ultimate fetal hemoglobin response to sickle cell patients (Nagel et al 1993, Rodgers et al 1993). Figure 4 shows the kinetics of the F-reticulocyte and HbF response to hydroxyurea alone and hydroxyurea alternating with Epo. These data have been subsequently substantiated in trials in Greece and Saudi Arabia. In addition, Epo therapy has been shown to be efficacious in a patient, with Hb Burke, on chronic dialysis (Kamata et al 1993).

Studies employing Epo in patients with β-thalassemia have led to somewhat different results. In these studies, Epo therapy is associated with an increase in the total hemoglobin in the absence of major toxic effects (Olivieri

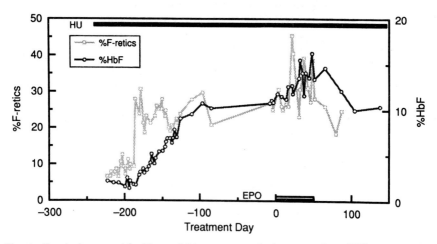

Fig. 4 F-reticulocyte and fetal hemoglobin response to hydroxyurea alone (HU) or combination hydroxyurea/erythropoietin therapy in a sickle cell patient. The hydroxyurea response on a fixed dose was monitored until a plateau for HbF and F-reticulocytes was achieved (treatment day –100). This dose was maintained until day 0 at which point erythropoietin was administered in an alternating fashion with hydroxyurea for about 50 days. Hydroxyurea was continued after the erythropoietin was discontinued, which was associated with a return to baseline in both the F-reticulocytes and the hemoglobin F percentages. (Adapted from Rodgers et al 1993; F-reticulocytes analysis performed by G Dover, MD, Johns Hopkins University).

et al 1992, Rachmilewitz et al 1995). Curiously, although the quantity of red blood corpuscles increased, there was no change in their quality, especially in the proportion of HbF (Olivieri et al 1992, Rachmilewitz et al 1995, Sher et al 1994). Nonetheless, an accelerated linear growth has been noted in seven pediatric patients receiving Epo alone (Rachmilewitz et al 1995). Combination therapy with Epo and hydroxyurea in thalassemia patients appears to be more advantageous than either therapy alone (Aker et al 1994, Loukopoulos et al 1993) with respect to HbF augmentation and an increased packed cell volume. Currently, the cost of erythropoietin still precludes its more extensive application in the setting of the hemoglobinopathies.

SHORT CHAIN FATTY ACIDS

Given the variability in response to the currently available agents, together with the short-term and uncertain long-term toxicities of the cytotoxic agents, a great deal of attention has been focused on expanding the list of available agents capable of stimulating HbF production. The butyrate analogues have emerged as likely candidates as they have been known for some time to be potent inducers of hematopoietic cell differentiation (Riggs et al 1977). Pertinent to potential effects of HbF induction, butyrate can modify histone acetylation (Riggs et al 1977) a process thought to be central to gene activation. More cogent, however, are findings that butyrate may interact with elements in the chicken ρ-globin gene promotor (Ginder et al 1984) and in the human γ-globin gene promoter in K562 cells (McDonagh & Nienhuis 1991). Elevated concentrations of butyric acid and other fatty acids in the maternal serum appear to be related to the elevated HbF levels present in infants born to poorly-controlled diabetic mothers (Perrine et al 1985). In addition, it has been reported very recently that individuals with congenital abnormalities in propionate metabolism also demonstrate a persistent high-level expression of HbF, even in the absence of anemia (Little et al 1995).

On the basis of these earlier observations, and preclinical studies which showed that arginine-butyrate infusions into the umbilical vein of sheep fetuses reversed the normal fetal-to-adult hemoglobin switch (Perrine et al 1983), a small pilot phase I/II study of intravenous butyrate was conducted in children with β-thalassemia and sickle cell disease (Perrine et al 1993). The preliminary data were quite promising with respect to γ-globin chain expression and hemoglobin levels in some patients in the absence of major toxicity. One patient with Hb Lepore was maintained on therapy for a more extended period and showed a very dramatic rise in hemoglobin level (Perrine et al 1993). A more recent trial involving 10 patients with either sickle cell disease or β-thalassemia, however, utilizing an almost identical protocol did not confirm these previous findings (Sher et al 1995). One patient who inadvertently was given a four-fold concentrated amount of butyrate suffered a grand mal seizure. Interestingly, specific neuropathological lesions have been demonstrated in baboons receiving extended infusions of butyrate at this slightly higher concentration, not related to the sodium content (Blau et al 1993). Therefore, given the equivocal efficacy in inducing HbF levels, the low therapeutic/toxic ratio and the requirement for a continuous infusion administration schedule, the practical application of this agent may be somewhat limited.

Nonetheless, it is now clear that many compounds with similar chemical structures to butyrate, collectively designated short chain fatty acids, have the capacity to stimulate HbF production in erythroid cell cultures (Constantoulakis et al 1989, Fibach et al 1993), animal models (Perrine et al 1985) and in patients with genetic disorders of urea metabolism (Dover et al 1992). The chemical structure of the related compound currently under investigation is shown in Figure 5. Recent trials with phenylbutyrate in sickle cell disease (Dover et al 1994) and β-thalassemia (Collins et al 1995) have confirmed its ability to augment HbF levels in the hemoglobinopathies. It is noted, however, that such therapy currently requires that patients take by mouth between 30–50 capsules each day, and not surprisingly drug compliance is a major factor related to the response rate (Dover et al 1994). A number of pharmaceutical companies and biotechnology firms are currently attempting to develop drugs within this class of agents which can be orally administered in a more concentrated form and with a longer biological half-life. As these searches are currently underway, it is hoped that the role of this group of agents, when used alone or in combination with existing agents in the treatment of the severe β-globin disorders, should soon be better appreciated.

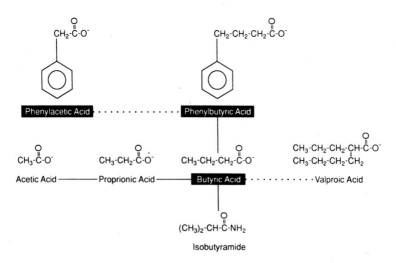

Fig. 5 Chemical structure of short chain fatty acids found to be capable of inducing fetal hemoglobin production in humans. Shaded compounds have been used in Phase I/II trials in patients with hemoglobinopathies.

CONCLUSION

Though the general medical care of patients with sickle cell disease and β-thalassemia has contributed to a longer life expectancy, generally acceptable, specific and non-toxic therapies are currently not available. While advances in bone marrow and hematopoietic stem cell transplantation makes these a viable curative treatment modality, this approach is currently limited by the availability of suitable donors and the expense of the procedure. Gene therapy directed at replacing or compensating for the defective β-globin allelles in the β-globin disorders remains a theoretically attractive, though currently non-feasible treatment option. Improvement in gene transfer methodologies and the ex vivo isolation and expansion of hematopoietic stem cells remains a formidable, though not insurmountable task. Until that time, therapies based on stimulating fetal hemoglobin synthesis by pharmacological means offer significant promise in favorably modifying the underlying pathogenic mechanisms in sickle cell disease and β-thalassemia.

KEY POINTS FOR CLINICAL PRACTICE

- Recent data derived from large prospective studies indicate a striking improvement in life expectancy in patients with sickle cell disease and β-thalassemia.

- A tremendous variability in morbidity exists among sickle cell patients, with the most severe patients, defined as those exhibiting three or more painful crises/year, accounting for less than 20% of the total patient population.

- Fetal hemoglobin levels correlate indirectly with pain rates among adults with sickle cell disease.

- Hydroxyurea therapy, by increasing fetal hemoglobin levels, appears to ameliorate the clinical course in most (75–80%) of adult sickle cell patients; it appears less effective in the treatment of β-thalassemia major.

- Hydroxyurea therapy should be restricted to severely affected sickle cell patients who should undergo periodic monitoring of blood counts and be fully informed of the uncertain long-term toxicities of this agent.

- Currently, there is only limited experience with hydroxyurea in pediatric and adolescent patients and therefore its use in these patients should be viewed as highly experimental, with eligible patients being referred to ongoing trials, where possible.

REFERENCES

Aker M, Perry D, Dover G, et al 1994 The effect of combined recombinant human erythropoietin and hydroxyurea on erythropoiesis in β-thalassemia intermedia. Blood 84 257a

Al-Khatti A, Papayannopoulou T, Knitter G et al 1988 Cooperative enhancement of F-cell formation in baboons treated with erythropoietin and hydroxyurea. Blood 72: 817–819

Bachir D, Galactleros F 1994 Potential alternatives to erythrocyte transfusion in hemoglobinopathies: hydroxyurea (HU), erythropoietin (EPO), butyrate derivatives, blood substitutes. Transf Clin Bio 1: 35–39

Beutler E 1961 The effect of methemoglobin formation in sickle cell disease. J Clin Invest 40: 1856–1871

Beutler E 1969 Effects of sex hormones on fetal hemoglobin levels. JAMA 207: 2284–2285

Blau CA, Constantoulakis P, Shaw CM et al 1993 Fetal hemoglobin induction with butyric acid: Efficacy and toxicity. Blood 81: 259

Brittenham G M, Griffith P M, Nienhuis A W et al 1994 Efficacy of deferoxamine in preventing complications of iron overload in patients with thalassemia major. N Engl J Med 331: 567–573

Bunn H F, Forget B G 1986 Hemoglobin: molecular, genetic and clinical aspects. W.B. Saunders Co, Philadelphia, PA

Charache S, Dover G, Smith K et al 1983 Treatment of sickle cell anemia with 5-azacytidine results in increased fetal hemoglobin production and is associated with non random hypomethylation of DNA around the gamma-delta-beta-globin gene complex. Proc Natl Acad Sci USA 80: 4842–4846

Charache S, Dover G, Moyer M et al 1987 Hydoxyurea-induced augmentation of fetal hemoglobin production in patients with sickle cell anemia. Blood 69: 109–116

Charache S, Dover G J, Moore R D et al 1992 Hydroxyurea: effects on hemoglobin F production in patients with sickle cell anemia. Blood 69: 2555–2565

Charache S, Terrin M L, Moore R D et al 1995 Effect of hydroxyurea on frequency of painful crises in sickle cell anemia. N Engl J Med 332: 1317–1322

Collins A F, Pearson H A, Giardina P et al 1995 Oral sodium phenylbutyrate therapy in homozygous beta thalassemia: a clinical trial. Blood 85: 43–49

Constantoulakis P, Knitter G, Stamatoyannopoulos G 1989 On the induction of fetal hemoglobin by butyrates: *in vivo* and *in vitro* studies with sodium butyrate and comparsion of combination treatment with 5-Aza C and Ara C. Blood 74: 1963–1971

De Ceulaer K, Gruber C, Hayes R J et al 1982 Medroxyprogesterone acetate and homozygous sickle cell disease. Lancet ii: 229–231

DeSimone J, Heller P, Hall I et al 1982 5 Azacytidine stimulates fetal hemoglobin synthesis in anemic baboons. Proc Natl Acad Sci USA 79: 4428–4431

Dover G J, Charache S, Boyer S H et al 1985 5-Azacytidine increases HbF production and reduces anemia in sickle cell disease: dose-response analysis of subcutaneous and oral dosage regimens. Blood 66: 527–532

Dover G J, Brusilow S, Samid D 1992 Increased fetal hemoglobin in patients receiving sodium-4-phenylbutyrate. N Engl J Med 327: 569–570

Dover G J, Brusilow S, Charache S 1994 Induction of fetal hemoglobin production in subjects with sickle cell anemia by oral sodium phenylbutyrate. Blood 84: 339–343

Dunbar C, Travis W, Kan Y W et al 1989 5-Azacytidine treatment in beta-thalassemic patients unable to be transfused due to multiple alloantibodies. Br J Hematol 72: 467–474

Fibach E, Prasanna P, Rodgers G P et al 1993 Enhanced fetal hemoglobin production by phenylacetate and 4-phenylbutyrate in erythroid precursors derived from normal donors and patients with sickle cell disease. Blood 82: 2203–2206

Fosburg M, Nathan D G 1990 Treatment of Cooley's anemia. Blood 76: 435–444

Fucharoen S, Siritanaratkul N, Winichagoon P et al 1996 Hydroxyurea increases HbF levels and improves the effectiveness of erythropoiesis in β-thalassemia/HbF disease. Blood: in press

Ginder G, Whitters M, Pohlman J 1984 Activation of a chicken-embryonic globin gene in adult erythroid cells by 5-azacytidine and sodium butyrate. Proc Natl Acad Sci USA 81: 3954–3958

Goldberg M A, Brugnara C, Dover G J et al 1990 Treatment of sickle cell anemia with hydroxyurea and erythropoietin. N Engl J Med 323: 366–372

Hajjar F M, Pearson H A 1994 Pharmacologic treatment of thalassemia intermedia with hydroxyurea. J Pediatr 125: 490–492

el-Hazmi M A, Warsy A S, al-Momen A et al 1992 Hydroxyurea for the treatment of sickle cell disease. Acta Haematol 88: 170–174

Kamata K, Sato N, Takahashi E 1993 High-dose erythroprotein for unstable hemoglobin Burke in a patient receiving hemodialysis. N Engl J med 328: 1498-1499

Lavelle D, DeSimone J, Heller P 1993 Fetal hemoglobin reactivation in baboon and man: a short perspective. Am J Hematol 42: 91–95

Ley T J 1991 The pharmacology of hemoglobin switching: of mice and men. Blood 15: 1146–1152

Ley T, Nienhuis A W 1985 Induction of hemoglobin F synthesis in patients with β-thalassemia. Annu Rev Med 36: 485–498

Ley T J, DeSimone J, Anagnou N et al 1982 5-Azacytidine selectively increases gamma-globin synthesis in a patient with β-thalassemia. N Engl J Med 307: 1469–1475

Ley T J, DeSimone J, Noguchi C T et al 1983 5-Azacytidine increases gamma-globin synthesis and reduces the proportion of dense cells in patients with sickle cell anemia. Blood 62: 370–380

Little JA, Dempsey NJ, Tuchman M et al 1995 Metabolic persistence of fetal hemoglobin. Blood 85: 1712-1718

Liu D P, Liang C C, Ao Z H et al 1990 Treatment of severe beta-thalassemia (patients) with myleran. Am J Hematol 33(1): 50–55

Lowrey C, Nienhuis A W 1993 Brief report: treatment with azacytidine of patients with end-stage beta-thalassemia. N Engl J Med 329: 845–848

Loukopoulos D, Vosakaridou E, Cozma G et al 1993 Effective stimulation of erythropoietins in thalassemia intermedia with r-hu-erythropoietin and hydroxyurea. Blood 82: 357a

McDonagh K T, Nienhuis A W 1991 Induction of the human gamma globin gene promoter in K562 cells by sodium butyrate: reversal repression by CCAAT displacement protein. Blood 78: 255a

McDonagh K T, Orringer E P, Dover G J et al 1990 Hydroxyurea improves erythopoiesis in a patient with homozygous beta-thalassemia. Clin Res 38: 346A

McDonagh K T, Dover G J, Donahue R E et al 1992 Hydroxyurea-induced HbF production in anemic primates: augmentation by erythropoietin, hematopoietic growth factors, and sodium butyrate. Exp Hematol 20: 1156–1164

de Montalembert M, Belloy M, Bernaudin F et al 1994 Clinical and hematological response of sickle cell children to treatment with hydroyurea. Blood 84: 219a

Nagel R L, Vichinsky E, Shah M et al 1993 F reticulocyte response in sickle cell anemia treated with recombinant human erythropoietin: a double-blind study. Blood 81: 9–14

Ohene-Frempong K, Horiuchi K, Bulgarelli W et al 1993 Hydroxyurea increases HBF production in children with sickle cell disease. Blood 82: 472a

Olivieri N F, Freedman M H, Perrine S P et al 1992 Trial of recombinant human erythropoietin: three patients with thalassemia intermedia. Blood 80: 3258–3260

Olivieri NF, Nathan DG, MacMillan JH et al 1994 Survival in medically treated patients with homozygous β-thalassemia. N Engl J Med 331: 544–578

Perrine S P, Rudolph A, Faller D V et al 1988 Butyrate infusions in the ovine fetus delay the biologic clock for globin gene switching. Proc Natl Acad Sci USA 85: 8540–8542

Perrine S P, Ginder G D, Faller D V et al 1993 A short-term trial of butyrate to stimulate fetal-globin-gene expression in the beta-globin disorders. N Engl J Med 328: 81–86

Perrine S P, Greene M F, Faller D V et al 1985 Delay in the fetal globin switch in infants of diabetic mothers. N Engl J Med 312: 334–338

Papayannoupoulou T, De Torrealba R, Veith R et al 1984 Arabinosylcytosime induces fetal hemoglobin in baboons by perturbing erythroid differentiation kinetics. Science 224: 617–619

Platt O S, Orkin S H, Dover G et al 1984 Hydroxyurea enhances fetal hemoglobin production in sickle cell anemia. J Clin Invest 74: 652–656

Rodgers G P 1994 Pharmacological modulation of fetal hemoglobin. In Embury S, Hebbel R, Mohandas N, Steinberg M (eds) Sickle cell disease: basic principles and clinical practice. New York Raven Press, pp 829–843

Rodgers GP, Dover GJ, Noguchi CT et al 1990 Hematologic responses of patients with sickle cell disease to treatment with hydroxyurea. N Engl J Med 322:1037-1045

Rodgers G P, Dover G J, Uyesaka N et al 1993 Augmentation by erythropoietin of the fetal-hemoglobin response to hydroxyurea in sickle cell disease. N Engl J Med 328: 73–80

Rachmilewitz E A, Aker M, Perry D et al 1995 Sustained increase in haemoglobin and RBC following long-term administration of recombinant human erythropoietin to patients with homozygous beta-thalassaemia. Br J Haematol 90: 341-345

Riggs M G, Whittaker R G, Neumann J R et al 1977 N-Butyrate causes histone modification in HeLa and Friend erythroleukemia cells. Nature 268: 462–464

Steingart R 1992 Management of patients with sickle cell disease. Med Clin North Am 76: 669–682

Serjeant G R, Serjeant B E 1993 Management of sickle cell disease; lessons from the Jamaican Cohort Study. Blood Rev 7: 137–145

Stamatoyannopoulos J A, Nienhuis A W 1992 Therapeutic approaches to hemoglobin switching: a treatment of hemoglobinopathies. Ann. Rev Med 43: 497–521

Sumoza A, Bissotti R S 1986 Treatment of sickle cell anemia with hydroxyurea: results in twenty-six patients. Blood 68: 67a

Scott J P, Robinson E, Hillery C A et al 1993 A study of hydroxyurea (HDU) treatment of severely affected children with sickle cell disease (SCD). Clin Res 41: 331a

Schechter A N, Rodgers G P 1995 Sickle cell anemia-basic research reaches the clinic. N Engl J Med 332: 1372–1374

Sher G D, Olivieri F A, McCusker P J et al 1994 Long-term treatment with recombinant human erythropoietin (rHuEpo) in thalassemia: Reduction in requirement for transfusion and chelation therapy. Blood 84: 258a

Sher G D, Ginder G D, Little J et al 1995 Extended therapy with intravenous arginine butyrate in patients with β-hemoglobinopathies. N Engl J Med 332: 1606–1610

Thein S L 1993 β-thalassemia. Balliere's Clinical Haematol 6: 151–175

Veith R, Galanello R, Papayannopoulou T et al 1985a Stimulation of F-cell production in patients with sickle cell anemia treated with cytarabine or hydroxyurea. N Engl J Med 313: 1571–1575

Veith R, Papayannopoulou T, Kuracho S et al 1985b Treatment of baboon with vinblastine: insights into the mechanisms of pharmacologic stimulation of HbF in the adult. Blood 66: 456–459

Voskaridou E, Kalotychou V, Loukopoulos D 1995 Clinical and laboratory effects of long-term administration of hydroxyurea to patients with sickle-cell/β-thalasemia. Br J Haematol 89: 479–484

Zeng Y T, Huang S Z, Ren Z R et al 1995 Hydroxyurea therapy in β-thalassemia intermedia: improvement in hematological parameters due to enhanced β-globin synthesis. Br J Haematol 90: 557-563

12

Human stem cell biology and therapy

K. Auditore-Hargreaves   M. Krieger   C. Jacobs   S. Heimfeld
R. J. Berenson

INTRODUCTION

The antigenic profile of human hematopoietic cells changes both quantitatively and qualitatively during the course of differentiation. This heterogeneity has been exploited to select specific subpopulations of cells, at various stages of lineage commitment, for use in a variety of research and clinical studies of hematopoiesis.

Although a cell surface marker unique to human hematopoietic stem cells has yet to be discovered, there are several markers shared by stem cells and more committed progenitor cells. Among these, the most widely studied is the CD34 antigen. The CD34 molecule is a 115 kDa glycoprotein present on about 1–3% of human bone marrow cells and detected in vitro on virtually all committed progenitor cells as well as more primitive progenitors, such as long-term, culture-initiating cells (LTC-IC) and high proliferative potential cells (HPP-CFC) (Civin et al 1984, Andrews et al 1986, Egeland et al 1991, Srour et al 1991, 1993).

Although in vitro data suggested that the CD34 antigen was expressed by colony-forming cells, in vivo studies were required to determine whether CD34 marked stem cells were capable of long-term hematopoietic reconstitution. Development of the anti-CD34 antibody 12.8 (Andrews et al 1986) was a critical step forward to in vivo testing because 12.8 cross-reacts with a non-human primate progenitor cell population (Berenson et al 1988). Experiments were subsequently carried out in baboons demonstrating that highly-enriched populations of autologous CD34+ marrow cells could restore hematopoiesis and lead to long-term recovery of bone marrow function in lethally irradiated baboons (Berenson et al 1988). Additional allogeneic transplant studies in baboons have confirmed these findings and evidenced that both short-term and long-term hematopoiesis is provided by transplanted, purified populations of CD34+ cells (Andrews et al 1992). Collectively, these data provided the first evidence that the CD34 antigen is expressed by true hematopoietic stem cells.

Many different methods of hematopoietic stem cell selection have been described in the literature (reviewed in Auditore-Hargreaves et al 1994). Some, like counterflow centrifugal elutriation, rely on differences in cell size and density to effect cell selection. However, most investigators use an anti-CD34 antibody alone (Berenson et al 1991, Law et al 1993, Briddell et al 1994, Marolleau et al 1994), or in combination with other cell surface markers (Okarma et al 1992, Reading et al 1994) to identify engrafting cell populations and separate them from non-engrafting cells. Over the last few years, CD34 selected cells have been used in a variety of clinical settings including allogeneic and autologous marrow and peripheral blood transplantation. In this chapter, we review clinical experience in CD34+ cell transplantation and also discuss other clinical applications of purified CD34+ cells that are emerging in gene therapy, solid organ transplantation, and autoimmunity.

AUTOLOGOUS STEM CELL TRANSPLANTATION

Rationale

In the autologous transplant setting, CD34+ selection has been used to reduce the tumor cell burden in a graft and to decrease the infusional toxicities that are observed when patients receive cryopreserved marrow or peripheral blood stem cells. Infusional toxicity is generally believed to be a result of the volume of dimethyl sulfoxide (DMSO) used to cryopreserve an autologous graft (Davis et al 1990, Stroncek et al 1991) and to cellular debris resulting from cryoinjury to red cells and granulocytes contained in the graft (Pinski & Maloney 1990, Stroncek et al 1991). Both the amount of cell debris and the amount of DMSO can be reduced by stem cell selection.

Volume reduction may be particularly important when peripheral blood rather than marrow is used as the source of stem cells (see below). The larger number of cells in a peripheral blood stem cell (PBSC) collection results in correspondingly larger product volumes for cryopreservation (Kessinger et al 1990) and reinfusion may expose the patient to as much as 10 g DMSO per kilogram of patient weight (Rowley et al 1994). Although the LD_{50} of DMSO in man is not known, 10 g/kg is in or above the range determined for other species.

Gene marking studies have shown definitively that reinfusion of tumor cells contributes to relapse in acute myelogenous leukemia (AML) and neuroblastoma (Brenner et al 1993). Additional studies using the neomycin resistance (*neo*) gene to mark CD34+ selected cells from patients with chronic myelogenous leukemia (CML) have also shown the presence of marked cells at the time of relapse in the leukemic population in marrow and peripheral blood (Khouri & Deisseroth 1995).

Although these studies did not establish the relative importance of tumor reinfused in the graft versus residual tumor in the patient, more recent studies indicate that reinfused tumor cells play a prominent role in relapse. Shpall and co-workers examined disease-free survival (DFS) among breast cancer patients with tumor detectable by immunocytochemistry in their marrow or pheresis products prior to CD34+ selection. They found a statistically significant increase in DFS in those patients whose grafts were purged to negativity by

CD34+ selection (n = 15), as compared to patients whose grafts still contained detectable tumor cells post CD34+ selection (n = 30). After almost 600 days follow-up, approximately 60% of patients in the first group were still alive and without evidence of disease, versus less than 10% of patients in the second group (Shpall et al 1994a)

Bone marrow

We recently completed a prospective, randomized multicenter Phase III study in patients with advanced breast cancer, in which we compared transplantation with autologous, CD34+ selected cells to transplantation with unselected, marrow buffy coat. The objectives of this study were two fold: first, to demonstrate that CD34+ selected cells are equivalent to unselected marrow in rate and pattern of engraftment, and second, to demonstrate that toxicity associated with reinfusion of the marrow is reduced by CD34+ selection.

The study used a continuous-flow affinity chromatography system to select CD34+ cells from marrow (Fig. 1). This technique utilizes a biotinylated, anti-CD34 antibody (12.8) to label stem and progenitor cells in a buffy coat, and a disposable, single-use column containing avidin-conjugated, polyacrylamide beads to capture the labeled cells. Bound cells are released from the beads, largely free of antibody, by gentle mechanical agitation. Clinical use of this technique has been facilitated by development of a computer-controlled instrument, the CEPRATE® SC Stem Cell Concentration System (CellPro, Inc.), that is capable of processing up to one hundred billion cells in approximately 2 hours. At the completion of the process, the CD34+ cells are contained in a volume of about 5 ml that can be cryopreserved in less than 1 g of DMSO.

A total of 92 eligible patients were randomized after bone marrow harvest to receive either an unselected buffy coat graft or a CD34+ selected graft. All patients received rHu-GCSF (Amgen) 10 μg/kg/day, post transplant. Engraftment, defined as ANC > 0.5×10^9 cells/L by Day 20 post transplant, was equivalent in both arms of the study. Toxicity, defined by specific cardiovascular endpoints, was significantly decreased in the CD34+ selected arm (Shpall et al 1993). Similarly, grade 3 or 4 adverse events, life-threatening complications, and medical interventions were decreased in the CD34+ selected arm, relative to the buffy coat arm (Shpall et al unpublished in preparation).

Peripheral blood

It has been known for about 20 years that circulating myeloid progenitor cells are recruited from the marrow to the periphery following chemotherapy. More recently, it was shown that administration of colony stimulating factors, such as G-CSF or GM-CSF, produced a similar effect, and that the combination of a colony stimulating factor and chemotherapy produced a still more

DIRECT AVIDIN-BIOTIN IMMUNOADSORPTION

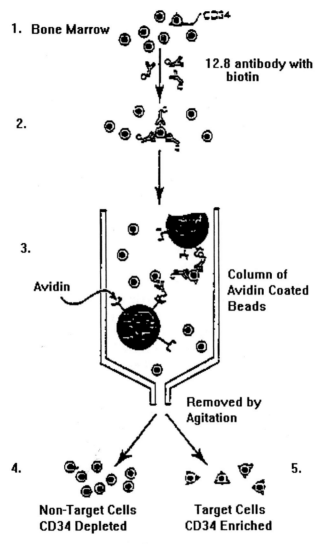

Fig. 1 Direct avidin–biotin immunoaffinity chromatography. A buffy coat is prepared from bone marrow (step 1), and the resultant cell suspension is incubated with a biotinylated, mouse monoclonal antibody to the CD34 antigen (Ab 12.8, step 2). The cell suspension is then passed through a column containing 40 ml of polyacrylamide beads to which avidin has been covalently attached (step 3). CD34+ cells adhere to the beads through the biotinylated antibody with which they are labeled, while CD34 negative cells flow through the column without binding (step 4). The contents of the column are agitated using a magnetically-driven stirring bar to release the bound CD34+ cells from the beads, and these cells are washed out of the column and collected (step 5).

Table 1 HLA-Matched transplants: Johns Hopkins experience

Patient Cohor	Days to ANC >500/ul	Days to Platelets >50,000/ul	RBC Units	Platelet Transfusions	Discharge Day	Cost	Survival (5 month follow-up
Unmanipulated (n=19)	25	30	29	22	37	$164,113	58%
Standard Elutriation (n=23)	21	48	17	14	28	NA	NA
Elutriation+ CD34 fraction (n=12)	18	24	16	8	23	$96,433	92%

Noga, Jones   median

profound mobilization. Thus, it is now routinely possible to collect a sufficient number of CD34+ cells from three or fewer phereses of a mobilized patient (Table 3).

In early clinical studies combining PBSC with marrow transplantation, hematologic recovery was observed to occur more rapidly than with marrow transplantation alone (Sheridan et al 1992). Subsequent studies employing PBSC alone (Jones et al 1994, Pettengell et al 1993), or CD34+ selected PBSC (Shpall et al 1992, Shpall et al 1994a,b) confirmed that the rate of neutrophil engraftment is approximately equivalent to that of marrow, while platelet engraftment is more rapid. It has been postulated that the faster engraftment seen with PBSC compared to marrow may reflect a higher content of more committed progenitors in mobilized blood.

Brugger and co-workers analyzed the engraftment kinetics of CD34+ selected PBSC in 21 patients with advanced malignancies, predominantly breast cancer and small-cell lung cancer, compared to 13 historical control patients who were transplanted with unselected PBSC. Both groups of patients were treated with high-dose VP16, ifosamide, carboplatin, and epirubicin, and both groups received post transplant growth factor. Patients in the CD34+ group received an average of 2.5×10^6 CD34+ cells/kg. As shown in Figure 2, the rate and pattern of engraftment of CD34+ selected PBSC is essentially identical to engraftment with unseparated PBSC. Patients reached an ANC > 500/µl by Day 12 and platelets > 50 000/µl by Day 15 (Brugger et al 1994).

It has been observed in a number of studies that platelet engraftment and, to a lesser extent, neutrophil engraftment are dependent on the number of CD34+ cells infused, engraftment being more rapid above a threshold CD34+ number. Schiller and co-workers (1994) noted that the threshold dose required to achieve prompt hematopoietic recovery was approximately 2×10^6 CD34+ selected PBSC/kg in multiple myeloma patients transplanted following myeloablative chemotherapy. This dose was readily achieved in their patient population with a median of two phereses (see Table 3).

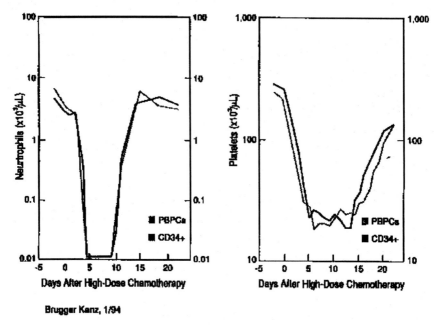

Fig. 2 Hematologic recovery: CD34+PBPC versus unseparated PBPC. Autologous peripheral blood progenitor cells (PBPC) were collected by apheresis from patients mobilized with G-CSF and chemotherapy. CD34+PBPC (n=15) were selected using the CEPRATE SC stem cell concentration system and the rate and pattern of engraftment compared to that of unseparated PBPC (n=13). All patients received G-CSF post transplant.

Table 3 presents data from several trials currently underway in the USA and Europe in which the CEPRATE SC is being used to select CD34+ cells from autologous PBSC collections. Both neutrophil and platelet engraftment occurred in a median of 15 days or less at the various sites. Different sites used different mobilization schemes, with the combination of chemotherapy plus growth factor generally superior to growth factor alone. However, adequate numbers of CD34+ cells could be collected in all cases, even in heavily pretreated patients, by performing multiple phereses. Thus far, patients transplanted with autologous CD34+ selected PBSC have demonstrated durable engraftment, with follow-up times in some cases as long as two years post transplant.

Tumor purging

In an autologous transplant, there is always a risk that tumor cells may contaminate the graft and lead to relapse if reinfused. Several studies have shown that tumor contamination of marrow and PBSC harvests occurs in patients with various types of solid tumors (Moss et al 1990, Ross et al 1993, Sharp et al 1992).

Other studies have suggested that PBSC are less frequently contaminated with tumor than are marrows and that when contamination does occur, the tumor burden is less in PBSC collections than in marrow (Ross et al 1993). Studies such as these have provided further impetus for a shift towards peripheral blood as the preferred source of stem cells.

Most studies of tumor involvement in the marrow or blood have relied on immunocytochemical methods to detect tumor cells. The sensitivity of these methods varies, but is generally between 10^{-4} and 10^{-6}, depending on the assay and the number of cells analyzed (Osborne et al 1991, Molino et al 1991). For solid-tumor micrometastases, antibodies to epithelial antigens and to cytokeratins have been widely employed as detection agents (Ross et al 1993, Pantel et al 1994, Mansi et al 1991).

Another methodology, developed by Ross and colleagues (1993), is a clonogenic assay for breast cancer cells. This assay may be more informative than simple immunocytochemistry with respect to the metastatic potential of the cells detected. Other groups have begun to use polymerase chain reaction (PCR) as a means of quantifying tumor cells burden in marrow and PBSC collections (Datta et al 1994, Traweek et al 1993, Gerhard et al 1994, Vescio et al 1994).

Franklin and colleagues at the University of Colorado have studied the question of tumor contamination in patients with advanced breast cancer (Franklin et al manuscript submitted). Using an immunocytochemical assay that they believe to have a sensitivity of 10^{-5}, they evaluated 210 bone marrow and 91 apheresis samples from women undergoing transplantation. Approximately 28% of marrow specimens and 15% of apheresis specimens were positive in their assay. Among patients with tumor detectable by this assay, the tumor burden was about 1 log less in peripheral blood than in marrow.

Selection of CD34+ cells results in significant depletion of tumor cells from the marrow or PBSC. Evaluating breast cancer patients with tumor contamination demonstrable by immunocytochemistry, Franklin and co-workers found that passive purging using the CEPRATE SC depleted tumor cells to less than the assay's limit of detection in 10/12 (83%) PBSC products and 4/21 (19%) marrow harvests. The efficiency of purging in PBSC may be related to the lower tumor burden generally seen in PBSC in this study.

Berenson and colleagues at UCLA undertook a study of CD34+ selection of PBSC in patients with multiple myeloma. Using a PCR assay to detect patient-specific rearrangements in the immunoglobulin V_H region of myeloma cells, they demonstrated that the CD34 antigen is not expressed on malignant plasma cells in multiple myeloma (Vescio et al 1995). They subsequently showed that CD34+ selection of PBSC resulted in a greater than 4 log reduction in the number of tumor cells contaminating the graft (Vescio et al 1994). On the basis of these results, we have recently undertaken a prospective, randomized, multicenter Phase III trial in multiple myeloma, the objective of which is to demonstrate that CD34+ selection of PBSC, using the CEPRATE SC, results in a reduction in tumor cell burden relative to unselected PBSC.

ALLOGENEIC STEM CELL TRANSPLANTATION

Rationale

Several different methods of T-cell depletion have been developed to prevent graft-versus-host-disease, including complement-mediated lysis, immuno-magnetic depletion, immunotoxins, E-rosetting, and counterflow centrifugal elutriation. More recently, CD34+ selection of donor marrow or peripheral blood has been used to provide a T-cell depleted graft for patients undergoing allogeneic transplantation.

CD34+ augmentation of elutriated marrow

Counterflow centrifugal elutriation is an effective method of T-cell depletion, but it suffers from several important clinical problems. Patients receiving elutriated grafts can experience delayed engraftment, increased incidence of graft failure, and mixed chimeric reconstitution that may lead to relapse (Noga et al 1994a,b). These problems are believed to result, at least in part, from the fact that a substantial fraction of stem and progenitor cells are contained in the lymphocyte-rich, small-cell fraction of the elutriated marrow. This fraction is normally discarded in the elutriation procedure since it contains the T-lymphocytes that contribute to GVHD.

Recently, Noga and co-workers at Johns Hopkins University have utilized the CEPRATE SC to salvage CD34+ cells from the elutriated, small-cell fraction (Noga et al 1994a,b). The CD34+ selected cells are given to the patient along with the lymphocyte-poor, large-cell fraction of the donor's marrow. Previously, this was the only cell fraction patients received. As shown in Table 2, using the CEPRATE SC to salvage CD34+ cells from the small-cell fraction results in a substantial increase in the total number of CD34+ cells provided to the patient, while still keeping the number of CD5+ T-cells in the graft low. Patients who received CD34+ augmented, elutriated marrow grafts engrafted earlier, required fewer blood product transfusions, experienced shorter hospital stays, and exhibited better survival after 5 months than patients who received standard elutriated grafts or unmanipulated grafts (Noga et al 1994a, Table 1).

Peripheral blood

Studies are currently underway at several clinical sites using CD34+ selected allogeneic PBSC, with or without bone marrow, to reconstitute hematopoiesis. In one such study, where unmanipulated bone marrow and CD34+ selected PBSC from matched, related donors were transplanted, 0/6 patients receiving

Table 2 CD34+ Augmentation of elutriated bone marrow

Cell Fraction	Total Nucleated Cells	% CD34+	CD34+ Cells/kg ($\times 10^6$)	CD5+ Cells/kg	CD5+ Cell Log Removal
Lymphocyte Enriched	4.6×10^9	5.5	2.5	2.2×10^7	–
Lymphocyte Enriched and CD34+ Selected	145×10^6	86	1.9	0.4×10^5	2.8
Lymphocyte Depleted	$2.2 \; 10^9$	1.9	0.7	0.6×10^5	–

Noga, Jones
Johns Hopkins

Table 3 CD34+ Peripheral blood progenitor cell transplant trials

Investigator (Site)	Disease	Mobilization (# Aphereses)	CD34+ Cells ($\times 10^6$/kg)	Days to Neutrophils >500/ul	Days to Platelet Recovery
Shpall (Colorado) n=34	Breast	G-CSF (3)	1.6	12	14
Spitzer (St. Louis) n=6	Breast	G-CSF (3)	1.3	10	10
Somlo (City of Hope) n=10	Breast	G-CSF (3)	1.1	11	14
Brugger, Kanz (Freiburg) n=15	Breast, Lung, Lymphoma	VIP+ G-CSF (1)	2.2	12	15
Schiller, Berenson (UCLA) n=15	Multiple Myeloma	CY+ Steroids+ G-CSF (2)	5.2	13	12
Watts, Linch (London) n=4	Lymphoma	CY+G-CSF (1)	>1.0	13	14

cyclosporine A and methotrexate prophylaxis developed serious (grade III–IV) acute GVHD (DiPersio et al 1994). Engraftment was equivalent to historical controls who received unmanipulated bone marrow and the same GVHD prophylaxis regimen. CD34+ selection using the CEPRATE SC was shown to result in a 3 log depletion of T-cells from PBSC in this study.

Although allogeneic transplantation with CD34+ selected bone marrow and/or PBSC appears promising, it will be necessary to evaluate larger numbers of patients over longer periods of time in order to ascertain rates of graft failure chronic graft versus host disease and disease relapse. It will also be important to evaluate CD34+ selected PBSC and/or bone marrow transplantation from mismatched-related and matched-unrelated donors, as success in these settings has the potential to greatly expand the donor pool.

EMERGING APPLICATIONS OF STEM CELL THERAPY

Gene therapy

Many genetic disorders that affect a single gene, such as severe combined immunodeficiency disease (SCID), Gaucher's disease, and β-thalassemia, can potentially be treated by gene-replacement therapy. Gene therapy has also been proposed as a treatment option for various malignancies and viral diseases.

Currently, the most widely used vectors in gene therapy protocols are retroviruses. A typical transfection using unselected marrow as the source of stem cells requires 80–100 L of retroviral supernatant. However, using CD34+ selected marrow as the targets for transfection, only about 1–2 L of retroviral supernatant are needed (Cassel et al 1993). This is an enormous practical advantage in the laboratory. The smaller culture volumes also lessen the possibility of contamination by reducing the amount of manipulation involved in a typical transfection.

The hematopoietic stem cell is in many ways the ideal target cell for gene therapy because it is capable both of self-renewal and of generating large numbers of mature cells. CD34+ cells have been used in many gene therapy protocols, including protocols for the treatment of Gaucher's disease (Nimgaonkar et al 1993), SCID (Kohn et al 1993), ovarian cancer, chronic myelogenous leukemia (CML), and breast cancer. The first two studies have been classic gene-replacement studies involving the glucocerebrosidase gene in one case and the adenosine deaminase gene in the other case. The latter three studies have involved transfecting CD34+ cells with the multidrug resistance (*mdr*) gene to render the patient's marrow resistant to high-dose chemotherapy with myelotoxic chemotherapeutic agents. CD34+ cells have also been used in numerous gene-marking studies in which a reporter gene, such as the gene encoding neomycin resistance, is transfected into cells to determine their fate post-transplantation (Deisseroth et al 1994).

Solid organ transplantation

The concept of using CD34+ cells, selected from marrow or PBSC, to induce tolerance to foreign MHC antigens in the recipient of a solid organ transplant has its roots in work performed 50 years ago in cattle and mice. These seminal studies showed that tolerance to donor allografts was enhanced by the development of mixed chimerism in the lymphoid compartment of the host animal. More recently, Starzl and colleagues have invoked the migration of leukocytes from solid organ transplants into recipient tissues, where they persist for long periods of time, to explain organ acceptance (Starzl et al 1992, 1993).

A number of investigators have attempted to induce tolerance in man to solid organ allografts by means of random donor blood transfusions, donor-specific blood transfusions (van Twuyver et al 1991) and donor bone marrow transfusions (Barber, 1990, Fontes et al 1994). While collectively these studies have demonstrated the establishment of mixed chimerism and hyporeactivity toward donor tissues, they have not generally shown an improvement in survival or a statistically significant decrease in rejection-free interval or incidence of rejection, relative to historical controls. In addition, some of these tolerance induction methods are not applicable to cadaveric donors and several have led to GVHD as a result of the introduction of immunocompetent lymphocytes into an immunosuppressed host.

We plan to initiate clinical studies shortly to test the feasibility of inducing tolerance to solid organ grafts by infusing donor CD34+ cells into an organ recipient during the peritransplant period. By utilizing CD34+ cells rather than unfractionated marrow, we expect to achieve several advantages. First, CD34+ cells can mediate a durable state of mixed chimerism because of their ability to engraft in the host, Second, because CD34+ cells can differentiate into all of the mature elements of the hematopoeitic system, they can mediate tolerance by any of a variety of mechanisms, including suppression (by T-cells or so-called natural suppressor cells) and clonal anergy. Third, the likelihood of eliciting GVHD is less than with unfractionated marrow, which contains alloreactive T-cells. If successful, this strategy could have a major impact on solid organ transplantation. Currently, more than 10 000 solid organ transplants are performed each year in the USA, the majority of these being kidney grafts. About 20% of kidney allografts fail within 1 year of transplant, increasing to 80% within 10 years, despite the administration of potent immunosuppressive agents. Furthermore, chronic administration of immunosuppressive drugs is highly undesirable from the standpoint of toxicity and increased risk of malignancy or infection in the recipient.

Autoimmunity

Autoimmune diseases are generally believed to result from autoreactive T- and B-lymphocytes. Removal of the offending clones by total lymphoid irradiation or by the administration of immunosuppressive agents often results in at least transient improvement in the disease.

By the same token, it is possible to effect long-term remission of autoimmune disease by myeloablation followed by stem cell rescue. Several investigators have reported patients who were cured of their autoimmune diseases following allogeneic bone marrow transplantation for other, co-existing conditions (Eedy et al 1990, Liu Yin & Jowitt 1992, Jacobs et al 1986).

The rationale for autologous transplantation in autoimmunity is less obvious but, we believe, more compelling. There is significantly less morbidity and mortality associated with autotransplantation than with allotransplantation, an important consideration given that autoimmune diseases, while severely debilitating, are rarely life-threatening. CD34+ selection of autologous marrow or PBSC eliminates the mature lymphocytes that can transfer the disease, while still enabling prompt hematopoietic reconstitution. Since reconstitution is probably oligoclonal, there is a good chance that the offending lymphoid clones will not be reconstituted following autologous CD34+ transplantation, even if there is an underlying stem cell defect in autoimmune disease, as Marmont (1992) has suggested. Furthermore, if induction of autoimmunity is also caused by an unknown stimulus (e.g. virus) in the patient's environment, and that stimulus is not present following reconstitution, autoimmunity should not manifest, regardless of whether or not the potentially autoreactive clones are reconstituted.

Recently, a patient with a 3-year history of persistently active myasthenia gravis (MG) received an autologous stem cell transplant for non-Hodgkin's lymphoma, using CD34+ cells selected with the CEPRATE SC (Salzman et al 1994). Following transplant, the patient achieved a sustained remission from MG and was withdrawn from all medications. The patient's MG was still in remission approximately 1 year post transplant, at which time the patient relapsed with NHL.

KEY POINTS FOR CLINICAL PRACTICE

- Transplanting CD34+ selected autologous marrow produces equivalent hematologic recovery to a marrow buffy coat and significantly reduces the frequency and severity of adverse events associated with marrow infusion.

- Rapid and durable hematologic recovery is achieved in patients transplanted for a variety of malignancies with CD34+ selected peripheral blood progenitor cells.

- CD34+ selection has been shown to result in the removal of up to 4 logs of tumor cells from bone marrow and peripheral blood in patients with breast cancer or multiple myeloma.

- CD34+ selection may be useful in allogeneic transplantation since selection leads to an approximate 3 log depletion of T-lymphocytes from bone marrow or aphereses.

- In transplants with elutriated allogeneic bone marrow, clinical results are dramatically improved when CD34+ cells selected from the lymphocyte-rich elutriated fraction are infused together with the lymphocyte-poor elutriated fraction that was the only fraction infused in the past.

- Early clinical studies have shown that retroviral genes can be introduced and stably expressed in CD34+ selected cells in vivo for at least 1 year post transplant.

REFERENCES

Andrews R G, Singer J W, Bernstein I D 1986 Monoclonal antibody 12-8 recognizes a 115 kd molecule present on both unipotent and multipotent hematopoietic colony-forming cells and their precursors. Blood, 67: 842

Andrews R G, Bryant E M, Bartelmez S H et al 1992 CD34+ marrow cells, devoid of T and B lymphocytes, reconstitute stable lymphopoiesis and myelopoiesis in lethally irradiated allogeneic baboons. Blood 80: 1693

Auditore-Hargreaves K, Heimfeld S, Berenson R J 1994 Selection and transplantation of hematopoietic stem and progenitor cells. Bioconjug Chem 5: 287

Barber W H 1990 Induction of tolerance to human renal allografts with bone marrow and antilymphocyte globulin. Transplant Rev 4: 68

Berenson R J, Andrews R G, Bensinger W I et al 1988 Antigen CD34+ marrow cells engraft lethally irradiated baboons. J Clin Invest 81: 951

Berenson R J, Bensinger W I, Hill R S et al 1991 Engraftment after infusion of CD34+ marrow cells in patients with breast cancer or neuroblastoma. Blood 77: 1717

Brenner M K, Rill D R, Holladay M S 1993 Gene marking to trace origin of relapse after autologous bone marrow transplantation. Lancet 341: 85

Briddell R, Shieh J-H, Stoney G et al 1994 Purification of CD34+ cells from mobilized peripheral blood using the Miltenyi MACS separation system. Blood 84 Suppl 1: 2918a

Brugger W, Henschler R Heimfeld S et al 1994 Positively selected peripheral blood CD34+ cells and unseparated peripheral blood progenitor cells mediate identical hematopoietic engraftment after high-dose chemotherapy. Blood 81: 2579

Cassel A, Cottler-Fox M, Doren, S et al 1993 Retroviral-mediated gene transfer into CD34-enriched human peripheral blood stem cells. Exp Hematol 21: 585

Civin C I, Strauss L C, Brovall C et al 1984 Antigenic analysis of hematopoiesis. III. A hematopoietic progenitor cell surface antigen defined by a monoclonal antibody raised against KG-1a cells. J Immunol 133: 157

Datta Y, Adams P, Drobyski W et al 1994 Sensitive detection of occult breast cancer by the reverse-transcriptase polymerase chain reaction. J Clin Oncol 12: 475

Davis J M, Rowley S D, Braine H G et al 1990 Clinical toxicity of cryopreserved bone marrow graft infusion. Blood 75: 781

Deisseroth A, Zu Z, Claxton D et al 1994 Genetic marking shows that Ph+ cells present in autologous transplant of chronic myelogenous leukemia (CML) contribute to relapse after autologous bone marrow transplantation in CML. Blood 83: 3068

DiPersio J, Martin B, Abboud C et al 1994 Allogeneic BMT using bone marrow and CD34 selected mobilized PBSC: Comparison to bone marrow alone and mobilized PBSC alone. Blood 84: 351

Eedy D J, Burrows D, Bridges J M et al 1990 Clearance of severe psoriasis after allogeneic bone marrow transplantation. Br Med J 300: 908

Egeland, T, Steen R, Quarstein H et al 1991 Myeloid differentiation of purified CD34+ cells after stimulation with recombinant human granulocytes-monocyte colony-stimulating factor (CSF), granulocyte-CSF, monocyte-CSF, and interleukin-3. Blood 78: 3192

Fontes P, Rao A S, Demetris A J et al 1994 Bone marrow augmentation of donor-cell chimerism in kidney, liver, heart, and pancreas islet transplantation. Lancet 344: 151

Gerhard M, Juhl H, Kalthoff H et al 1994 Specific detection of carcinoembryonic antigen-expressing tumor cells in bone marrow aspirates by polymerase chain reaction. J Clin Oncol 12: 725

Jacobs P, Vincent M D, Martell R W 1986 Prolonged remission of severe refractory rheumatoid arthritis following allogeneic bone marrow transplantation for drug-induced aplastic anaemia. Bone Marrow Transplant 1: 237

Jones H M, Jones S A, Watts M J et al 1994 Development of a simplified single apheresis approach for peripheral blood progenitor cell transplantation in previously treated patients with lymphoma. J Clin. Oncol. 12: 661

Kessinger A, Schmit-Pokorny K, Smith D et al 1990 Cryopreservation and infusion of autologous peripheral blood stem cells. Bone Marrow Transplant 5: 25

Khouri I F, Deisseroth A B 1995 Genetic modification of hematopoietic stem cells for therapy of solid tumors and hematopoietic neoplasms. In Levitt D, Mertelsman R (eds) Hematopoietic stem cells: biology and therapeutic applications. Marcel Dekker, New York, p 219

Kohn D B, Weinberg K, Parkman R et al 1993 Gene therapy for neonates with adenosine deaminase (ADA)-deficiency (SCID) by retroviral-mediated transfer of the human ADA cDNA into umbilical cord CD34+ cells. Blood 82: 315

Law P, Ishizawa, L, van de Ven C et al 1993 Immunomagnetic positive selection and colony culture of CD34+ cells from blood. J Hematother 2: 247

Liu-Yin J A, Jowitt S N 1992 Resolution of immune-mediated diseases following allogeneic bone marrow transplantation for leukaemia. Bone Marrow Transplant 9: 31

Mansi J, Easton D, Berger U et al 1991 Bone marrow micrometastases in primary breast cancer: Prognostic significance after 6 years' follow-up. Eur J Cancer 27: 1552

Marmont A M 1992 Autoimmunity and allogeneic bone marrow transplantation. Bone Marrow Transplant 9: 1

Marolleau J P, Mullen M, Law P et al 1994 CD34+ selection with Isolex 300 device: Application to multiple cycles of high dose chemotherapy in lymphomas. Blood 84 (Suppl 1): 370a

Molino A, Colombatti M, Bonetti F et al 1991 A comparative analysis of three different techniques for the detection of breast cancer cells in bone marrow. Cancer 67: 1033

Moss T J, Ross A A (1992) The risk of tumour cell contamination in peripheral blood stem cell collections. J Hematotherapy 1: 225–230

Moss T J, Sanders D G, Lasky L D et al 1990 Contamination of peripheral blood stem cell harvests by circulating neuroblastoma cells. Blood 76: 1879

Nimgaonkar M, Bahnson A, Boggs S et al 1993 G-CSF primed peripheral blood stem cells as targets for gene therapy in Gaucher disease. Exp Hematol 21: 1160

Noga S J, Berenson R, Davis J et al 1994a CD34+ stem cell augmentation of T cell depleted allografts reduces engraftment time, GVHD, and length of hospitalization. Brit J Haematol 87: 41

Noga S J, Davis J, Schepers K et al (1994b) The clinical use of elutriation and positive stem cell selection columns to engineer the lymphocyte and stem cell composition of the allograft. Prog Clin Biol Res 398: 317

Okarma T, Lebkowski J, Schain L et al 1992 The AIS Cellector: A new technique for stem cell purification. In Worthington-White D, Gee A P, Gross S (eds) Advances in bone marrow purging and processing. Wiley-Liss, New York, p 449

Osborne M, Wong G, Asina S et al 1991 Sensitivity of immunocytochemical detection of breast cancer cells in human bone marrow. Cancer Res 51: 2706

Pantel K, Felber E, Schlimok G 1994 Detection and characterization of residual disease in breast cancer. J Hematother 3: 315

Pettengell R, Morgenstern G R, Woll P J et al 1993 Peripheral-blood progenitor-cell transplantation in lymphoma and leukemia using a single apheresis. Blood 82: 3770

Pinski S L, Maloney J D 1990 Adenosine: a new drug for acute termination of supraventricular tachycardia. Cleve Clin J Med 57(4): 383–384

Reading C, Sasaki D, Leemhuis T et al 1994 Clinical scale purification of CD34+Thy-1+Lin- stem cells from mobilized peripheral blood by high speed fluorescence-activated cell sorting for use as an autograft for multiple myeloma patients. Blood 84 (Suppl 1): 1581a

Ross A A, Cooper B W, Lazarus H M et al 1993 Detection and viability of tumor cells in peripheral blood stem cell collections from breast cancer patients using immunocytochemical and clonogenic assay techniques. Blood 82: 2605

Rowley S D, Bensinger W I, Gooley T A et al 1994 Effect of cell concentration on bone marrow and peripheral blood stem cell cryopreservation. Blood 83: 2731

Salzman D, Tami J, Jackson C et al 1994 Clinical remission of myasthenia gravis (MG) in a patient after high dose therapy and autologous transplantation with CD34+ stem cells (SC). Blood 84: 808.

Schiller G, Rosen L, Vescio R et al 1994 Threshold dose of autologous CD34 positive peripheral blood progenitor cells (PBPC) required for engraftment after myeloablative treatment for multiple myeloma. Blood 84: 813

Sharp JG, Kessinger A, Vaughan WP et al 1992 Detection and clinical significance of minimal tumor cell contamination of peripheral stem cell harvests. Int J Cell Cloning 10: 92

Sheridan W P, Begley C G, Juttner C A et al 1992 Effect of peripheral-blood progenitor cells mobilized by filgrastim (G-CSF) on platelet recovery after high-dose chemotherapy. Lancet 339: 640

Shpall E J, Jones R B, Franklin W et al 1992 CD34+ marrow and/or peripheral blood progenitor cells (PBPCs) provide effective hematopoietic reconsitution of breast cancer patients following high-dose chemotherapy with autologous hematopoietic progenitor cell support. Blood 80 (Suppl 1): 24

Shpall, EJ, Ball, ED, Champlin, RE, et al. (1993) A prospective randomized phase III study using the CEPRATE® SC stem cell concentrator to isolate CD34+ hematopoietic progenitors for autologous marrow transplantation after high dose chemotherapy. Blood 82: (Suppl 1): 83a

Shpall E J, Franklin W, Jones R et al (1994a) Transplantation of CD34+ marrow and/or peripheral blood progenitor cells (PBPC) into breast cancer patients following high-dose chemotherapy. Blood 84 (Suppl 1): 396

Shpall E J, Jones R B, Franklin W et al 1994b Transplantation of enriched CD34+ autologous marrow into breast cancer patients following high-dose chemotherapy: Influence of CD34+ peripheral blood progenitors and growth factors on engraftment. J Clin Oncol 12: 28

Srour E F, Brandt J E, Briddell R A, et al 1991 Human CD34+, HLA-DR-bone marrow cells contain progenitor cells capable of self-renewal, multilineage differentiation, and long-term in vitro hematopoiesis. Blood Cells 17: 287

Srour E F, Brandt J E, Bridell R A et al 1993 Long-term generation and expansion of human primitive hematopoietic progenitor cells in vitro. Blood 81: 661

Starzl T E, Demetris A J, Murase N et al 1992 Cell migration, chimerism and graft acceptance. Lancet 339: 1579

Starzl T E, Demetris A J, Trucco M et al 1993 Cell migration and chimerism after whole organ transplantation. The basis of graft acceptance. Hepatology 17: 1127

Stroncek D F, Fautsch S K, Lasky L C et al 1991 Adverse reactions in patients transfused with cryopreserved marrow. Transfusion 31: 521

Traweek S, Liu J, Battifora H 1993 Keratin gene expression in non-epithelial tissues. Detection with polymerase chain reaction. Am J Pathol 142: 1111

Van Twuyver E, Mooijaart R J D, Ten Berge I J M, et al 1991 Pretransplantation blood transfusion revisited. New Engl J Med 17: 1210

Vescio R, Cao J, Hong C, et al 1994 CD34-positive CEPRATE selection leads to a 4–5 log reduction in tumor burden in myeloma PBC autografts based on PCR and Poisson distribution. Blood 84 (Suppl 1): 1580

Vescio R A, Hong C H, Cao J et al 1995 The hematopoietic stem cell antigen, CD34, is not expressed on the malignant cells in multiple myeloma. Blood 84: 3283

13

Gene transfer into human hemopoietic progenitor cells

M. K. Brenner   J. M. Cunningham   B. P. Sorrentino
H. E. Heslop

Most of the applications of somatic gene transfer in hematological disease involve the transfer of new genes to hemopoietic progenitor cells. Although disorders such as hemophilia A and B may be responsive to gene transfer and expression in heterologous tissues, most malignant and non-malignant abnormalities of marrow-derived cells will be corrected by transduction of hemopoietic stem cells (HSC) or their progeny. Hemopoietic stem cells are appealing targets for gene transfer, since their genetic modification could be effective in a variety of malignant and non-malignant disorders. As well as their suitability as targets for a wide range of clinical applications, the use of HSC for gene transfer is attractive because of their logistical characteristics. Both marrow and peripheral blood progenitor cells are readily obtained, manipulated, and returned to the host. Moreover, in principle, successful gene transfer into a single pluripotent stem cell could be sufficient to repopulate each individual with modified cells for their entire life span. In almost every other type of somatic gene therapy, transfer is required to a vast number of cells which may be spread over a wide anatomical area.

However, to take full advantage of these characteristics, there is a need to use vectors which permanently integrate in hemopoietic stem cell DNA and are therefore present in all the progeny of this cell (Hughes et al 1992). At present, retroviruses are the only integrating vectors approved for clinical use (Anderson 1990, Miller 1992). One of the characteristics of these vectors is that integration occurs almost exclusively in cells which are progressing through cell cycle. Since most mammalian HSC are in G_0, the efficiency of gene transfer into these cells is generally far below the levels that would be expected to produce benefit in the great majority of gene therapy settings (Anderson 1990, Miller 1992, Smith 1992, Schuening et al 1991, Van Beusechem et al 1992). In animal models, a number of techniques have been shown to induce HSC to cycle and thereby increase the efficiency of retroviral-mediated gene transfer (Hughes et al 1992, Rill et al 1992a). These include prior treatment of the animal with cycle-specific cytotoxic drugs (Wieder et al 1991), or in vivo/ex vivo exposure to hemopoietic growth factors (Otsuka et al 1991a,b, Stoeckert Jr et al 1990, Dick et al 1991). At present, however, the human stem cell has not been precisely identified, and there are no assays which can directly analyze their number or activity. It has therefore been impossible to devise preclinical experiments which show how well retroviruses transfer genes to human stem cells, and whether manipulation of those stem cells enhanced their susceptibility to retroviral-mediated gene transfer. This has been a major constraint on the development of therapeutic protocols. No clinical gene transfer study can be entirely devoid of risk, and when the probability of benefit is unknown and likely to be small, then the risk benefit ratio becomes unacceptably high (Smith 1992, Anderson 1990, Miller 1992, Cornetta et al 1991). On the other hand, until human studies are performed, it is impossible to make an accurate assessment of the true risks and the true probability of success.

One way of resolving this impasse has been to develop clinical protocols in which even a low efficiency of gene transfer would potentially be of benefit. One example is ADA gene transfer (Blaese et al 1995). In these studies it was anticipated that the ADA gene-corrected population would initially be in an extreme minority, but would ultimately expand because they would have a selective growth advantage over unmodified cells. A more widely applicable example is to use gene transfer simply as a means of marking hemopoietic progenitor cells prior to transplantation, in order to track their subsequent fate in vivo (Rill et al 1992a,b Brenner et al 1993a,b), and to detect contaminating tumorigenic cells. In this instance, the purpose of gene transfer is not to correct a defect in hemopoietic progenitor cells, but rather to improve the **process** of progenitor cell transplantation. As a by-product of these studies, information should be generated which will facilitate true gene therapy protocols.

GENE MARKING OF HEMOPOIETIC PROGENITOR CELLS

Source of relapse after autologous bone marrow transplantation

While autologous bone marrow transplantation appears to improve survival in many malignant diseases, including acute myeloid leukemia, relapse remains the major cause of treatment failure (Appelbaum & Buckner 1986, Burnett et al 1984, Goldstone et al 1986, Shpall & Jones 1994). The possibility that reinfused leukemic cells may contribute to relapse has led to extensive evaluation of techniques for purging marrow to eliminate residual malignant cells, although it has been unclear whether such maneuvers are necessary (Rill et al 1992a,b, De Fabritiis et al 1989, Shpall & Jones 1994, Brugger et al 1994, Santos et al 1989). One way of resolving this issue is to mark the marrow at the time of harvest and then find out if the marker gene is present in malignant cells at the time of a subsequent relapse (Brenner et al 1993b, O'Shaughnessy et al 1993, Deisseroth et al 1991).

Studies to address these issues using bone marrow of patients with AML and neuroblastoma began at St. Jude in September 1991 and January 1992, respectively and closed in March 1993. Nucleated bone marrow ($>1.5 \times 10^8$ cells/kg of body weight) was taken from the posterior iliac crest and two-thirds were cryopreserved immediately. The remaining third was separated on a

Ficoll gradient to produce a mononuclear cell fraction that was transduced with either the LNL6 or the closely related G1N retroviral vector for 6 hours. Both these vectors encode the neomycin resistance gene (neo^R) which can subsequently be detected in transduced cells by polymerase chain reaction PCR or because it confers resistance to the neomycin analogue G418. At the time of transplantation, both transduced and unmanipulated marrow cells were thawed and reinfused through each patient's central venous line.

To assess the efficiency of gene transfer and expression in marrow progenitor cells both pre-and post-transplantation, we obtained mononuclear cells from peripheral blood or bone marrow, separated them on Ficoll-Hypaque gradients and cultured them in methylcellulose. Transduced cells were cultured with or without G418. PCR was used to detect the transferred Neo^R gene in individual colonies or in bulk populations. The PCR-amplified products were analyzed by gel electrophoresis (1.5% agarose) and Southern blotting with a ^{32}P-labeled neo-specific probe. Semiquantitative PCR was also used, with 25 cycles of amplification corresponding to linear signal strength.

In the AML study, four of twelve patients relapsed. To definitively prove that the marker gene is in leukemia cells it is necessary to have a collateral leukemia specific marker to show both this marker and the marker gene in the same cell. For example, in one of the AML patients who relapsed, the malignant blasts co-expressed CD34 and CD56, a combination not found on normal hemopoietic cells. The blasts also had a complex t(1:8:21) translocation, resulting in generation of an AML1/ETO fusion transcript that could be identified by PCR (Miyoshi et al 1991, Erickson et al 1992). We were therefore able to sort blasts expressing CD34 and CD56, and show co-expression in a single clonogenic cell of both a leukemia-specific marker (the AML:ETO fusion protein) and the transferred neomycin gene (Brenner et al 1993a). In three patients, the malignant cells contained the marker gene, while the fourth patient was uninformative. PCR showed that his marrow mononuclear cells had low levels of neo^R but no blast colonies grew in G418. Since his blasts did not have a leukemia-specific marker, the source of the PCR signal could not be determined.

In the neuroblastoma study (Rill et al 1994), five patients relapsed, and gene-marked neuroblastoma cells were detected in four cases. In these patients, identification of marked neuroblastoma cells was confirmed by detecting co-expression of the neuroblastoma-related antigen GD2 together with the transferred marker gene. Four of the neuroblastoma patients relapsed in their marrow, but the fifth had disease recurrence in an extramedullary site in his liver. Biopsy of this extramedullary site showed the presence of gene-marked neuroblasts.

Similar results have been obtained at MD Anderson Hospital in adult patients receiving autologous BMT for chronic myeloid leukemia (Deisseroth et al 1994). These data showed definitively that marrow harvested in apparent clinical remission may contain residual tumorigenic cells and that these cells can contribute to disease recurrence at both medullary and extramedullary sites. The implication is that effective purging will be necessary, although perhaps not sufficient, for improving the outcome of ABMT.

Gene transfer to normal cells

Two of the 21 patients in the first generation St. Jude studies died (of disease progression and sepsis) within 21 days of transplantation. In the remaining 19 patients, there were no indications that laboratory manipulation of marrow specimens had adversely affected engraftment. None of the patients has shown evidence of malignant transformation or other complications that could be attributed to the gene transfer process. The presence of the gene in hemopoietic progenitor cells in vivo was confirmed by clonogenic assays that showed gene-marked progenitor cells in 15/19 patients at 1 month after autologous BMT. The marker gene continued to be detected and expressed for up to 3 years in the mature progeny of marrow precursor cells, including peripheral blood T and B-cells and neutrophils. It was also detected in lymphoblastoid cell lines and in cytotoxic T-cell lines derived from these patients. The level of transfer varied and was highest in marrow clonogenic hemopoietic progenitors. In peripheral blood cells, expression was variable between the different lineages and was higher by an order of magnitude in myeloid cells than in T-lymphocytes. The lowest level of expression was seen in B-lymphocytes. These levels of transfer are higher than predicted from animal models and may be attributed to the fact that marrow was harvested during regeneration after intensive chemotherapy, when a higher than normal proportion of stem cells are in cycle.

These data also support a substantial contribution to marrow reconstitution from autologous transplants and suggest that this contribution includes long-lived multipotent stem cells. Similar patterns of transfer have been seen in adults receiving gene-marked marrow, although levels of transfer were somewhat lower than in myeloablated children (Dunbar 1994). In these adult studies, both peripheral blood and marrow-derived stem cells were shown to be able to contribute to long-term reconstitution. These results have implications for the design of future gene therapy protocols.

Purging Studies

We have begun second generation studies of marrow purging using two gene markers to compare either marrow purging versus no purging, or two different purging techniques. We are using two closely related vectors, G1N and LNL6, which can be discriminated by virtue of the differing fragment sizes they produce after PCR amplification. In the AML study, one-third of the marrow is frozen unpurged as a safety backup. The remaining marrow is split into two aliquots which are marked with G1Na or LNL6 and then randomly assigned to purging with 4HC or IL2. At the time of transplant both aliquots are reinfused. If the patient should subsequently relapse, detection of either marker will show if either of these purging techniques is effective. Fourteen patients have been treated on this protocol as of April 1995. One has relapsed with unmarked cells, and transfer has been seen into normal progenitors in most recipients, albeit at a lower level than in the studies using unpurged marrow. A similar protocol for neuroblastoma has recently opened.

Ex vivo expansion studies

Genetic marking could also be used to determine directly which ex vivo or in vivo combination of cytokines will increase the entry of long-term marrow repopulating cells into cell cycle and thereby reduce the period of marrow hypoplasia and immunodeficiency that follows autologous stem cell transplantation. In humans, it certainly appears possible to use growth factors such as IL-1, IL-3 and stem cell factor to increase the numbers of hemopoietic progenitor cells by 10- to 50-fold, and to increase the efficiency of gene transfer to levels in excess of 50% (Otsuka et al 1991a,b, Stoeckert Jr et al 1990, Dick et al 1991). Unfortunately, it is not certain that such ex vivo data will be reflected by results in vivo. In primate and human studies, transplantation of marrow treated ex vivo with the growth factor combinations shown to greatly augment both progenitor numbers and gene transfer rates have been followed by disappointingly low levels of long-term gene expression in vivo. The likeliest explanation for this apparent paradox is that many of the growth factors intended only to induce cycling in marrow stem cells also induce their differentiation and the loss of their self renewal capacity.

Without any proven ex vivo surrogate method for studying the effects of growth factors on stem cell expansion and transducibility, it is possible to use the marker-gene technique to evaluate whether any increase in progenitor cell numbers and transducibility produced by growth factor combinations and cell culture devices ex vivo has an effect in vivo. By using two distinguishable vectors to mark each patient's marrow, we can compare treatment regimens **within** a patient. Because each patient acts as their own control, it should be possible to discern the effects of any given growth factor regimen on stem cells, even in a cohort as small as 10 patients. This technique can also be used to compare the reconstitution of peripheral blood and marrow-derived hemopoietic progenitor cells (Dunbar 1994).

Is gene transfer to hemopoietic progenitor cells safe?

One of the major concerns regarding the use of long-lived marrow progenitor cells for retrovirus-mediated gene transfer or therapy is that insertional mutagenesis will occur (Cornetta et al 1991). This event could occur at the time of initial vector exposure to the vector, or subsequently, if wild-type retrovirus contaminates the vector, or is formed by recombination. This concern has been given extra weight following the discovery of thymomas in monkeys injected with a vector contaminated with wild-type virus (Donahue et al 1992). In the clinical studies reported here, helper-free vector was used, and no evidence has been obtained for any recombinational events with endogenous retroviral sequences that have generated infectious virus. But although no events to date have occurred which are attributable to mutagenesis, all patients will have prolonged follow up and genetic analysis of any tumors which do appear within the next 15 years.

MODIFICATION OF THE DRUG SENSITIVITY OF THE PROGENITOR CELLS

There would be two potential advantages for patients if hemopoietic stem cells could be rendered resistant to one or more cytotoxic drugs. As a primary therapeutic benefit, it might enable them to resist the myelosuppressive effects of cytotoxic drugs during cancer therapy, allowing longer or more intensive therapy that might cure a higher proportion of patients (Murphy et al 1993, Levin & Hryniuk 1987, Levin et al 1993). Of more generic importance, drug resistance genes could behave as a dominant selectable marker and thereby offer a strategy to compensate for the small proportion of primate stem cells that are modified with currently available protocols (Brenner et al 1993a, Bodine et al 1993, Sorrentino et al 1992). Building on the observation that murine hematopoietic cells expressing the human multidrug resistance (MDR1) gene can be positively selected with post-transplant taxol treatment (Sorrentino et al 1992), Gottesman and colleagues have recently shown that bicistronic vectors containing the MDR1 gene allow selection of cells expressing a second linked therapeutic gene (Aran et al 1994). These studies suggest that selectable vectors could be used to overcome the low transduction efficiency that limits stem cell-directed gene therapy for non-malignant genetic diseases such as sickle cell anemia and thalassemia (Gottesman et al 1994).

Mechanisms of drug resistance

The study of cytotoxic drug resistance in cancer cells has revealed the operation of diverse genetic mechanisms. This increased understanding of drug resistance has not only produced strategies to circumvent acquired resistance in tumor cells (Salmon et al 1991, Gottesman & Pastan 1989), it has also suggested gene therapy approaches to protect normal host tissues from the toxicity of chemotherapy. Molecular mechanisms of drug resistance include increased expression of normal cellular genes, decreased expression of cellular gene products that are essential for drug-induced cytotoxicity, and acquired mutations leading to structurally altered gene products. Table 1 catalogs several examples for each of these mechanisms.

Preclinical studies

The first eukaryotic drug resistance gene to be transferred to reconstituting bone marrow cells was a methotrexate-resistant rodent dihydrofolate reductase

Table 1. Suggested gene therapy approaches to protect chest tissues from chemotherapy

Mechanism of drug resistance	Gene	Drugs	References
Increased expression of structurally normal gene products	Human multidrug resistance 1	Wide variety of naturally occuring cytotoxic compounds	Pastan & Gottesman 1991, Chen et al 1986, Roninson et al 1986
	Dihydrofolate reductase	Methotrexate	Tyler-Smith & Alderson 1981, Flintoff et al 1982
	Cytosolic aldehyde dehydrogenase	cyclophosphamide	Yoshida et al 1993, Radin et al 1991
	Alkylguanine alkyltransferases	Nitrosoureas	Pegg et al 1983, Robins et al 1983 Allay et al 1995
Decreased expression of gene products essential for cytotoxicity	Topoisomerase II	Epipodophyllotoxins, anthracyclines	Takano et al 1991, Kasahara et al 1992
	Topoisomerase I	Camptothecin, CPT-11	Sugimoto et al 1990, Eng et al 1990
	Deoxycytidine kinase	Arabinosylcytosine	Drahovsky & Kreis 1970, Richel et al 1990, Stegmann et al 1993
Acquired mutations resulting in structurally gene products	Dihydrofolate reductase	Methotrexate	McIvor & Simonsen 1990, Simonsen & Levinson 1983, altered Blakley et al 1993
	Topoisomerase II	Epipodophyllotoxins, anthracyclines	Bugg et al 1991
	Topoisomerase I	Camptothecin, CPT-11	Andoh et al 1987, Benedetti et al 1993, Gromova et al 1993

(MDHFR) gene. These studies showed that mice transplanted with cells transduced with a MDHFR-containing retroviral vector were protected from methotrexate-induced myelosuppression and had increased survival following methotrexate administration (Corey et al 1990, Williams et al 1987). Later experiments have suggested that methotrexate can be used to select for murine hemopoietic cells expressing transferred MDHFR genes (Vinh & McIvor 1993, Zhao et al 1994). These initial studies were done with a rodent DHFR gene containing a leucine to arginine mutation in the 22nd codon. Recent work has shown that human DHFR variants containing mutations in other codons may be much more active in conferring antifolate resistance (Banerjee et al 1994, Li et al 1994, H T Spencer, S E H Sleep, S K Chandaru, M Webb, R L Blakely, B P Sorrentino unpublished). One of these variants has successfully been used for ex-vivo selection of CD34+ peripheral blood progenitor cells obtained from cancer patients (Flasshove et al 1995), suggesting that preinfusion expansion and selection of drug resistant cells can be used to increase the number of gene-modified cells administered to the patient.

Transfer of the human MDR1 gene to hemopoietic cells has also been described. P-glycoprotein, the product of the MDR1 gene, functions as a drug efflux pump and confers resistance to a wide variety of naturally occurring chemotherapeutics (Pastan & Gottesman 1991). The feasibility of using the MDR1 gene to protect hemopoietic cells has been demonstrated by transgenic mouse experiments (Mickisch et al 1991a,b). In addition, retroviral transfer of MDR1 to murine clonogenic progenitors produced drug resistance in vitro (McLachlin et al 1990). In murine transplant experiments, mice transplanted with MDR1-transduced cells showed attenuation of taxol-induced myelosuppression (Sorrentino et al 1992, Hanania et al 1993, Hanania & Deisseroth 1994). In taxol-treated animals, the proportion of circulating leukocytes transduced with the MDR1 virus increased with drug treatment, suggesting that cells expressing the transferred MDR1 gene can be dominantly selected in vivo with taxol (Sorrentino et al 1992, Podda et al 1992). Human progenitor cells have also been rendered taxol resistant after transduction of CD34+ bone marrow cells, showing that these vectors are feasible for clinical use (Ward et al 1994). Recent work has shown that expression of these first generation MDR1 vectors is attenuated by aberrant RNA splicing, suggesting that further vector modifications may lead to even greater levels of resistance (Sorrentino et al 1995).

The experiments with MDR1 and mutant DHFR-containing vectors demonstrate the principle that drug resistance genes can be used to attenuate drug-induced myelosuppression and can act as dominant selectable markers for genetically altered hemopoietic cells. It is probable that other drug resistance genes may function in an analogous fashion. DNA-methylguanine methyltransferases (MGMT) are enzymes that repair DNA damage done by the nitrosoureas, a class of cancer chemotherapeutic alkylating agents. MGMT vectors have been shown to attenuate the severe and prolonged myelosuppression which is the dose limiting toxicity of nitrosoureas such as BCNU. Recent work has shown that retroviral vectors containing a MGMT cDNA protected murine hematopoietic cells from BCNU toxicity in vitro (Allay et al 1995). Furthermore, periodic infusions of MGMT transduced cells into nonablated recipient mice partially protected against BCNU-induced cytopenias (Moritz et al 1995), showing that gene therapy-mediated protection of hematopoiesis is possible outside the transplant setting. Preliminary data suggests that some of the other drug resistance genes listed in Table 1 are useful for generating drug-resistant hemopoietic cells.

Clinical trials

Based on the preclinical studies described above, three trials proposing transfer of the MDR1 gene transfer to bone marrow or peripheral blood stem cells from adult cancer patients have been approved by the National Institutes of Health Recombinant DNA Advisory Committee. The MDR1 vector will be transferred to hemopoietic cells in the setting of autologous bone marrow transplantation. Patients will be treated with taxol after transplantation as clinically indicated. The endpoints of these trials are: 1. to test if MDR1 gene transfer results in toxicity specific to gene transfer; 2. to test if the MDR1 vector can be transferred to human hemopoietic stem cells; 3. To test if MDR1 can be used as a dominant selectable marker in vivo; 4. To test if MDR1 gene transfer will result in amelioration of taxol-induced myelosuppression.

Clinical application of drug resistance gene transfer has several potential pitfalls. The low stem cell transduction efficiencies observed with current clinical protocols predict that amelioration of drug-induced myelosuppression will not occur unless dramatic in vivo selection can be enacted. Other methods to increase the transduction efficiency of pluripotent repopulating stem cells will probably be required for successful application of this approach. A second potential limitation is the risk of transferring drug resistance genes to tumor cells that contaminate the marrow graft. This possibility could theoretically result in a drug resistant relapse. The current protocols exclude patients with documented bone marrow metastases determined by marrow biopsy and bone scan. However, these conventional methods cannot detect low levels of tumor cells in bone marrow (Leslie et al 1990). Despite these considerations, it is not known if clinical vectors would transduce breast cancer cells, or if transduction of tumor cells would have significant clinical consequences. For example, breast cancer relapse after standard autologous transplant is associated with a uniformly poor prognosis, and drugs not affected by P-glycoprotein expression could be used as palliative therapy if the MDR1 gene were transferred to tumor cells at relapse. A final potential limitation is that non-hematopoietic drug toxicity could limit dose-escalation and in vivo selection, even if high degrees of hematopoietic resistance were achieved. Some of the systems developed to date were chosen based on relatively specific hematopoietic toxicity of the associated drug. For example, MDR1 transgenic mice tolerate four- to five-fold increases in taxol dose without significant non-hematopoietic toxicity (Mickisch et al 1991a). In the DHFR system, toxicity in other organ systems may be related to the degree of bone marrow suppression. Mice containing DHFR-modified bone marrow cells were also protected from methotrexate-induced gastrointestinal toxicity (Zhao et al 1994). Prevention of severe leukopenia and thrombocytopenia is presumed to allow more rapid recovery from mucositis and associated gut ulcerations.

GENE TRANSFER TO MODULATE IMMUNOCYTE FUNCTION

Genetic modification of the function of effector cells derived from marrow could have an impact on autoimmune disease, infective illness and malignancy. Initial interest has focussed on the last of these two areas because it has been in these conditions that the potential therapeutic role of the immune system

(Kolb et al 1990, Riddell et al 1992, Rosenberg et al 1986) makes the risk: benefit ratio most attractive. Immunocytes may be altered by changing their effector function or by modifying their receptor specificity.

Therapy of malignant disease

Altered function of effector cells. One way of increasing the antitumor activity of immunocytes is to increase the levels of cytotoxic cytokines (such as TNF) which they produce at local tumor sites. This approach is being evaluated in studies with tumor infiltrating lymphocytes (TILs). The problems with this strategy are that it has been difficult to persuade TIL cells to secrete high levels of cytokines, and that only scanty data support the belief that reinfused human TIL cells selectively home to tumor sites. In addition, the transduced cytokine gene may act as an autocrine growth factor for the TILs, resulting in uncontrolled growth. The first patients to receive therapy with cytokine-transduced TIL were treated at the National Institute of Health in January 1991 in a Phase I dose escalation study. Patients received TNF-transduced TILs either alone or in conjunction with IL-2, in doses from 10^8 to 3×10^{11} cells. The first six patients have shown few side effects and one patient has had a sustained response (Rosenberg 1992a).

Altered specificity of effector cells. A long-term aim of tumor immunology has been to identify tumor-specific antigens which might be a target for specific responses. Over the last few years, the molecular basis of antigen recognition by cytotoxic T-lymphocytes (CTL) has been elucidated (Townsend & Bodmer 1989). The demonstration that CTL recognize processed intracellular proteins presented as short peptide fragments in conjunction with MHC molecules on the cell surface, raised the possibility that internal proteins unique to the malignant clone may act as tumor-specific antigens for CTL. Several human malignancies indeed contain novel proteins such as mutated oncogenes or fusion proteins generated by chromosomal translocations (Brenner & Heslop 1991, Melief & Kast 1993). Other tumors may express immunogenic proteins encoded by Epstein-Barr or papilloma viruses. Finally, even normal proteins can elicit CTL responses if they are expressed in very high quantities, for example the MAGE protein in melanoma cells (van Der Bruggen et al 1991).

If a tumor is to be recognized by CTL several conditions must be met. First, the tumor must contain a unique antigen that is a target for recognition. Second, the antigen must be processed and expressed in sufficient quantity to induce immune responses to the peptide. Finally, the peptide/MHC complex must be recognizable within the T-cell repertoire of the individual and it must be possible to amplify the signal by exogenous help or co-stimulatory signals. If tumor cells do indeed express weakly immunogenic peptides, it may be possible to enhance the capacity of the immunocyte to recognize the tumor cell target by transfection with appropriate antigen-specific T-cell receptors.

Therapy of viral and malignant disease

One example of the potential for a combination cell therapy and gene transfer approach is apparent in the response of Epstein-Barr virus (EBV)-related immunoblastic lymphoma to infusion of gene-modified cytotoxic T-lymphocytes. EBV is a herpes virus that infects the majority of individuals and persists in an asymptomatic state by a combination of chronic replication in the mucosa and latency in peripheral blood B-cells (Straus et al 1992). These EBV-infected B-cells are highly immunogenic and normally susceptible to killing by specific cytotoxic T-lymphocytes. However, patients who are severely immunocompromised after organ grafting may develop EBV-driven lymphoproliferation. This complication occurs in 1–30% of allograft recipients, depending on the organ transplanted and the degree of associated immunosuppression. Until recently, the disease responded (variably) only to withdrawal of immunosuppression, often with attendant loss of the transplanted organ. After bone marrow transplantation, when immunosuppression is particularly severe and prolonged, the disease almost always had a fatal progression regardless of intervention. We are evaluating the use of EBV-specific CTL in therapy. These specific T-cells are generated by culturing donor T-cells with donor-derived EBV-infected lymphoblastoid cell lines (Heslop et al 1994). To determine whether these cells persist, whether they are active, and whether they cause adverse effects, they are marked with the neomycin resistance gene before administration. As of November 1995, 20 patients have been enrolled on this protocol. The neo^R gene was detected in peripheral blood lymphocytes for 18 weeks or more after injection of gene-marked cells, and in EBV-specific CTL lines regenerated from these patients for up to 15 months (Rooney et al 1995).

We also have evidence for efficacy of the infused CTL. In four patients, it has been possible to show anti-viral activity in vivo, with a dramatic fall in EBV DNA following infusion, and the development of a circulating anti-EBV cytotoxic T-cell response. One patient received CTL as therapy rather than prophylaxis. He presented with fevers and cervical, hilar and retroperitoneal lymphadenopathy, and biopsy showed immunoblastic lymphoma with positive immunofluorescence staining for EBNA1 and LMP. Administration of CTL was associated with resolution of the lymphadenopathy over a 6-week period and he remains in remission 14 months later (Rooney et al 1995). Therefore, a limited number of T-cells infusions may be adequate to establish and maintain cellular immunity against EBV after bone marrow transplantation. It should be possible to use a similar approach in other malignancies where tumor-specific antigens have been identified. Further genetic modification of the CTL, by modifying their receptor specificity or the cytokines they produce (see above), may increase the effectiveness of the approach.

GENETIC MODIFICATION OF TUMOR CELLS ISOLATED FROM MARROW; GENERATION OF TUMOR VACCINES

While conditions have been identified under which the immune system is able to eradicate malignant disease (Kolb et al 1990, Rosenberg et al 1986, Rosenberg 1992b), it has been suggested that the more general failure of the system to perform this function can be attributed to the poor immunogenicity of most tumors. For example, even if tumors do express immunogenic determinants on their surface (see above), there may be insufficient activation of immune system effector cells. In an attempt to enhance immune recognition, investigators have evaluated the effect of transducing tumor cells with cytokine genes or with allogeneic MHC molecules (Nabel et al 1993) or with B7.1 (Chen et al 1992, Townsend & Allison 1993), a co-stimulatory molecule which activates cytotoxic T-cells after engaging their surface CD28 or CTLA4 ligands.

In a number of different murine model systems, transfection of tumor cell lines with these molecules has augmented immunogenicity. Injection of neoplastic cells in doses that would normally establish a tumor results instead in the recruitment of immune system effector cells and the eradication of injected tumor cells (Tepper et al 1989, Golumbek et al 1991, Fearon et al 1990, Gansbacher et al 1990, Dranoff et al 1993, Colombo et al 1991, Colombo & Forni 1994). In many cases the animal is then resistant to challenges by further local injections of non-transduced parental tumor. The transduced tumor has therefore acted like a vaccine. In some models, established, non-transduced, parental tumors at distant sites are also eradicated (Fearon et al 1990, Gansbacher et al 1990).

There are several potential problems in translating this approach to human marrow-derived tumors. First, one recent study has suggested that the same effect is attained if tumor cells are admixed with non-specific adjuvants such as *C. parvum* (Hock et al 1993). Since adjuvant-dependent cancer immunotherapy has had limited success in treating human cancer, there is a concern that the cytokine gene-transfer model in animals will translate no better than any other rodent tumor immunotherapy model. Another risk is that the transferred growth factor may act as an autocrine growth factor for marrow-derived tumor. For example, expression of the IL-2 gene in a murine T-cell line results in autocrine growth in vitro and tumorigenicity in vivo in immunodeficient mice (Yamada et al 1993). Finally, it may only be possible to grow, transduce and select cytokine-secreting tumor cells from the marrow of a small minority of patients with malignant disease. In all other patients the approach would have to be modified, using, for example, cytokine-transduced patient fibroblasts co-injected with autologous tumor, or cytokine-transduced allogeneic but partially HLA-matched tumor cells. While all these alternatives are effective in mice, their relevance to human disease again remains questionable. As of November 1995, the available approaches are being evaluated in more than 30 different clinical trials. Table 2 outlines our tumor/cytokine combinations used in current trials.

SINGLE GENE DEFECTS

A number of single gene defects of hemopoietic cells may be amenable to gene therapy. These include the hemoglobinopathies, the immunodeficiencies, the

Table 2. Current cytokine gene therapy vaccination studies

Tumor	Cytokine
Melanoma	TNF, IL–2, γ-interferon, IL–7, IL–4, GMCSF
Neuroblastoma	IL–2, γ-interferon
Renal cell carcinoma	GMCSF, IL–2
Small cell lung cancer	IL–2
Colon cancer	IL–2
Glioblastoma	IL–2
Prostate cancer	GMCSF, IL–2 and γ-interferon
Breast cancer	IL–2

Table 3. Current gene therapy protocols using hemopoietic cells for inherited genetic disorders

1. Gaucher disease
2. Chronic granulomatous disease
3. Fanconi anemia
4. Hunter syndrome
5. Adenosine deaminase deficiency

lipidoses, the mucopolysaccharidoses, chronic granulomatous disease, Fanconi anemia and inborn errors of metabolism. Table 3 shows diseases for which gene therapy protocols, using hemopoietic cells as the target, are currently underway. All may be corrected, at least in part, in tissue culture cell lines or murine systems (Wei et al 1994, Walsh et al 1994, Karlsson 1991) and clinical success has been reported for ADA deficiency (Blaese et al 1995). We will use the hemoglobinopathies and Gaucher disease to illustrate progress and problems in these areas.

Despite rapid progress in our understanding of the molecular pathogenesis of sickle cell disease (SCD) and β-thalassemia, chronic transfusion, iron chelation and infection prophylaxis continue to be the mainstay of treatment (McDonagh et al 1992, Bunn 1994). Nonetheless the majority of patients with β-thalassemia die in early adulthood, and cerebrovascular and other vasoocclusive manifestations of sickle cell disease (SCD) continue to have a significant impact on morbidity and premature mortality (Bunn 1994). Studies of pharmacological agents that elevate fetal hemoglobin (HbF) show promise (Rodgers et al 1990). However, in many patients these agents fail to stimulate adequate levels of HbF and the long-term efficacy and safety remain unknown. Gene replacement utilizing allogeneic bone marrow transplantation has gained increasing acceptance as a curative option but is only available to a minority of patients with a matched sibling donor (Lucarelli et al 1987, Ferster et al 1992).

An alternative approach is the genetic transfer of a corrective globin gene to hematopoietic stem cells (HSCs). For SCD, a γ-gene is preferable in view of its positive effects on the prevention of sickle hemoglobin polymerization. Patient data, in vitro polymerization studies, and animal models indicate that 20–30% HbF expression with a transduced γ-globin gene will be required to significantly ameliorate the SCD phenotype (Bunn 1994, Rodgers et al 1990). In β-thalassemia, 20% expression from a transduced β-globin gene will probably be curative. Understanding the normal regulation of the genes of the human β-globin locus, the development of vector systems able to efficiently deliver the gene to stem cells, and a high level of tissue-specific expression of the transduced gene in erythroid progenitors are required to achieve these effects. Advances made in these areas have been substantial and have guided the studies of gene transfer described below.

The individual β-globin-like genes (ε, $^G\gamma$, $^A\gamma$, δ, β) are arranged in a linear array over a 70 kb interval on chromosome 11 (Fig. 1) (Stamatoyannopoulos & Nienhuis 1994). Studies in transgenic mice have demonstrated that the promoters directly adjacent to these genes, and the β-enhancer, contain all the necessary elements to allow correct developmental and tissue-specific expression of the globin genes (Kollias et al 1986). However, these sequences alone are insufficient for high-level expression. Deletions upstream of the globin genes in certain (γδβ)°-thalassemias completely ablate expression although the individual genes remain structurally unaffected. Characterization of these deletions resulted in the identification of a powerful tissue-specific enhancer region, the locus control region, or LCR, which is required for high-level expression of the β-globin like genes (Orkin 1990, Grosveld et al 1987). Further dissection of the LCR identified four core sequences, termed hypersensitivity sites 1–4 (HS1–4), which are sufficient for high-level expression. Interestingly, individual sites linked to the β-globin gene have also been shown to induce levels of expression almost equivalent to that of the endogenous murine β-globin gene in transgenic mice (Fraser et al 1990).

Gene transfer of globin sequences to HSCs has been predominantly explored utilizing viral vectors (Miller 1992, Nienhuis et al 1993, Morgan & Anderson 1993). Many laboratories have focussed on retroviruses as a delivery system despite the problems associated with transduction of large numbers of stem cells and subsequent transgene expression. Recent data suggests that adeno-associated virus (AAV), a non-pathogenic parvovirus, may provide an alternative approach. Results with each of these systems are summarized below.

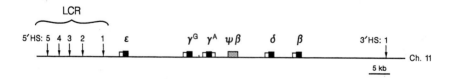

Fig. 1. Structure of the human β-globin locus on chromosome 11. Filled boxes indicate the positions of the active genes of the locus. The hatched box represents the position of the Ψβ pseudogene. Open boxes denote the ε $^G\gamma$, $^A\gamma$ and β promoters and the 3′ $^A\gamma$ regulatory element. The β-globin IVSII enhancer is not shown. The positions of the 5′ DNase I hypersensitivity sites (1–5) of the locus control region (LCR) and the single 3′ DNase I hypersensitivity site are also depicted.

Studies with recombinant retroviral vectors containing selectable markers (Nienhuis et al 1993), the subsequent availability of improved vectors and packaging cell lines (Miller & Rosman 1989, Armentano et al 1987) and the demonstration of HSC transduction (Williams et al 1986) stimulated the evaluation of constructs containing either the β- or γ-globin gene. Transduction of tissue culture cells, and murine and human HSCs utilizing ecotropic or amphotropic retroviruses, demonstrated both the feasibility and problems of this approach. Initial experiments employed an ecotropic retrovirus containing a 3 kb genomic fragment of the β-gene and its adjacent cis-acting regulatory sequences. Only retroviral constructs containing the globin gene in the reverse orientation were functional and allowed normal viral production. Infection of the murine erythroleukemia cell line MEL resulted in single-copy proviral integration and expression levels of less than 0.1% of endogenous β-globin (Cone et al 1987). Similar results were obtained with an amphotropic vector containing a γβ-hybrid globin cassette, although 10% expression of the transgene was obtained (Karlsson et al 1987). Subsequent experiments in a mouse bone marrow transplant model showed transgenic expression levels of less than 5%. Infectivity was low (less than 20% of reconstituted animals) although all transduced animals showed trilineage long-term engraftment (Dzierzak et al 1988). Studies evaluating the efficiency of infection and expression of a β-globin construct in human erythroid progenitors, the ultimate target of all gene therapy strategies, revealed low levels of infectivity (<0.1%) and 5% expression of the transgene.

The problems of low retroviral titer and low infectivity of HSCs were addressed with improvements in stem cell isolation and viral titer (Bodine et al 1989, Bender et al 1989). However, globin transgene expression remained unchanged. An explanation for low transduced gene expression became apparent with the identification of the LCR and its role in high-level expression. Studies with recombinant retroviruses containing varying size fragments of the individual or linked HSs to the β- or γ-gene revealed relatively high-level expression in MEL cells (Novak et al 1990), particularly with HS2β constructs. However, a major obstacle has been the difficulty in the consistent manufacture of high titer unrearranged producer cell lines for use in primary cells. Where transduction has been achieved, less than 1% expression is observed in animal transplant studies. Recently, several groups have reported retroviral constructs containing the HS1–4 or HS2–4 of the LCR and a human β-globin gene that has been altered to reduce recombination. Transgene expression of up to 70% in MEL cells and relatively high expression in mice has been reported (Plavec et al 1993). Although encouraging, reproduction of these results in non-human primates and human bone marrow is awaited.

The difficulties inherent to retroviral gene transfer have stimulated interest in other vector systems, particularly AAV. This defective parvovirus is a single-stranded 4675 nucleotide DNA virus which is bordered by inverted terminal repeat (ITR) sequences of 145 nucleotides. Wild-type AAV is a dependovirus as it requires adeno or herpes virus gene products, provided by co-infection, for packaging. The virus has two known states, latent and lytic. The virus integrates preferentially into chromosome 19 with the establishment of a latent state (Samulski et al 1991). Infection of the cell with adenovirus or herpes simplex virus results in reactivation and lysis. The virus has a broad host range but is not associated with any disease state. Five serotypes have been identified, with AAV-2 studied most (Nienhuis et al 1993). Recombinant AAV(rAAV) particles, containing a Neo^R selectable marker, first demonstrated the ability of this virus to infect hematopoietic cells with high transduction efficiency (80%) (Hermonat & Muzyczka 1984). Subsequently, primary mouse (Zhou et al 1993), human hematopoietic (Goodman et al 1994) and cord blood progenitor cells (Miller et al 1994) have been transduced with rAAV. Goodman and colleagues have shown that CD34+ selected rhesus or human stem cells can be transduced with a β-galactosidase-containing virus (Goodman et al 1994). These cells showed high levels of expression of the transgene, suggesting its usefulness for hemopoietic stem cell-targeted gene transfer. Recombinant AAV was demonstrated to integrate randomly as 1–3 unrearranged tandem copies in these studies. Hence, AAV has the advantages of lack of pathogenicity, the ability to transduce and integrate into quiescent hemopoietic stem cells (Goodman et al 1994), and the apparent lack of interference from flanking viral sequences. However, the vector has significant practical disadvantages, including lack of an efficient producer cell system and the capacity to package only a limited quantity of DNA (<5 kb).

The above limitations notwithstanding, the study of AAV as a delivery system for globin genes suggests considerable promise. Initial experiments utilizing a HS2^{A}γNeo^R gene construct demonstrated expression levels 40–110% of the endogenous gene in K562 erythroleukemia cells (Walsh et al 1992, Miller et al 1993). Genomic analysis demonstrated a single randomly integrated copy of an unrearranged provirus per cell. These encouraging results led several laboratories to investigate the expression of similar constructs in erythroid progenitors (Zhou et al 1993). A construct containing core fragments of HS2, 3 and 4 and the ^{A}γ gene (v432^{A}γ) without a selectable marker gives high-level expression in human BFU-E (Miller et al 1994). Further studies in mice and non-human primates will allow an appropriate assessment of this system's potential.

Future progress in hemoglobinopathies

Clearly, there are a number of requirements for further advances in gene transfer for correction of hemoglobinopathies:

1. Improved vector technology. This may include the use of selectable markers other than drug resistance genes and viral pseudotyping to modify the tropism and infectivity of retroviruses (Yee et al 1994, Kasahara et al 1994). Improvement of the packaging of AAV may increase its usefulness;

2. A broader understanding of the role of the cis-acting elements and trans-acting factors in globin gene regulation;

3. Improved stem cell isolation/transduction (Moritz et al 1993, Cassel et al 1993).

Metabolic storage diseases

Metabolic storage diseases, a large group of monogenic diseases, have also been the focus of much effort in gene therapy. Although amenable to allogeneic BMT, lack of donors and significant morbidity secondary to GvHD has limited the use of this approach (Krivit et al 1993, Karlsson 1991). We will use Gaucher's disease as a paradigm for the problems associated with this disease.

Gaucher's disease, an autosomally recessive inherited condition, is the commonest lysosomal storage disease. It is caused by glucocerebrosidase (GC) deficiency which predominantly affects macrophage metabolism. Three clinical forms (Types I-III) have been identified, all of which are associated with significant morbidity and mortality. Although recombinant enzyme replacement is available, it is extremely expensive (Beutler 1993). Correction of enzyme deficiency by gene transfer was first demonstrated in skin fibroblasts (Correll et al 1989), and then in human lymphoblastoid cell lines and bone marrow cultures (Karlsson 1991). More recently, long-term reconstitution of mice with HSCs containing GC expressing retroviral constructs has been achieved (Karlsson 1991). However, long-term expression in all lineages has been reported by some but not all groups.

The effects of transduction on GC levels has also been assessed in vivo. Neurological damage caused by this disease necessitates that the defect must be corrected in circulating macrophages and CNS microglia. Recently, mice transduced with a GC-containing virus demonstrated expression in both cell types (Krall et al 1994), an observation that is important not only for Gaucher's disease but also for other diseases (such as Hurler syndrome) in which enzyme delivery to the CNS is crucial. However, the required level of gene expression to correct these diseases requires further study. Recently, the in vitro correction of the enzyme defect with returned vectors, in human hematopoietic cells from patients with Gaucher's disease has been reported (Xu et al 1994), and clinical trials using these vectors have begun. The use of variant retroviral backbones and the AAV system has also been investigated (Wei et al 1994). Preliminary results of these studies suggest that they may provide alternative approaches to this problem.

CONCLUSION

By combining some of the strategies outlined in this chapter, it is possible to make the most of the imperfect systems currently available for transducing hemopoietic progenitor cells. For example, gene-marking studies are helping to reveal how best to prepare and manipulate marrow progenitor cells for gene transfer, while co-transfection of drug resistance genes has the potential to provide an in vivo dominant selectable marker for cells transduced with the gene of interest. Similarly, co-transfection of cytokine genes may provide a subsequent selective advantage for transduced cells in vivo. However, there remains little doubt that the full potential of hemopoietic stem cell therapy will be realized only after the development of improved gene transfer systems, with an improved understanding of gene regulation in hemopoietic stem cells and their mature progeny.

KEY POINTS FOR CLINICAL PRACTICE

- Gene marking studies have provided useful biological information on the contribution of marrow to relapse after autologous bone marrow transplantation, and the biology of normal reconstitution following this procedure.

- Gene marking studies of adoptively transferred cytotoxic T-lymphocytes have demonstrated that these cells can persist for a significant period of time.

- Transfer of drug resistance genes into hemopoietic progenitors may allow more intensive chemotherapy to be administered and may also serve as a dominant selective marker to allow selection of transduced cells.

- Immunogenicity of tumor cells may be enhanced by a transfection with cytokine genes or with co-stimulatory molecules which enhance T-cell activation, and this strategy is currently being explored in a number of clinical trials.

- Gene transfer into hemopoietic cells is currently being used as therapy for single-gene disorders involving hematopoietic cells.

- Correction of hemoglobinopathies by gene transfer requires improved knowledge of globin gene regulation and increased efficiency of gene transfer to hemopoietic stem cells.

ACKNOWLEDGEMENTS

This work was supported in part by NIH grants CA 20180, CA 61384, Cancer Center Support CORE Grant CA 21765, and by the American Lebanese Syrian Associated Charities (ALSAC). We would like to thank all our clinical and laboratory co-workers who made these studies possible; Genetic Therapy, Inc. for providing the clinical grade vectors; and Nancy Parnell for word processing.

REFERENCES

Allay J A, Dumenco L L, Liu L et al 1995 Retroviral transduction and expression of the human alkyltransferase cDNA provides nitrosourea resistance to hemopoietic cells. Blood: 85: 3342-51

Anderson K C, Weinstein H J 1990 Transfusion-associated graft-versus-host disease. N Engl J Med 323: 315–321

Andoh T, Ishii K, Suzuki Y et al 1987 Characterization of a mammalian mutant with a camptothecin-resistant DNA topoisomerase I. Proc Natl Acad Sci USA 84: 5565

Appelbaum F R, Buckner C D 1986 Overview of the clinical relevance of autologous bone marrow transplantation. Clin Haematol 15: 1–18

Aran J M, Gottesman M M, Pastan I 1994 Drug-selected coexpression of human glucocerebrosidase and P-glycoprotein using a bicistronic vector. Proc Natl Acad Sci USA 91: 3176–3180

Armentano D, Yu S, Kantoff P W et al 1987 Effects of internal virus sequences on the utility of retroviral vectors. J Virol 61: 1747–1750

Banerjee D, Schweitzer B I, Volkenandt M et al 1994 Transfection with a cDNA encoding a Ser31 or Ser34 mutant human dihydrofolate reductase into Chinese hamster ovary and mouse marrow progenitor cells confers methotrexate resistance. Gene 139: 269

Bender M A, Gelinas R E, Miller A D 1989 A majority of mice show long-term expression of a human β-globin gene after retrovirus transfer into hematopoietic stem cells. Mol Cell Biol 9: 1426–1434

Benedetti P, Fiorani P, Capuani L et al 1993 Camptothecin resistance from a single mutation changing glycine 363 of human DNA topoisomerase I to cysteine. Cancer Res 53: 4343

Beutler E 1993 Gaucher disease as a paradigm of current issues regarding single gene mutations of humans. Proc Natl Acad Sci USA 90: 5384–5390

Blaese RM, Culver KW, Miller AD et al 1995 T-Lymphocyte directed gene therapy for ADA SCID: itial trial results after 4 years. Science 270: 475-80

Blakley R L, Appleman J R, Chunduru S K et al 1993 Mutations of human dihydrofolate reductase causing decreased inhibition by methotrexate. In: Ayling J E, Nair M J, Baugh C M (eds) Chemistry and biology of pteridines and folates. Plenum Press, New York, p 473

Bodine D M, Karlsson S, Nienhuis A W 1989 Combination of interleukins 3 and 6 preserves stem cell function in culture and enhances retrovirus-mediated gene-transfer into hematopoietic stem cells. Proc Natl Acad Sci USA 86: 8897–8901

Bodine D M, Moritz T, Donahue R E et al 1993 Long-term in vivo expression of a murine adenosine deaminase gene in rhesus monkey hematopoietic cells of multiple lineages after retroviral mediated gene transfer into CD34+ bone marrow cells. Blood 82: 1975–1980

Brenner M K, Heslop H E 1991 Graft-versus-host reactions and bone marrow transplantation. Curr Opin Immunol 3: 752–757

Brenner M K, Rill D R, Holladay M S et al 1993a Gene marking to determine whether autologous marrow infusion restores long-term haemopoiesis in cancer patients. Lancet 342: 1134–1137

Brenner M K, Rill D R, Moen R C et al 1993b Gene-marking to trace origin of relapse after autologous bone marrow transplantation. Lancet 341: 85–86

Brugger W, Bross K J, Glatt M et al 1994 Mobilization of tumor cells and hematopoietic progenitor cells into peripheral blood of patients with solid tumors. Blood 83: 636–640

Bugg B Y, Danks M K, Beck W T et al 1991 Expression of a mutant DNA topoisomeras II in CRF-CEM human leukemic cells selected for resistance to teniposide. Proc Natl Acad Sci USA 88: 7654

Bunn H F 1994 Sickle hemoglobin and other hemoglobin mutants. In: Stamatoyannopoulos G, Nienhuis A W, Majerus P J, Varmus H (eds) The molecular basis of blood diseases. W B Saunders, Philadelphia, pp 207–256

Burnett A K, Tansey P, Watkins R et al 1984 Transplantation of unpurged autologous bone-marrow in acute myeloid leukaemia in first remission. Lancet 2: 1068–1070

Cassel A, Cottler-Fox M, Doren S et al 1993 Retroviral-mediated gene transfer into CD34-enriched human peripheral blood stem cells. Exp Hematol 21: 585–591

Chen C J, Chin J E, Ueda K et al 1986 Internal duplication and homology with bacterial transport proteins in the mrdl (P-glycoprotein) gene from multidrug-resistant human cells. Cell 47: 381

Chen L, Ashe S, Brady W A et al 1992 Costimulation of antitumor immunity by the B7 counterreceptor for the T lymphocyte molecules CD28 and CTLA-4. Cell 71: 1093–1102

Colombo M P, Forni G 1994 Cytokine gene transfer in tumor inhibition and tumor therapy: where are we now? Immunol Today 15: 48–51

Colombo M P, Ferrari G, Stoppacciaro A et al 1991 Granulocyte colony-stimulating factor gene transfer suppresses tumorogenicity of a murine adenocarcinoma in vivo. J Exp Med 173: 889–897

Cone R D, Weber-Benarous A, Baorto D et al 1987 Regulated expression of a complete human beta-globin gene encoded by a transmissible retrovirus vector. Mol Cell Biol 7: 887–897

Corey C A, DeSilva A D, Holland C A et al 1990 Serial transplantation of methotrexate-resistant bone marrow: protection of murine recipients from drug toxicity by progeny of transduced stem cells. Blood 75: 337

Cornetta K, Morgan R A, Anderson W F 1991 Safety issues related to retrovirus-mediated gene transfer in humans. Hum Gene Ther 2: 5–14

Correll P H, Fink J K, Brady R O et al 1989 Production of human glucocerebrosidase in mice after retroviral gene transfer into multipotential hematopoietic progenitor cells. Proc Natl Acad Sci USA 86: 8912–8916

De Fabritiis P, Ferrero D, Sandrelli A et al 1989 Monoclonal antibody purging and autologous bone marrow transplantation in acute myelogenous leukemia in complete remission. Bone Marrow Transplant 4: 669–674

Deisseroth A B, Kantarjian H, Talpaz M et al 1991 Autologous bone marrow transplantation for CML in which retroviral markers are used to discriminate between relapse which arises from systemic disease remaining after preparative therapy versus relapse due to residual leukemia cells in autologous marrow: A pilot trial. Hum Gene Ther 2: 359–376

Deisseroth A B, Zu Z, Claxton D et al 1994 Genetic marking shows that Ph+ cells present in autologous transplants of chronic myelogenous leukemia (CML) contribute to relapse after autologous bone marrow transplant in CML. Blood 83: 3068–3076

van Der Bruggen P, Traversari C, Chomez P et al 1991 A gene encoding an antigen recognized by cytolytic T lymphocytes on a human melanoma. Science 254: 1643–1647

Dick J E, Kamel-Reid S, Murdoch B et al 1991 Gene transfer into normal human hematopoietic cells using in vitro and in vivo assays. Blood 78: 624–634

Donahue R E, Kessler S W, Bodine D et al 1992 Helper virus induced T cell lymphoma in nonhuman primates after retroviral mediated gene transfer. J Exp Med 176: 1125–1135

Drahovsky D, Kreis W 1970 Studies on drug resistance. II. Kinase patterns in P815 neoplasms sensitive and resistant to 1-beta-D-arabinofuranosylcytosine. Biochem Pharmacol 19: 940

Dranoff G, Jaffee E, Lazenby A et al 1993 Vaccination with irradiated tumor cells engineered to secrete murine GM-CSF stimulates potent, specific, and long lasting anti-tumor immunity. Proc Natl Acad Sci USA: 90: 3539-43

Dunbar C E 1994 Hematopoietic stem cells as targets for gene therapy. Marrow Transplant Rev 4: 26–29

Dzierzak E A, Papayannopoulou T, Mulligan R C 1988 Lineage-specific expression of a human beta-globin gene in murine bone marrow transplant recipients reconstituted with retrovirus-transduced stem cells. Nature 331: 35–41

Eng W K, McCabe F L, Tan K B et al 1990 Development of a stable camptothecin-resistant subline of P388 leukemia with reduced topoisomerase I content. Mol Pharmacol 38: 471

Erickson P, Gao J, Chang K et al 1992 Identification of breakpoints in t(8;21) AML and isolation of a fusion transcript with similarity to Drosophila segmentation gene runt. Blood 80: 1825–1831

Fearon E R, Pardoe D M, Itaya T et al 1990 Interleukin-2 production by tumor cells bypasses T helper function in the generation of an antitumor response. Cell 60: 397–403

Ferster A, De Valck C, Azzi N et al 1992 Bone marrow transplantation for severe sickle cell anaemia. Br J Haematol 80: 102–105

Flasshove M, Banerjee D, Mineishi S et al 1995 Ex vivo expansion and selection of human CD34+ peripheral blood progenitor cells after introduction of a mutated dihydrofolate reductase cDNA via retroviral gene transfer. Blood 85: 566

Flintoff W F, Weber M K, Nagainis C R et al 1982 Overproduction of dihydrofolate reductase and gene amplification in methotrexate-resistant Chinese hamster ovary cells. Mol Cell Biol 2: 275

Fraser P, Hurst J, Collis P et al 1990 DNaseI hypersensitive sites 1, 2 and 3 of the human β-globin dominant control region direct position-independent expression. Nucl Acids Res 18: 3503–3508

Gansbacher B, Zier K, Daniels B et al 1990 Interleukin 2 gene transfer into tumor cells abrogates tumorigenicity and induces protective immunity. J Exp Med 172: 1217–1224

Goldstone A H, Anderson C C, Linch D C et al 1986 Autologous bone marrow transplantation following high dose chemotherapy for the treatment of adult patients with acute myeloid leukaemia. Br J Haematol 64: 529–537

Golumbek P T, Lazenby A J, Levitsky H I et al 1991 Treatment of established renal cancer by tumor cells engineered to secrete interleukin-4. Science 254: 713–716

Goodman S, Xiao X, Donaheu R E et al 1994 Recombinant adeno-associated virus-mediated gene transfer into hematopoietic progenitor cells. Blood 84: 1492–1500

Gottesman M M, Pastan I 1989 Clinical trials of agents that reverse multidrug-resistance. J Clin Oncol 7: 409

Gottesman M M, Germann U A, Aksentijevich I et al 1994 Gene transfer of drug resistance genes. Implications for cancer therapy. Ann N Y Acad Sci 716: 126

Gromova I I, Kjeldsen E, Svejstrup J Q et al 1993 Characterization of an altered DNA catalysis of a camptothecin-resistant eukaryotic topoisomerase I. Nucl Acids Res 21: 593

Grosveld F, vanAssenfeldt B, Greaves D R et al 1987 Position independant high level expression of the human β-globin gene in transgenic mice. Cell 51: 975–985

Hanania E G, Deisseroth A B 1994 Serial transplantation shows that early hematopoietic precursor cells are transduced by MDR-1 retroviral vector in a mouse gene therapy model. Cancer Gene Ther 1: 21–25

Hanania E, Fu S, Roninson I et al 1993 cDNA for the multidrug resistance (MDR-1) gene in a transcription unit of a safety modified retrovirus confers in vivo resistance to taxol on early precursor cells in a mouse transplant model and on long-term culture initiating cells in long-term human marrow culture. Blood 82 (Suppl. 1): 216a

Hermonat P, Muzyczka N 1984 Use of adeno-associated virus as a mammalian DNA cloning vector: transduction of neomycin resistance into mammalian tissue culture cells. Proc Natl Acad Sci USA 81: 6466–6470

Heslop H E, Brenner M K, Rooney C M et al 1994 Administration of neomycin-resistance-gene-marked EBV-specific cytotoxic T lymphocytes to recipients of mismatched-related or phenotypically similar unrelated donor marrow grafts. Hum Gene Ther 5: 381–397

Hock H, Dorsch M, Kunzendorf U et al 1993 Vaccinations with tumor cells genetically engineered to produce different cytokines: Effectivity not superior to a classical adjuvant. Cancer Res 53: 714–716

Hughes P F D, Thacker J D, Hogge D et al 1992 Retroviral gene transfer to primitive normal and leukemia hematopoietic cells using clinically applicable procedures. J Clin Invest 89: 1817–1824

Karlsson S 1991 Treatment of genetic defects in hematopoietic cell function by gene transfer. Blood 78: 2481–2492

Karlsson S, Papayannopoulo T, Schweiger S G et al 1987 Retroviral-mediated transfer of genomic globin genes leads to regulated production of RNA and protein. Proc Natl Acad Sci USA 84: 2411–2415

Kasahara K, Fujiwara Y, Sugimoto Y et al 1992 Determinants of response to the DNA topoisomerase II inhibitors doxorubicin and etoposide in human lung cancer cell lines. J Natl Cancer Inst 84: 113

Kasahara N, Dozy A M, Kan Y W 1994 Tissue-specific targeting of retroviral vectors through ligand-receptor interactions. Science 266: 1373–1376

Kolb H J, Mittermuller J, Clemm C et al 1990 Donor leukocyte transfusions for treatment of recurrent chronic myelogenous leukemia in marrow transplant patients. Blood 76: 2462–2465

Kollias G, Wrighton N, Hurst J et al 1986 Regulated expression of human gamma-, beta-and hybrid gamma beta-globin genes in transgenic mice: manipulation of the developmental expression patterns. Cell 46: 89–94

Krall W J, Challita P M, Perlmutter L S et al 1994 Cells expressing human glucocerebrosidase from a retroviral vector repopulate macrophages and central nervous system microglia after murine bone marrow transplantation. Blood 83: 2737–2748

Krivit W, Shapiro E, Hoogerbrugge P M et al 1993 Bone marrow transplantation treatment for storage diseases. Bone Marrow Transplant 11 (Suppl): 87–101

Leslie D S, Johnston W W, Daly L et al 1990 Detection of breast carcinoma cells in human bone marrow using fluorescence-activated cell sorting and conventional cytology. Am J Clin Pathol 94: 8

Levin L, Hryniuk W M 1987 Dose intensity analysis of chemotherapy regimens in ovarian carcinoma. J Clin Oncol 5: 756

Levin L, Simon R, Hryniuk W 1993 Importance of multiagent chemotherapy regimens in ovarian carcinoma: dose intensity analysis. J Natl Cancer Inst 85: 1732

Li M X, Banerjee D, Zhao S C et al 1994 Development of a retroviral construct containing a human mutated dihydrofolate reductase cDNA for hematopoietic stem cell transduction. Blood 83: 3403-3408

Lucarelli G, Galimberti M, Polchi P et al 1987 Marrow transplantation in patients with advanced thalassemia. N Engl J Med 316: 1050-1056

McDonagh K, Nienhuis A W 1992 The thalassemias. In: Nathan D G, Oski F A (eds) Hematology of infancy and childhood. W B Saunders, Philadelphia, pp 783-897

McIvor R S, Simonsen C C 1990 Isolation and characterization of a variant dihydrofolate reductase cDNA from methotrexate-resistant murine L5178Y cells. Nucl Acids Res 18: 7025

McLachlin J R, Eglitis M A, Ueda K et al 1990 Expression of a human complementary DNA for the multidrug resistance gene in murine hematopoietic precursor cells with the use of retroviral gene transfer. J Natl Cancer Inst 82: 1260

Melief C J, Kast W M 1993 Potential immunogenicity of oncogene and tumor supressor gene products. Curr Opin Immunol 5: 709-713

Mickisch G H, Licht T, Merlino G T et al 1991a Chemotherapy and chemosensitization of transgenic mice which express the human multidrug resistance gene in bone marrow: efficacy, potency, and toxicity. Cancer Res 51: 5417

Mickisch G H, Merlino G T, Galski H et al 1991b Transgenic mice that express the human multidrug-resistance gene in bone marrow enable a rapid identification of agents that reverse drug resistance. Proc Natl Acad Sci USA 88: 547

Miller A D 1992 Human gene therapy comes of age. Nature 357: 455-460

Miller A D, Rosman G J 1989 Improved retroviral vectors for gene transfer and expression. Biotechniques 7: 980-990

Miller J L, Walsh C E, Ney P A et al 1993 Single-copy transduction and expression of human gamma-globin in K562 erythroleukemia cells using recombinant adeno-associated virus vectors: the effect of mutations in NF-E2 and GATA-1 binding motifs within the hypersensitivity site 2 enhancer. Blood 82: 1990-1906

Miller J L, Donahue R E, Seller S E et al 1994 Recombinant adeno-associated virus (rAAV) mediated expression of a human gamma-globin gene in human progenitor derived erythroid cells. Proc Natl Acad Sci USA 91: 10183-7

Miyoshi H, Shimizu K, Kozu T et al 1991 t(8;21) breakpoints on chromosome 21 in acute myeloid leukemia are clustered within a limited region of a single gene, AML 1. Proc Natl Acad Sci USA 88: 10431-10435

Morgan R A, Anderson W F 1993 Human gene therapy. Annu Rev Biochem 62: 191-217

Moritz T, Keller D C, Williams D A 1993 Human cord blood cells as targets for gene transfer: potential use in genetic therapies of severe combined immunodeficiency disease. J Exp Med 178: 529-536

Moritz T, Mackay W, Glassner B J et al 1995 Retroviral-mediated expression of a DNA repair protein in bone marrow protects hematopoietic cells from nitrosourea-induced toxicity in vitro and in vivo. Cancer Res:

Murphy D, Crowther D, Renninson J et al 1993 A randomised dose intensity study in ovarian carcinoma comparing chemotherapy given at four week intervals for six cycles with half dose chemotherapy given for twelve cycles. Ann Oncol 4: 377

Nabel G J, Nabel E G, Yang Z Y et al 1993 Direct gene transfer with DNA-liposome complexes in melanoma: expression, biologic activity, and lack of toxicity in humans. Proc Natl Acad Sci USA 90(23): 11307-11311

Nienhuis A W, Walsh C E, Liu J 1993 Viruses as therapeutic gene transfer vectors. In: Young N S (ed) Viruses and bone marrow. Marcell Decker Inc, New York, pp 353-414

Novak U, Harris E A S, Forrester W et al 1990 High-level β-globin expression after retroviral transfer of locus activation region-containing human β-globin gene derivatives into murine erythroleukemia cells. Proc Natl Acad Sci USA 87: 3386-3390

Orkin S H 1990 Globin gene regulation and switching: circa 1990. Cell 63: 665-672

Otsuka T, Thacker J D, Eaves C J et al 1991a Differential effects of microenvironmentally presented interleukin 3 versus soluble growth factor on primitive human hematopoietic cells. J Clin Invest 88: 417-422

Otsuka T, Thacker J D, Hogge D E 1991b The effects of interleukin 6 and interleukin 3 on early hematopoietic events in long-term cultures of human marrow. Exp Hematol 19: 1042-1048

Pastan I, Gottesman M M 1991 Multidrug resistance. Annu Rev Med 42: 277

Pegg A E, Wiest L, Foote R S et al 1983 Purification and properties of 06-methylguanine-DNA transmethylase from rat liver. J Biol Chem 258: 2327

Plavec I, Papayannopoulou T, Maury C et al 1993 A human β-globin gene fused to the human β-globin locus control region is expressed at high levels in erythroid cells of mice engrafted with retrovirus-transduced hematopoietic stem cells. Blood 81: 1384–1392

Podda S, Ward M, Himelstein A et al 1992 Transfer and expression of the human multiple drug resistance gene into live mice. Proc Natl Acad Sci USA 89: 9676

Radin A I, Zhoa X, Woo T H et al 1991 Structure and expression of the cytosolic aldehyde dehydrogenase gene in cyclophosphamide-resistant murine leukemia L 1210 cells. Biochem Pharmacol 42: 1933

Richel D J, Colly L P, Arkesteijn G J et al 1990 Substrate-specific deoxycytidine kinase deficiency in 1-beta-D-arabinofuranosylcytosine-resistant leukemic cells. Cancer Res 50: 6515

Riddell S R, Watanabe K S, Goodrich J M et al 1992 Restoration of viral immunity in immunodeficient humans by the adoptive transfer of T cell clones. Science 257: 238–241

Rill D R, Moen R C, Buschle M et al 1992a An approach for the analysis of relapse and marrow reconstitution after autologous marrow transplantation using retrovirus-mediated gene transfer. Blood 79: 2694–2700

Rill D R, Buschle M, Foreman N K et al 1992b Retrovirus mediated gene transfer as an approach to analyze neuroblastoma relapse after autologous bone marrow transplantation. Hum Gene Ther 3: 129–136

Rill D R, Santana V M, Roberts W M et al 1994 Direct demonstration that autologous bone marrow transplantation for solid tumors can return a multiplicity of tumorigenic cells. Blood 84: 380–383

Robins P, Harris A L, Goldsmith I et al 1983 Cross-linking of DNA induced y chlorethylnitrosourea is presented by 06-methylguanine-DNA methyltransferase. Nucl Acids Res 11: 7743

Rodgers G P, Dover G J, Noguchi C T et al 1990 Hematologic responses of patients with sickle cell disease to treatment with hydroxyurea. N Engl J Med 322: 1037–1045

Roninson I B, Chin J E, Choi K G et al 1986 Isolation of human mdr DNA sequences amplified in multidrug-resistant KB carcinoma cells. Proc Natl Acad Sci USA 83: 4538

Rooney C M, Smith C A, Ng C Y C et al 1995 Use of gene-modified virus-specific T lymphocytes to control Epstein-Barr virus-related lymphoproliferation. Lancet 345: 9–13

Rosenberg S A 1992a Gene therapy for cancer. JAMA 268: 2416–2419

Rosenberg S A 1992b The immunotherapy and gene therapy of cancer. J Clin Oncol 10: 180–199

Rosenberg S A, Spiess P, Lafreniere R 1986 A new approach to the adoptive immunotherapy of cancer with tumor-infiltrating lymphocytes. Science 233: 1318–1321 Salmon S E, Dalton W S, Grogan T M et al 1991 Multidrug-resistant myeloma: laboratory and clinical effects of verapamil as a chemosensitizer. Blood 78: 44

Samulski R J, Zhu X, Xiao X et al 1991 Targeted integration of adeno-associated virus (AAV) into human chromosome 19. EMBO J 10: 3941–3950

Santos G W, Yeager A M, Jones R J 1989 Autologous bone marrow transplantation. Annu Rev Med 40: 99–112

Schuening F G, Kawahara K, Miller A D et al 1991 Retrovirus-mediated gene transduction into long-term repopulating marrow cells of dogs. Blood 78: 2568–2576

Shpall E J, Jones R B 1994 Release of tumor cells from bone marrow. Blood 83: 623–625

Simonsen C C, Levinson A D 1983 Isolation and expression of an altered mouse dihydrofolate reductase cDNA. Proc Natl Acad Sci USA 80: 2495

Smith C 1992 Retroviral vector-mediated gene transfer into hematopoietic cells: Prospects and issues. J Hematother 1: 155–166

Sorrentino B P, Brandt S J, Bodine D et al 1992 Selection of drug-resistant bone marrow cells in vivo after retroviral transfer of human MDR1. Science 257: 99–103

Sorrentino B P, McDonagh K T, Woods D et al 1995 Expression of retroviral vectors containing the human MDR1 cDNA in hematopoietic cells of transplanted mice. Blood: In press

Stamatoyannopoulos G, Nienhuis A W 1994 Hemoglobin switching. In: Stamatoyannopoulos G, Nienhuis A W (eds) The Molecular basis of blood diseases. W B Saunders, Philadelphia, pp 107–156

Stegmann A P, Honders M W, Kester M G et al 1993 Role of deoxycytidine kinase in an in vitro model for Ara-C and DAC-resistance: substrate-enzyme interactions with deoxycytidine, 1-beta-D-arabinofuranosylcytosine and 5-aza-2'-deoxycytidine. Leukemia 7: 1005

Stoeckert C J Jr, Nicolaides N C, Haines K M et al 1990 Retroviral transfer of genes into erythroid progenitors derived from human peripheral blood. Exp Hematol 18: 1164–1170

Straus S E, Cohen J I, Tosato G et al 1992 Epstein-Barr virus infections: Biology, pathogenesis and management. Ann Intern Med 118: 45–58

Sugimoto Y, Tsukahara S, Oh-hara T et al 1990 Decreased expression of DNA topoisomerase I in camptothecin-resistant tumor cell lines as determined by a monoclonal antibody. Cancer Res 50: 6925

Takano H, Kohno K, Ono M et al 1991 Increased phosphorylation of DNA topoisomerase II in etoposide-resistant mutants of human cancer KB cells. Cancer Res 51: 3951

Tepper R I, Pattengale P K, Leder P 1989 Murine interleukin-4 displays potent anti-tumor activity in vivo. Cell 57: 503–512

Townsend A, Bodmer H 1989 Antigen recognition by class I-restricted T lymphocytes. Annu Rev Immunol 7: 601–624

Townsend S E, Allison J P 1993 Tumor rejection after direct costimulation of CD8+ T cells by B7-transfected melanoma cells. Science 259: 368–370

Tyler-Smith C, Alderson T 1981 Gene amplification in methotrexate-resistant mouse cells. I. DNA rearrangement accompanies dihydrofolate reductase gene amplification in a T-cell lymphoma. J Mol Biol 153: 203

Van Beusechem V W, Kukler A, Heidt P J et al 1992 Long-term expression of human adenosine deaminase in rhesus monkeys transplanted with retrovirus-infected bone-marrow cells. Proc Natl Acad Sci USA 89: 7640–7644

Vinh D B, McIvor R S 1993 Selective expression of methotrexate-resistant dihydrofolate reductase (DHFR) activity in mice transduced with DHFR retrovirus and administered methotrexate. J Pharmacol Exp Ther 267: 989

Walsh C E, Liu J M, Xiao X et al 1992 Regulated high level expression of a human gamma-globin gene introduced into erythroid cells by an adeno-associated virus vector. Proc Natl Acad Sci USA 89: 7257–7261

Walsh C E, Grompe M, Vanin E et al 1994 A functionally active retrovirus vector for gene therapy in Fanconi anemia group C. Blood 84: 453–459

Ward M, Richardson C, Pioli P et al 1994 Transfer and expression of the human multiple drug resistance gene in human CD34+ cells. Blood 84: 1408–1414

Wei F F, Wei F, Samulski R J et al 1994 Expression of the human glucocerebridase and arylsulfatase genes in murine and patient primary fibroblasts transduced by an adeno-associated virus vector. Gene Therapy 1: 261–268

Wieder R, Cornetta K, Kessler S W et al 1991 Increased efficiency of retrovirus-mediated gene transfer and expression in primate bone marrow progenitors after 5-fluorouracil-induced hematopoietic suppression and recovery. Blood 77: 448–455

Williams D A, Orkin S H, Mulligan R C 1986 Retrovirus-mediated transfer of human adenosine deaminase gene sequences into cells in culture and into murine hematopoietic cells in vitro. Proc Natl Acad Sci USA 83: 2566–2570

Williams D A, Hsieh K, DeSilva A et al 1987 Protection of bone marrow transplant recipients from lethal doses of methotrexate by the generation of methotrexate-resistant bone marrow. J Exp Med 166: 210

Xu L, Stahl S K, Dave H P et al 1994 Correction of the enzyme deficiency in hematopoietic cells of Gaucher patients using a clinically acceptable retroviral supernatant transduction protocol. Exp Hematol 22: 223–230

Yamada G, Kitamura Y, Sonoda H et al 1993 Retroviral expression of the human IL-2 gene in a murine T cell line results in cell growth autonomy and tumorigenicity. EMBO J 6: 2705–2709

Yee J K, Miyanohara A, LaPorte P et al 1994 A general method for the generation of high titer, pantropic retroviral vectors: Highly efficient infection of primary hepatocytes. Proc Natl Acad Sci USA 91: 9564–9568

Yoshida A, Dave V, Han H et al 1993 Enhanced transcription of the cytosolic ALDH gene in cyclophosphamide resistant human carcinoma cells. Adv Exp Med Biol 328: 63

Zhao S C, Li M X, Banerjee D et al 1994 Long-term protection of recipient mice from lethal doses of methotrexate by marrow infected with a double-copy vector retrovirus containing a mutant dihydrofolate reductase. Cancer Gene Therapy 1: 27–33

Zhou S Z, Li O, Stamatoyannopoulos G et al 1993 Adeno-associated virus 2-mediated gene transfer in murine hematopoietic progenitor cells. Exp Hematol 21: 928–933

Index

Acetylcholinesterase deficiency, PNH cells, 145
Aclarubicine, 122
Acute lymphoblastic leukaemia (ALL)
  alternative donor BMT, 201, 202-203
  apoptosis, 2, 3, 5, 58
  Bcl 2 expression, 10-11
  childhood
    bone marrow transplantation, 55-58, 201, 202-203
    cytogenetics, 49
    drug sensitivity, 49
    immunophenotyping, 48
    late effects of treatment, 58-59
    minimal residual disease, 52-53
    prognostic factors, 46-49
    risk groups, 46-48
    survival, 45-46
    treatment, 45, 50-59
  growth factor support for chemotherapy, 23
  B-ALL, 55
  CNS-directed, 53-54, 59
  induction, 50
  infants, 55
  intensification, 50-51
  maintenance therapy, 51-52
  minimal residual disease, 52-53
Acute myeloid leukaemia (AML)
  growth factor support for chemotherapy, 23
  paroxysmal nocturnal haemoglobinuria, 139-140
Acute myeloid leukaemia (AML) in elderly
  biological characteristics, 127-128
  myelodysplasia and, 127
  smouldering variant, 130-131
  treatment, 119-136
    age-related problems, 126-127
    alternative donor BMT, 201-202
    alternatives to conventional induction, 128-131
    conventional induction, 120-126
    correlation between age and results, 120-121, 128
    differentiating agents, 128-130
    disease-free survival rates, 124, 125
    palliative, 131
    post-remission, 123-124
    prognostic models, 131
    resistance, 123
    toxicity reduction, 121-123
    variations in study results, 124-126
    wait and see strategy, 130-131
Adenosine deaminase deficiency, gene therapy, 275
Adreno-associated virus, 276, 277-278
Alglucerase
  Gaucher disease treatment, 106-110
  unwanted effects, 107-109
ALL *see* Acute lymphoblastic leukaemia
AML *see* Acute myeloid leukaemia
Amsacrine, 122
Anaemia
  aplastic
    anti-thymocyte globulin treatment, 204
    growth factor therapy, 24
  fanconi
    alternative donor BMT, 204
    gene therapy, 275
  Gaucher disease, 92-93, 94
  multiple myeloma, growth factor therapy, 24
  paroxysmal nocturnal haemoglobinuria, 139, 140, 153-154
    alternative donor BMT, 204
  sickle cell *see* Sickle cell disease
Angiotensin converting enzyme, Gaucher disease, 94
Anisocytosis, measurement, 160, 175
Anthracedione, AML in elderly, 122
Anthracyclines
  AML in elderly, 120, 121
  cardiac toxicity, 59
  resistance, molecular mechanisms, 269
Anti-lymphocyte globulin, paroxysmal nocturnal haemoglobinuria, 141
Anti-thymocyte globulin (ATG), severe acquired aplastic anaemia, 204
Anticoagulation system, 215, 216-217
Anticoagulation therapy
  paroxysmal nocturnal haemoglobinuria, 141
  pregnancy, 142
  thromboembolic disease, 214, 223-226
Antithrombin
  deficiency, 220-222
  structure, 221-222
Apoptosis, 1
  biochemical events, 4-5
  detection and measurement, 12-14
    DNA fragmentation assay, 12-13

287

288 INDEX

flow cytometry, 13-14
inducers, 1-3
morphologic events, 3-4
and oncogenesis, 10-12
regulation, 1-19
  cell proliferation regulators and, 7-8
  in lympho-haematopoiesis, 8-10
  molecular, 5-7
AraC see Cytosine arabinose
Asparaginase, childhood ALL, 50
Autoimmune disorders
  Gaucher disease, 93
  stem cell transplantation, 257-258
5-Aza-2'-deoxycitidine, AML in elderly, 129
5-Azacytidine (5-Aza C), fetal haemoglobin stimulation, 232-234

B lymphocytes, apoptosis, 9
bcl-2
  apoptosis regulation, 6-7, 9, 10-11
  oncogenesis, 10-11
Bcl-x, apoptosis regulation, 6-7
BCNU
  chronic lymphocytic leukaemia, combination therapy, 70
  toxicity, gene therapy, 270
Bestatin, AML in elderly, 124
Biologic response modifiers, chronic lymphocytic leukaemia, 76
Blood cell count/counters
  automated, 160-176
    aperture-impedance system, 161-162
    calibration, 179-182
    controls, 182-183
    development, 160-166
    evaluation, 186-188
    external quality assessment, 183-185
    flagging, 175
    light-scatter, 161, 163
    light-scatter system, 161, 163
    method, 166-171
    modern instruments, 176-179
    'new' parameters, 175
    sheath-flow technique, 165, 167
    thresholding, 165, 166
  semi-automated, 161
  history, 159-160
  see also under various cell types
Blood transfusion, paroxysmal nocturnal haemoglobinuria, 140-141
BMT see Bone marrow transplantation
Bone
  disorders/pain, Gaucher disease, 88-89
  management, 103, 104
  Erlenmeyer flask deformity, 88-89
Bone marrow transplantation (BMT)
  acute lymphoblastic leukaemia
    after relapse, 56-58
    first remission, 55-56
  alternative (unrelated) donor, 191-211

acute leukaemias/myelodysplasia, 201-204
bone marrow failure, 204
chronic leukaemias/myeloma, 199-201
donor selection/searching, 195-199
genetic disorders, 205-206
HLA typing and matching, 195-197
patient selection, 192-195
survival following, 192-193
chronic lymphocytic leukaemia, 76-78
  allogeneic transplants, 76-77
  autologous transplants, 77-78
elutriated marrow, CD34+ augmentation, 254, 255
Gaucher disease, 104-105
growth factor support for chemotherapy
  allogeneic transplantation, 34-40
  autologous transplantation, 25-30
paroxysmal nocturnal haemoglobinuria, 141-142
relapse, gene marking studies, 264-267
selected CD34+ cells, 248, 249, 253
  autoimmunity, 257-258
  gene therapy, 256
  organ transplantation, 256-257
  selection technique, 249, 250
Budd-Chiari syndrome, paroxysmal nocturnal haemoglobinuria, 138, 142
Butyrate analogues, fetal haemoglobin stimulation, 233, 241-242

c-myc
  apoptosis regulation, 7, 12
  oncogenesis, 11-12
CAMPATH-1 antigen deficiency, PNH cells, 145
Camptothecin
  apoptosis induction, 3
  resistance, molecular mechanisms, 269
Cancer, gene therapy, 272-275
Carboplatin, AML in elderly, combination therapy, 130
CD14 deficiency, 145
CD16 (γRIII) deficiency, 145, 147, 149
CD24 deficiency, 145
CD34+ cells, 247-248
  allogeneic transplantation, 254-256
    augmented elutrated grafts, 254
    peripheral blood cells, 254-256
  augmentation of elutriated marrow, 254, 255
  autoimmune disease therapy, 258
  autologous transplantation, 248-249
    bone marrow cells, 249
    cell selection by continuous-flow affinity chromatography, 249, 250
    peripheral blood cells, 249-252
  gene therapy, 256
  solid organ transplantation, 256-257
CD34, 247

CD55, 143-144
  deficiency, 144, 145, 147
CD58 (LFA-3) deficiency, 145, 147
CD59 deficiency, 144, 145, 147, 148, 149-150
CD67 deficiency, 145
CD73 deficiency, 145
CDw52 deficiency, 145
ced genes, apoptosis regulation, 5-6
Central nervous system disorders, Gaucher disease, 92
Chititriosidase activity, Gaucher disease, 94
Chlormabucil, chronic lymphocytic leukaemia, in combination with prednisone, 70
2-chloro-2′-deoxyadenosine (2CdA), apoptosis induction, 3
Chronic lymphocytic leukaemia (CLL), 65
  alternative donor BMT, 200, 201
  apoptosis, 2, 3
  definitions, 65
    'active' disease, 67-68
    'smouldering' disease, 68
    staging, 65-66
  treatment, 65-81
    biologic response modifiers, 76
    bone marrow transplantation, 76-78
    conventional, 70
    monoclonal antibodies/immunotoxins/ radioimmunoconjugates, 78
    nucleoside analogues, 71-76
    response criteria, 66
    timing, 66-67, 68-69
Chronic myeloid leukaemia (CML), alternative donor BMT, 199-200
Cladribine, 71
  adverse effects, 75
  chronic lymphocytic leukaemia, 75
  structure, 71
CLL *see* Chronic lymphocytic leukaemia
Coagulation disorders, Gaucher disease, 93
Coagulation system, 215, 216
Colony-stimulating factors *see* Growth factors; *names of specific factors*
Complement lysis sensitivity test, 143
Complement sensitivity, paroxysmal nocturnal haemoglobinuria, 143-144
Cord blood transplants, 206-207
Coronary angioplasty, use of hirudin/Hirulog ™i, 225-226
Coumarins, 223
CPT-11 resistance, molecular mechanisms, 269
Cyanmethaemoglobin, quantitation, 160, 176
Cyclophosphamide
  chronic lymphocytic leukaemia
    bone marrow transplant conditioning, 77
    combination therapy, 70
  combination therapy
    B-ALL, 55

chronic lymphocytic leukaemia, 77
resistance, molecular mechanisms, 269
Cyclosporin, graft versus host disease prophylaxis in CLL, 77
Cyclosporin A, paroxysmal nocturnal haemoglobinuria, 141
Cytokine gene therapy, 272, 274-275
Cytokines, fetal haemoglobin stimulation, 233, 239-241
Cytosine arabinoside (AraC; Cytarabine)
  AML in elderly, 120, 123, 124
    combination therapy, 130
    low density AraC, 128-129
  childhood ALL
    B-ALL, 55
    combination therapy, 51, 55
  chronic lymphocytic leukaemia, combination therapy, 70
  fetal haemoglobin stimulation, 233, 234
  resistance, molecular mechanisms, 269
Cytotoxic drugs, apoptosis induction, 2-3
Cytoxan, bone marrow transplant conditioning, 77

Daunorubicin
  AML in elderly, 121-122
    combination therapy, 130
  childhood ALL, 50
Decay accelerating factor (DAF; CD55), 143-144
  deficiency, 144, 145, 147
Decitabine, AML in elderly, 129
Dexamethasone, childhood ALL, CNS-directed treatment, 54
Difluoromethylornithine (DFMO), apoptosis regulation, 7
DNA fragmentation assay, apoptosis, 12-14
Doxorubicin
  childhood ALL, 50
  chronic lymphocytic leukaemia, combination therapy, 70
Drug resistance
  genes, 268
  transfer, 268-271
  mechanisms, 268-270

E2F, apoptosis regulation, 7
Ecto-5′-nucleotidase deficiency, PNH cells, 145
Endonucleases, apoptosis, 4
Enzyme replacement therapy, Gaucher disease, 94, 105-111
  effect on lung disorders, 90
  unwanted effects, 107-109
Epipodophyllotoxins, 59
  resistance, molecular mechanisms, 269
Epirubicin, AML in elderly, combination therapy, 130
Epstein-Barr virus (EBV)
  infection, apoptosis regulation, 9

malignant disease, cytotoxic T-lymphocyte
    therapy, 273
Erythrocytes *see* Red cells
Erythropoietin
  apoptosis regulation, 10
  clinical use
    after allogeneic bone marrow
      transplantation, 38
    after autologous bone marrow
      transplantation, 30
    conventional therapy, 24
    fetal haemoglobin stimulation, 233, 240
    high-dose therapy, 30
    myelodysplasia, 24
Etoposide
  AML in elderly, 123
    combination therapy, 130
  apoptosis induction, 3

Factor V abnormality, 218
  tests, 220
Factor IX deficiency, Gaucher disease, 93
Factor XI deficiency, Gaucher disease, 93
FAs/Apo1 ligation, apoptosis regulation, 4
  T lymphocytes, 8
Fatty acids, short chain, fetal haemoglobin
    stimulation, 233, 241-242
FcγIII *see* CD16
Fetal haemoglobin stimulation, 231-246
  cytokines, 233, 239-241
  early studies, 232-234
  hydroxyurea, 233, 234-239
  short chain fatty acids, 233, 241-242
Fibrinolysis, 215, 216-217
Flow cytometry
  apoptosis, 13-14
  paroxysmal nocturnal haemoglobinuria
    diagnosis, 147
Fludarabine, 71
  adverse effects, 72, 73
  AML in elderly, combination therapy, 130
  chronic lymphocytic leukaemia, 71-75
    bone marrow transplantation, 77
    combination therapy, 73
  structure, 71

Gaucher disease, 83-118
  alternative donor BMT, 206
  clinical management, 103-105
    organ transplantation, 104-105
    surgery, 103-104
  clinical manifestations, 83-95
    age of onset, 84-86
    bone, 88-89, 103, 104
    central nervous system, 92
    growth, 91-92
    gynaecological, 94
    haematological, 92-93, 103
    heart, 90-91
    immune system, 93

  kidney, 90
  liver, 87-88, 103
  lung, 89-90
  obstetric, 94
  skin, 91
  spleen, 86-87
enzyme replacement therapy, 94, 105-111
  effect on lung disorders, 90
  unwanted effects, 107-109
gene therapy, 256, 275, 279
molecular biology, 95-103
  glucocerebrosidase gene
    polymorphisms, 102-103
  glucocerebrosidase genes and cDNA,
    95-101
  saporin C and A, 102
type I
  age of onset, 84-85
  clinical management, 86-87, 88, 89-90,
    92, 94
  molecular biology, 95-100, 101
  treatment, 104-105, 106, 108
type II
  age of onset, 85-86
  clinical management, 89, 90, 91, 92
  molecular biology, 96-100, 101
type III
  age of onset, 86
  clinical management, 87, 88, 90, 91, 92
  molecular biology, 96-97, 99-100, 101
  treatment, 105, 108
Gene therapy
  CD34+ cells in, 256
  cytotoxic drug resistance, 268-270
  gene transfer studies, 263-286
  malignant disease, 272-274
    virus-related, 273
  safety, 267-268
  single gene defects, 274-278
Gene transfer to haemopoietic progenitor
    cells, 263-268
  adreno-associated virus as vector, 276,
    277-278
  drug resistance genes, 268-271
  gene marking studies, 264-267
  immunocyte function modulation,
    271-273
  retrovirus vectors, 263-264, 276
Genes
  and apoptosis regulation, 5-7
  drug resistance, 268
  transfer, 268-271
Glucocerebrosidase
  assay, 83
  replacement therapy, 94, 105-111
Glucocerebrosidase genes
  and cDNA, Gaucher disease, 95-101
  fusion genes and recombinations, 101
  mutations, 95-101, 102-103
  polymorphisms, 102-103

Glucocorticoids, apoptosis induction, 2-3
Glycosylphosphatidylinositol (GPI) anchors, 146, 150
  biosynthesis, 150-151
  block, 151, 152
  paroxysmal nocturnal haemoglobinuria, 145, 151, 152
Graft versus host disease (GVHD)
  alternative donor BMT, 200
  bone marrow tansplantation for CLL, 77
  effect of growth factors, 34, 35, 37, 38
Granulocyte colony stimulating growth factor (G-CSF), clinical use, 21
  acute leukaemia, 23
  acute myeloid leukaemia, 122
  after bone marrow transplantation
    allogeneic, 35-37
    autologous, 27-29
  conventional therapy, 22-24
  high-dose therapy, 25
  lymphomas, 22-23
  myelodysplasia, 24
  peripheral blood stem cell mobilisation, 31, 32, 33-34, 38-40
  side-effects, 21-22
Granulocyte-macrophage colony stimulating growth factor (GM-CSF),
  clinical use, 21-22
  acute leukaemia, 23
  acute myeloid leukaemia, 122
  after bone marrow transplantation
    allogeneic, 34-35, 36
    autologous, 25-27
  conventional therapy, 23-24
  fetal haemoglobin stimulation, 233
  high-dose therapy, 25
  myelodysplasia, 24
  peripheral blood stem cell mobilisation, 32, 33
  side-effects, 22
Granulomatous disease, chronic, gene therapy, 275
Growth factors
  apoptosis regulation, 2
  haemopoiesis, 9-10
  clinical use, 21-44
    after allogeneic transplantation, 34-40
    after autologous bone marrow transplantation, 25-30
    AML in elderly, 122-123, 124
    future developments, 40
    peripheral blood stem cell mobilization and transplantation, 30-34
    in support of conventional therapy, 22-24
    in support of high-dose therapy, 24-25
  effect on stem cell expansion/transducibility, 267
  fetal haemoglobin stimulation, 233, 239-241
Growth retardation, Gaucher disease, 91-92

Haemoglobin, fetal see Fetal haemoglobin
Haemoglobinometry, 160, 176, 178
Haemoglobinopathies
  alternative donor BMT, 205-206
  gene therapy, 275-279
Haemoglobinuria, paroxysmal nocturnal see Paroxysmal nocturnal haemoglobinuria
Ham test, paroxysmal nocturnal haemoglobinuria diagnosis, 143, 147, 150
Heart disorders, Gaucher disease, 90-91
Heparin, 223
  binding site on antithrombin, 222
  thromboembolic disease, 214, 223-224
Hepatomegaly, Gaucher disease, 87
Hexamethylene bisacetamide (HMBA), AML in elderly, 129-130
Hirudin, thromboembolic disease, 214, 224-226
Hirulog ™, 224-226
HLA haplotypes, frequency in various ethnic groups, 198
HLA typing and matching
  alternative donor BMT, 195-197, 199
  partially HLA matched family donors, 197-198
Homologous restriction factor (HRF) deficiency, PNH cells, 145
Human chorionic gonadotrophin (HCG), fetal haemoglobin stimulation, 232, 233
Hunter syndrome, gene therapy, 275
Hurler's disease, alternative donor BMT, 206
Hydroxyurea, fetal haemoglobin stimulation, 233
  Multicenter Study, 237-239
  phase I/II trials, 234-237
Hypercholesterolaemia, Gaucher disease, 94
Hypergammaglobulinaemia, Gaucher disease, 93

Idarubicin, 122
IL-1b-converting enzyme (ICE), apoptosis regulation, 6
Imiglucerase, 109-111
Immune system disorders, Gaucher disease, 93-94
Immunodeficiencies, inherited
  alternative donor BMT, 205
  gene therapy, 256
Immunoglobulins, Gaucher disease, 93
Immunophenotyping, childhood ALL, 48
Immunosuppressive therapy, paroxysmal nocturnal haemoglobinuria, 141
Immunotoxins, conjugated
  childhood ALL, 58
  chronic lymphocytic leukaemia, 78
Inborn errors of metabolism, alternative donor BMT, 206

Interferon alpha-2b, chronic lymphocytic leukaemia, 76
Interleukin-2 (IL-2)
 AML in elderly, 124
 chronic lymphocytic leukaemia, 76
Interleukin-3 (IL-3)
 fetal haemoglobin stimulation, 233
 mobilisation of peripheral blood stem cells, 33
 supporting high-dose therapy after autologous bone marrow transplant, 29-30
International Marrow Unrelated Search and Transplant (IMUST) Study, 191, 194, 196

JMH antigen deficiency, PNH cells, 145
Joint disorders, Gaucher disease, 88
 management, 104

Kidney disorders, Gaucher disease, 90

Leucocytes, counting, 177-178, 179, 180
 differential, 160, 171-172
 total cells, 170-171, 177-178
Leukaemias
 acute
  alternative donor BMT, 201-203
  growth factor support for chemotherapy, 23
 chronic, alternative donor BMT, 199-201
 paroxysmal nocturnal haemoglobinuria, 139-140
 see also specific leukaemias
LFA-3 *see* CD58
Liver disorders, Gaucher disease, 87-88
 management, 103
Liver transplantation, Gaucher disease, 104
Lung disorders, Gaucher disease, 89-90
Lymphocyte function-associated antigen-3 (LFA-3) deficiency, PNH cells, 145
Lymphocytes
 B type *see* B lymphocytes
 T type *see* T lymphocytes
Lymphomas, growth factor support for chemotherapy, 22

Melphalan, CLL combination therapy, 70
Membrane inhbitor of reactive lysis (MIRL; CD59) deficiency, 144, 145, 147, 148, 149-150
Mercaptopurine, childhood ALL, 52, 58
 combination therapy, 51, 52
Metabolic storage disease, gene therapy, 275, 279
Methotrexate
 childhood ALL, 52
  B-ALL, 55
  CNS-directed treatment, 53-54
  combination therapy, 51

fetal haemoglobin stimulation, 233
graft versus host disease prophylaxis in CLL, 77
resistance, molecular mechanisms, 268-269
Minimal residual disease, acute lymphoblastic leukaemia, 52-53
Mitoxantrone, AML in elderly, 122, 130
 in combination with etoposide, 130
Monoclonal antibodies, CLL treatment, 78
Monocyte-macrophage colony stimulating growth factor (M-CSF), 29, 37-38
Multidrug resistance (MDR1) gene, 268, 269
 transfer to haemopoietic cells, 270-271
Myelodysplasia (MDFS)
 alternative donor BMT, 203-204
 growth factor therapy, 24
Myeloma
 alternative donor BMT, 200, 201
 Gaucher disease, 93
 growth factor therapy, 24
 stem cell transplantation, selected CD34+ cells, 253-254
Myleran, fetal haemoglobin stimulation, 233, 234
Myocardial infarction treatment, use of hirudin/Hirulog TMî, 225-226

Neutrophil alkaline phosphatase deficiency, PNH cells, 145
Neutrophils, paroxysmal nocturnal haemoglobinuria, 149-150
Nitrosourea
 resistance, molecular mechanisms, 269
 toxicity, gene therapy, 270
Nucleoside analogues, 71
 chronic lymphocytic leukaemia, 71-76

Oncogenesis, apoptosis and, 10-12
Oral contraceptives
 activated protein C and, thrombosis risk, 219
 paroxysmal nocturnal haemoglobinuria, 143
Ornithine decarboxylase (ODC), apoptosis regulation, 7
Osteomyelitis, Gaucher disease, 88, 89

p53
 apoptosis regulation, 7-8
 oncogenesis, 10
Paroxysmal nocturnal haemoglobinuria (PNH), 137-158
 associated conditions, 139-140
 aplastic anaemia, 139, 140, 153-154
 biochemical defect, 150-151
 clinical features, 137-143
 complement sensitivity, 143-144
 complications, 138-139
 diagnosis, 143, 147-150

glycosylphosphatidylinositol (GPI) anchor, 150
management, 140-143
membrane defect, 144-146
molecular defect, 151-153
pathophysiology, 153-154
pregnancy in, 142-143
Pentostatin, 71
adverse effects, 76
chronic lymphocytic leukaemia, 75-76
structure, 71
Peripheral blood stem cell transplantation (PBSCT)
allogeneic, selected CD34+ cells, 254-256
autoimmunity, 258
autologous, 248, 353
selected CD34+ cells, 249-252, 253-254
growth factor support, 22
Phenylbutyrate, fetal haemoglobin stimulation, 242
Phosphatase, acid, Gaucher disease and, 94
PIG-A, 151-153
mutations, paroxysmal nocturnal haemoglobinuria (PNH), 153
PITSLRE protein kinase activity, and apoptosis, 14
Platelets
counting, 168-170, 177
volume distribution measurement, 175
PNH *see* Paroxysmal nocturnal haemoglobinuria
Pokeweed antiviral protein, CLL immunotoxin therapy, 78
Prednisolone, childhood ALL, 54
combination therapy, 52
Prednisone, CLL combination therapy, 70, 73
Pregnancy
Gaucher disease and, 94
in paroxysmal nocturnal haemoglobinuria, 142-143
Progesterone, fetal haemoglobin stimulation, 232, 233
Protein C, 217
activated (APC), resistance, 218-220
deficiency, 217-218
and thrombosis formation, 213-214, 217-220
Protein S defects, 219
Pseudo-osteomyelitis, Gaucher disease, 88, 89
Pseudomonas exotoxin, CLL immunotoxin therapy, 78

Radioimmunotherapy, chronic lymphocytic leukaemia, 78
Reactive oxygen species, in apoptosis, 14
Red cells
counting, 168, 177
measurements

haemoglobin concentration, 173-174
haemoglobin distribution, 175
indices, 160, 172-174
sizing, 160, 177
volume, 172-174
volume distribution, 175
paroxysmal nocturnal haemoglobinuria, 143-144, 147-149
Reticulocytes, counting, 160
automated, 178, 179, 1716
Retinoic acid, AML in elderly, 129
Ricin, CLL immunotoxin therapy, 78

Saporin, CLL immunotoxin therapy, 78
Saposin, Gaucher disease, 102
Serpins, 220-222
Sickle cell disease, 231
bone marrow transplantation, 205-206
fetal haemoglobin stimulation, 231-232
early studies, 232-234
erythropoietin, 240
hydroxyurea, 234-239, 240
short chain fatty acids, 241-242
gene therapy, 275-276
Skin disorders, Gaucher disease, 90
Splenomegaly, Gaucher disease, 86-87
Stem cell transplantation
allogeneic, 254-256
CD34+ augmented marrow, 254
peripheral blood cells, 38-40, 192, 207, 254-256
autologous, 248-254
bone marrow cells, 248, 249
gene marking studies, 264-267
peripheral blood cells, 248, 249-252
tumour purging, 252-254, 266-267
gene transfer into, 263-268
drug resistance studies, 268-271
gene marking studies, 264-267
immunocyte function modulation, 271-273
safety of, 267-268
see also Gene therapy
organ transplantation, 256-257
autoimmunity, 257-258
Stem cells
biology, 247-248
drug resistance, modification, 268
effect of growth factors, 30-34, 267
peripheral blood, mobilisation and transplantation after high-dose chemotherapy, 30-34
umbilical cord blood, 206

T lymphocytes
cytotoxic
antigen recognition, 272
EBV-related lymphoproliferation, 273
deficiencies, Gaucher disease and, 93

immature, apoptosis, 8-9
β-Thalassaemia, 231
   alternative donor BMT, 205
   chelation therapy, 231
   fetal haemoglobin stimulation, 231-232
      early studies, 232-234
      erythropoietin, 240
      hydroxyurea, 237, 241
      short chain fatty acids, 241-242
   gene therapy, 256, 275, 276
Thioguanine
   AML in elderly, 124
   childhood ALL, 52, 58
Thrombin, 215, 216-217
   inhibitors, 223-226
Thrombocytopenia, Gaucher disease, 92, 94
Thrombosis
   formation, control of, 213, 215-217
   genetic defects and, 213, 217-222
      antithrombin deficiency, 220-222
      protein C, 217-220
   inhibitors, 214, 223-226
   paroxysmal nocturnal haemoglobinuria, 138-139, 142, 143
   treatment, 142
Topoisomerase inhibitors, apoptosis induction, 3

Transplantation
   bone marrow *see* Bone marrow transplantation
   human umbilical cord blood, 206-207
   organ, selected CD34+ stem cells, 256-257
   see also under names of specific organs
Tumour cells, cytokine-transduced, 274

Umbilical cord blood transplants, 206-207
Urokinase-type plasminogen activator deficiency, PNH cells, 145
Vinblastine, fetal haemoglobin stimulation, 233, 234
Vincristine
   AML in elderly, combination therapy, 130
   childhood ALL, combination therapy, 52
   CLL combination therapy, 70
Vp16, AML in elderly, combination therapy, 130

Warfarin, thromboembolic disease, 214
White cells *see* Leucocytes

Zorubicine, 122